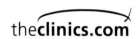

CHILD AND ADOLESCENT PSYCHIATRIC CLINICS OF NORTH AMERICA

Attention Deficit Hyperactivity Disorder

GUEST EDITORS
Luis Augusto Rohde, MD, PhD
Stephen V. Faraone, PhD

CONSULTING EDITOR
Harsh K. Trivedi, MD

April 2008 • Volume 17 • Number 2

SAUNDERS

An Imprint of Elsevier, Inc.
PHILADELPHIA   LONDON   TORONTO   MONTREAL   SYDNEY   TOKYO

W.B. SAUNDERS COMPANY
A Division of Elsevier Inc.

Elsevier Inc. • 1600 John F. Kennedy Boulevard • Suite 1800 • Philadelphia, Pennsylvania 19103-2899

http://www.childpsych.theclinics.com

CHILD AND ADOLESCENT PSYCHIATRIC CLINICS	Volume 17, Number 2
OF NORTH AMERICA	ISSN 1056–4993
April 2008	ISBN-13: 978-1-4160-5865-6
Editor: Sarah E. Barth	ISBN-10: 1-4160-5865-6

The ideas and opinions expressed in *Child and Adolescent Psychiatric Clinics of North America* do not necessarily reflect those of the Publisher. The Publisher does not assume any responsibility for any injury and/or damage to persons or property arising out of or related to any use of the material contained in this periodical. The reader is advised to check the appropriate medical literature and the product information currently provided by the manufacturer of each drug to be administered to verify the dosage, the method and duration of administration, or contraindications. It is the responsibility of the treating physician or other health care professional, relying on independent experience and knowledge of the patient, to determine drug dosages and the best treatment for the patient. Mention of any product in this issue should not be construed as endorsement by the contributors, editors, or the Publisher of the product or manufacturers' claims.

Child and Adolescent Psychiatric Clinics of North America (ISSN 1056-4993) is published quarterly by Elsevier Inc., 360 Park Avenue South, New York, NY 10010-1710. Months of issue are January, April, July, and October. Business and Editorial Offices: 1600 John F. Kennedy Boulevard, Suite 1800, Philadelphia, PA 19103-2899. Customer Service Offices: 6277 Sea Harbor Drive, Orlando, FL 32887-4800. Periodicals postage paid at New York, NY and additional mailing offices. Subscription prices are $220.00 per year (US individuals), $344.00 per year (US institutions), $113.00 per year (US students), $250.00 per year (Canadian individuals), $406.00 per year (Canadian institutions), $136.00 per year (Canadian students), $279.00 per year (international individuals), $406.00 per year (international institutions), and $136.00 per year (international students). International air speed delivery is included in all *Clinics* subscription prices. All prices are subject to change without notice. **POSTMASTER:** Send address changes to *Child and Adolescent Psychiatric Clinics of North America*, Elsevier Periodicals Customer Service, 6277 Sea Harbor Drive, Orlando, FL 32887-4800. **Customer Service: 1-800-654-2452 (US). From outside the United States, call 1-407-563-6020. Fax: 1-407-563-8521. E-mail: JournalsCustomerService-usa@elsevier.com.**

Child and Adolescent Psychiatric Clinics of North America is covered in *Index Medicus, ISI, SSCI, Research Alert, Social Search, Current Contents*, and *EMBASE/Excerpta Medica*.

Printed in the United States of America.

CONSULTING EDITOR

HARSH K. TRIVEDI, MD, Director of Adolescent Services and Site Training Director, Bradley Hospital Assistant Professor of Psychiatry and Human Behavior (Clinical), Brown Medical School Consulting Editor, Child and Adolescent Psychiatric Clinics of North America East Providence, Rhode Island

CONSULTING EDITOR EMERITUS

ANDRE'S MARTIN, MD, MPH

FOUNDING CONSULTING EDITOR

MELVIN LEWIS, MBBS, FRCPsych, DCH

GUEST EDITORS

LUIS AUGUSTO ROHDE, MD, PhD, Professor of Adolescent Psychiatry, Attention Deficit Hyperactivity Disorder Outpatients Program, Child and Adolescent Psychiatric Division. Hospital de Clínicas de Porto Alegre, Federal University of Rio Grande do Sul, Porto Alegre, Brazil

STEPHEN V. FARAONE, PhD, Director, Medical Genetics Research, Professor of Psychiatry, Neuroscience and Physiology; Director, Child and Adolescent Psychiatry Research, State University of New York Upstate Medical University, Syracuse, New York

CONTRIBUTORS

KEVIN M. ANTSHEL, PhD, Assistant Professor of Psychiatry, Department of Psychiatry & Behavioral Sciences, State University of New York Upstate Medical University, Syracuse, New York

RUSSELL BARKLEY, PhD, Clinical Professor of Psychiatry, Medical University of South Carolina, Charleston, South Carolina; and Research Professor of Psychiatry, Department of Psychiatry & Behavioral Sciences, State University of New York Upstate Medical University, Syracuse, New York

JOSEPH BIEDERMAN, MD, Chief of Pediatric Psychopharmacology Research Unit, Massachusetts General Hospital; Professor of Psychiatry, Harvard Medical School, Boston, Massachusetts

OSCAR BUKSTEIN, MD, Western Psychiatric Institute and Clinic, University of Pittsburgh School of Medicine, Pittsburgh, Pennsylvania

GEORGE BUSH, MD, Associate Professor, Department of Psychiatry, Harvard Medical School; Assistant Director of Psychiatric Neuroimaging Research, Department of Psychiatry, Massachusetts General Hospital; MIT/HMS/MGH Athinoula A. Martinos Center for Functional and Structural Biomedical Imaging (Massachusetts Institute of Technology, Harvard Medical School and Massachusetts General Hospital), Charlestown; and Massachusetts General Hospital, Clinical and Research Program in Pediatric Psychopharmacology, Boston, Massachusetts

FRANCISCO X. CASTELLANOS, MD, Department of Child and Adolescent Psychiatry, New York University School of Medicine, and Nathan S. Kline Institute for Psychiatric Research, Orangeburg; and NYU Child Study Center, New York, New York

STEPHEN V. FARAONE, PhD, Director, Medical Genetics Research, Professor of Psychiatry, Neuroscience and Physiology; Director, Child and Adolescent Psychiatry Research, State University of New York Upstate Medical University, Syracuse, New York

CATHRYN A. GALANTER, MD, Assistant Professor of Clinical Psychiatry, Division of Child and Adolescent Psychiatry, Columbia University/New York State Psychiatric Institute, New York, New York

LAURENCE L. GREENHILL, MD, Ruane Professor of Clinical Psychiatry, Columbia University, Research Psychiatrist II, Department of Psychiatry, New York State Psychiatric Institute, Columbia University, New York, New York

RENATA R.F. GONCALVES, MA, Department of Psychiatry, Federal University of Rio Grande do Sul, Brazil

PETER JENSEN, MD, The REACH Institute, Resource for Advancing Children's Health, New York, New York

CHRISTIAN KIELING, MD, Department of Psychiatry, Federal University of Rio Grande do Sul, Brazil

CHRISTOPHER J. KRATOCHVIL, MD, Associate Professor of Psychiatry and Pediatrics, University of Nebraska Medical Center, Omaha, Nebraska

ELLEN LEIBENLUFT, MD, Senior Investigator and Chief, Section on Bipolar Spectrum Disorders, Emotion and Development Branch, Mood and Anxiety Disorders Program, National Institute of Mental Health, Bethesda, Maryland

JAMES J. McGOUGH, MD, Professor of Clinical Psychiatry, Division of Child and Adolescent Psychiatry, University of California Los Angeles Semel Institute for Neuroscience and Human Behavior; and Director, University of California Los Angeles Child and Adolescent Psychopharmacology Program and ADHD Clinic; and University of California Los Angeles Medical Plaza, Los Angeles, California

ERIC MICK, ScD, Assistant Professor, Department of Psychiatry, Massachusetts General Hospital and Harvard Medical School, Boston, Massachusetts

JOEL NIGG, PhD, Department of Psychology, Michigan State University, East Lansing, Michigan

GUILHERME POLANCZYK, MD, ADHD Program, Child and Adolescent Psychiatric Division, Hospital de Clinicas de Porto Alegre, Porto Alegre, RS, Brazil

KELLY POSNER, PhD, Assistant Professor of Psychology in Psychiatry, Research Scientist IV, Division of Child and Adolescent Psychiatry, Columbia University/New York State Psychiatric Institute, New York, New York

LUIS AUGUSTO ROHDE, MD, PhD, Professor of Adolescent Psychiatry, ADHD Outpatient Program, Division of Child and Adolescent Psychiatry, Hospital de Clínicas de Porto Alegre, Federal University of Rio Grande do Sul, Rua Ramiro Barcelos, Porto Alegre, RS, Brazil

JOSEPH A. SERGEANT, PhD, Department of Neuropsychology, Clinical Neuropsychology, Vrije Unviersiteit Amsterdam, Amsterdam, Netherlands

THOMAS J. SPENCER, MD, Associate Chief of Pediatric Psychopharmacology Research Unit, Massachusetts General Hospital; and Associate Professor of Psychiatry, Harvard Medical School, Boston, Massachusetts

EDMUND J.S. SONUGA-BARKE, PhD, School of Psychology, Institute for Disorder on Impulse and Attention, University of Southampton, Highfield, Southampton, United Kingdom; Child Study Center, New York University, New York; and Social, Genetic, Developmental Psychiatry Centre, Institute of Psychiatry, University of London, London, United Kingdom

MARK A. STEIN, PhD, Professor, Department of Psychiatry, Institute for Juvenile Research, University of Illinois at Chicago; and Director of HALP Clinic and ADHD Research Center, University of Illinois at Chicago, Chicago, Illinois

CLAUDIA M. SZOBOT, MD, Attention-Deficit/Hyperactivity Disorder Outpatient Clinic, Hospital de Clínicas de Porto Alegre (HCPA), Federal University of Rio Grande do Sul (UFRGS); Center for Drug and Alcohol Research HCPA, UFRGS; Programa de Déficit de Atenção/Hiperatividade (PRODAH), Hospital de Clínicas de Porto Alegre. Rua Ramiro Barcelos, Porto Alegre, Brazil

ROSEMARY TANNOCK, PhD, Neuroscience and Mental Health Research Program, The Hospital for Sick Children, Toronto, Ontario, Canada

BRIGETTE S. VAUGHAN, APRN, University of Nebraska Medical Center, Omaha, Nebraska

BENEDETTO VITIELLO, MD, Chief of the Child and Adolescent Treatment and Preventive Intervention Research Branch, Division of Services and Intervention Research, National Institute of Mental Health, Bethesda; and Adjunct Professor of Psychiatry, John Hopkins University, Baltimore, Maryland

ERIK WILLCUTT, PhD, Department of Psychology, University of Colorado, Boulder, Colorado

Cover artwork Courtesy of Socorro Rivera G., Mexico City, Mexico

CONTENTS

> Epidemiologic data on attention deficit hyperactivity disorder (ADHD) are essential for planning health services and implementing strategies of detection and early intervention, with possible substantial benefits on public health. This article addresses methodological aspects of prevalence studies, recent findings on the prevalence of ADHD in childhood and adolescence based on a systematic review, current findings on the persistence of the disorder over time and prevalence in adulthood, and factors associated with ADHD. Evidence from the reviewed literature indicates the importance of methodological aspects in the understanding of epidemiologic findings and the necessity of large-scale cross-national studies. Moreover, governments clearly must direct attention to childhood mental disorders to guarantee a healthy future for their countries.

> Results of behavioral genetic and molecular genetic studies have converged to suggest that both genetic and nongenetic factors contribute to the development of attention deficit hyperactivity disorder (ADHD). Family, twin, and adoption studies provide

compelling evidence that genes play a strong role in mediating susceptibility to ADHD. In contrast to a handful of genome-wide scans conducted thus far, many candidate gene studies of ADHD have produced substantial evidence implicating several genes in the etiology of the disorder. Yet, even these associations are small and consistent with the idea that the genetic vulnerability to ADHD is mediated by many genes of small effects. These small effects emphasize the need for future candidate gene studies to implement strategies that will provide enough statistical power to detect such small effects.

article focuses on (1) population-based studies examining ADHD and bipolar disorder or ADHD and co-occurring irritability, (2) the co-occurrence and prospective relationships of ADHD and bipolar disorder in clinical samples, (3) phenomenology and assessment of bipolar disorder and ADHD, (4) treatment of comorbid ADHD and bipolar disorder, (5) family and genetic studies of ADHD and bipolar disorder, and (6) pathophysiologic comparisons between children with ADHD and irritability and bipolar disorder. We draw on the research to make clinical recommendations and highlight important directions for future research.

Attention deficit hyperactivity disorder (ADHD) is a common neurodevelopmental disorder with a childhood onset of symptoms and impairment. Although it is most frequently identified during elementary school years, epidemiologic data suggest that the onset of ADHD frequently occurs earlier, with presentation as young as 3 years of age. Early identification, however, allows consideration of appropriate interventions. Many data are available on safe and efficacious treatment options for school-aged children who have ADHD; however, little is known about the use of these modalities in preschoolers and, ultimately, the long-term effects of early treatment. Recognition of the preschool presentation of ADHD, appropriate differential diagnosis, and identification of comorbid conditions, and a developmental perspective on the course and potential outcomes of the disorder may guide treatment planning. Newly available data on the safety and efficacy of pharmacotherapy and psychosocial intervention for preschoolers who have ADHD may help clinicians make treatment decisions for these young children and their families.

In this article the authors reflect on the role of executive function (EF) deficits and delay aversion (DAv) in the diagnosis of attention deficit hyperactivity disorder (ADHD). The authors, empirical review shows clearly that EF deficits and DAv are implicated in ADHD, although neither is necessary for ADHD nor specific to it. The constructs are somewhat dissociable from one another so that each may represent a distinctive feature associated with an ADHD subsample. The authors argue that neither EF deficits nor DAv add much value to the diagnosis of ADHD as it is currently conceptualized, but may be crucial in helping to partition heterogeneity in the condition, leading to the refinement of ADHD nosology.

effects, improve long-term tolerability, and thus contribute to long-term treatment compliance and improved effectiveness. Early ADHD pharmacogenetic studies have focused predominantly on catecholamine pathway genes and response to methylphenidate. Future efforts will also examine a wider range of stimulant and nonstimulant medications on a range of outcome measures and durations. Based on these studies, the potential for personalizing ADHD treatment in clinical practice will be determined.

FORTHCOMING ISSUES

RECENT ISSUES

ELSEVIER
SAUNDERS

Child Adolesc Psychiatric Clin N Am
17 (2008) xv–xvi

CHILD AND
ADOLESCENT
PSYCHIATRIC CLINICS
OF NORTH AMERICA

Foreword
Focusing In

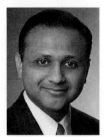

Harsh K. Trivedi, MD
Consulting Editor

"New Study Shows Children Can Outgrow ADHD"

   —*Hartford Courant (December 3, 2007)*

"Stimulants for ADHD may cause mild heart symptoms"

   —*Reuters (December 10, 2007)*

"19% of ADHD patients get too many drugs."

   —*Sydney Morning Herald (December 6, 2007)*

In the past 7 years since the last issue on attention deficit hyperactivity disorder (ADHD) was published in *Child and Adolescent Psychiatric Clinics of North America*, there has been much progress in our understanding of the disorder. From neurobiologic studies that help to elucidate the pathophysiology of ADHD, to prevalence studies that further our understanding of its progression through the life cycle, to molecular genetic studies that identify genes that may underlie its etiology—indeed, any one of these discoveries would be considered a significant advance in the field.

In addition to our professional curiosities regarding this disorder, there has been much interest from the popular media and the general public about it. In any given week, one can usually spot a headline or two about ADHD

1056-4993/08/$ - see front matter © 2008 Elsevier Inc. All rights reserved.
doi:10.1016/j.chc.2008.01.001   *childpsych.theclinics.com*

in the local newspaper, Internet blog, or nightly news broadcast. For parents and youth there continue to be questions, for example, regarding the meaning of this diagnosis, its implications for present and future functioning, and the safety and efficacy of prescribed treatments.

In developing this issue about ADHD, the difficult task was this: How do we do justice to the multiple areas of interest (understanding that each article in this issue could easily be the focus of an entire issue) while ensuring that the final product is reflective of the current evidence base (and accurately provides a synopsis of major advances)? To meet this high bar while also delivering clinically relevant and practical content to inform patient care is no small feat.

I am grateful to Luis Augusto Rohde and Stephen Faraone. They have intricately chiseled at this topic, while working with two different Consulting Editors, to create an issue that delivers along all of these fronts. I also thank each of the outstanding contributors for sharing their expertise in this ever-evolving field. If this issue is any indication of the advances that will occur in the upcoming years, I can only imagine what the next issue on ADHD will look like as we continue focusing in.

Harsh K. Trivedi, MD
Bradley Hospital
Brown Medical School
1011 Veterans Memorial Parkway
East Providence, RI 02915, USA

E-mail address: harsh_trivedi@brown.edu

ELSEVIER
SAUNDERS

Child Adolesc Psychiatric Clin N Am
17 (2008) xvii–xix

CHILD AND
ADOLESCENT
PSYCHIATRIC CLINICS
OF NORTH AMERICA

Preface

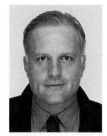 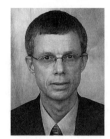

Luis Augusto Rohde, MD, PhD   Stephen V. Faraone, PhD
Guest Editors

When the former editor of *Child and Adolescent Psychiatric Clinics of North America*, Andrés Martin, contacted us to serve as guest editors for an issue on attention deficit hyperactivity disorder (ADHD), our first reaction was a mix of honor and apprehension.

We felt honor, because this is a key disorder for all of us who devote our lives to work with children and adolescents suffering with mental health problems. ADHD is highly prevalent in clinical settings and poses dilemmas for its diagnosis and treatment. A recent report documented the high prevalence of the disorder in all continents, even in epidemiologic samples [1]. Moreover, because ADHD is one of the best investigated child mental health disorders [2], the work of clinicians can be informed by a large body of research.

We felt apprehension, because the selection of topics to be included would be a challenge. To give readers a sense of the vast scientific literature on this disorder, we conducted an electronic search on PUBMED (www.pubmed.gov) for articles written in the last 5 years, using only the term ADHD. Immediately, more than 3600 abstracts appeared on the screen! Since the last *Child and Adolescent Psychiatric Clinics of North America* issue that focused on ADHD published more than 5 years ago, the field has advanced along several fronts. The diagnosis of ADHD has been progressively more and more accepted in different cultures, and our understanding of its etiology and neurobiology has advanced through studies of molecular genetics, neuropsychology, and neuroimaging. Clinical practice has been transformed by the development of new nonstimulants and extended release stimulants, which provide clinicians with new options for treating the disorder.

To face this task, we decided that this issue should have a double mission: presenting to our readers the most updated research findings, and discussing the most relevant clinical dilemmas that we face when taking care of children and adolescents who have ADHD. To achieve this mission, the first group of articles addresses basic aspects of the disorder. Drs. Polanczyk and Jensen provide an overview of the worldwide epidemiology of ADHD in children and adolescents. Drs. Mick and Faraone translate the exciting new findings on molecular genetics of ADHD, which progressively are helping us understand that the ADHD clinical phenotype is the result of a complex interplay between genetic susceptibility and a myriad of environmental factors. Drs. Kieling, Gonçalves, Tannock, and Castellanos address the neurobiology of the disorder by integrating data from studies suggesting alterations in specific brain areas and the clinical phenotype.

In the second group of articles, hot clinical topics are discussed extensively. Drs. Szobot and Bukstein present neurobiologic and developmental data that support the coexistence of ADHD and substance use disorder; these data also suggest clinical interventions for patients who have these dual diagnoses. Drs. Galanter and Leibenluft propose an innovative clinical approach to disentangle the frontiers between ADHD and bipolar disorder, and they present data on the comorbidity in both epidemiologic and clinical samples. Drs. Greenhill, Posner, Vaughan, and Kratochvil discuss an emerging new area of interest, the diagnosis and treatment of ADHD in preschoolers. In the next two articles, Drs. Sonuga-Barke, Sergeant, Nigg, and Willcutt describe modern neuropsychological understandings of the disorder with an emphasis on the nosological implications of these concepts, and Dr. Bush shows how to integrate neuroimaging findings into everyday clinical practice. Finally, Dr. Rohde discusses the pitfalls in our current clinical ADHD nosology.

The last set of articles addresses advances in the treatment of the disorder. Drs. Antshel and Barkley provide an overview of psychosocial treatment approaches to ADHD, focusing on the two that have received the greatest research support: parent training in child behavior management, and teacher training in classroom management. Drs. Biederman and Spencer describe psychopharmacologic interventions for the disorder and guide clinicians on how to choose among the different options. Dr. Vitiello describes data that help clinicians to better understand the risk of using medications, specifically regarding two areas of recent concern: physical growth and cardiovascular function. Drs. Stein and McGough present emerging new pharmacogenomic data on ADHD that may allow for a more personalized treatment in the near future.

The soul of this issue, however, resides much more on the stellar group of contributors, rather than on the topics chosen. The contributors are among the world's leading experts, both researchers and clinicians, in the field. We are very grateful for their suggestions on the table of contents, their availability to work on this project, and their willingness to share their wisdom and expertise. In addition, we note the extraordinary work done by our publishers at Elsiever, Sarah Barth and Lisa Richman, the inestimable insights from the former editor, Andrés Martin, on the areas of clinical interest to be addressed, and the perseverance and advice of the new consulting editor, Harsh K. Trivedi, who kept us on task during his term.

At the end of the day, we are confident that this issue will be valuable for all mental health professionals who work with children and adolescents and who face, in their everyday practice, the enormous clinical challenges and dilemmas faced when caring for youths suffering from ADHD.

Luis Augusto Rohde, MD, PhD
Attention Deficit Hyperactivity Disorder Outpatient Program
Child and Adolescent Psychiatric Division
Hospital de Clínicas de Porto Alegre
Federal University of Rio Grande do Sul
Rua Ramiro Barcelos 2350 – Room # 2101
Porto Alegre, Brazil 90035-003

E-mail address: lrohde@terra.com.br

Stephen V. Faraone, PhD
Medical Genetics Research
Departments of Psychiatry, Neuroscience and Physiology
Child and Adolescent Psychiatry Research
State University of New York Upstate Medical University
750 East Adams Street
Syracuse, NY 13210, USA

E-mail address: faraones@upstate.edu

References

[1] Polanczyk G, Horta B, Lima M, et al. The worldwide prevalence of attention-deficit hyperactivity disorder: a systematic review and meta-regression analysis. Am J Psychiatry 2007; 164(6):942–8.
[2] Goldman LS, Genel M, Bezman RJ, et al. Diagnosis and treatment of attention-deficit/hyperactivity disorder in children and adolescents. Council on Scientific Affairs, American Medical Association. JAMA 1998;279(14):1100–7.

ELSEVIER
SAUNDERS

Child Adolesc Psychiatric Clin N Am
17 (2008) 245–260

CHILD AND
ADOLESCENT
PSYCHIATRIC CLINICS
OF NORTH AMERICA

Epidemiologic Considerations in Attention Deficit Hyperactivity Disorder: A Review and Update

Guilherme Polanczyk, MD[a],*, Peter Jensen, MD[b]

[a]ADHD Program, Child and Adolescent Psychiatric Division, Hospital de Clinicas de Porto Alegre, Rua Ramiro Barcelos, 2350, Porto Alegre, RS, Brazil, 90035-003
[b]The REACH Institute, Resource for Advancing Children's Health, 71 West 23rd Street, 8th Floor, New York, NY 10010, USA

Epidemiology is the study of the distribution of a particular disease in the population and the factors associated to it. Epidemiologic data are essential for planning health services and implementing strategies of detection and early intervention, with possible substantial benefits on public health. Epidemiology can also provide insight into the etiology of the disorder, its natural history, and risk factors [1]. The merging of epidemiology, genetics, developmental psychology, and psychiatry has generated new knowledge on risk factors for psychiatric disorders [2,3]. Moreover, consideration of cultural aspects may provide a more thorough characterization of experiencing a mental disorder and its treatment, with potential benefits in improving provision of care.

This article reviews the current literature and summarizes current findings on the epidemiology of attention deficit hyperactivity disorder (ADHD). It is composed of four sections: (1) a brief review of methodological aspects of prevalence studies of ADHD in childhood and adolescence; (2) recent findings on the prevalence of ADHD in childhood and adolescence; (3) current

Funding sources: This work was supported by a research grant from Conselho Nacional de Desenvolvimento Científico e Tecnológico (CNPq, Brazil) (Grant MCT/CNPq 02/2006 - Universal). Dr. Polanczyk holds a doctoral fellowship, Coordenação de Aperfeiçoamento de Pessoal de Nível Superior (CAPES), Ministry of Education, Brazil.

Conflict of interest: Dr. Jensen currently receives investigator-initiated grants from Ortho-McNeil Pharmaceutical, Inc. and unrestricted educational grants from Pfizer Inc., Eli Lilly and Company, and Ortho-McNeil Pharmaceutical, Inc.; participates in speakers' bureaus for UCB Pharma, psychCME, CME Outfitters, and the Neuroscience Education Institute; and consults with Best Practice, Inc., Janssen Pharmaceutica, Inc., Novartis, and UCB Pharma. Dr. Polanczyk has no conflict of interest to declare.

* Corresponding author.
E-mail address: gvp.ez@terra.com.br (G. Polanczyk).

findings on the persistence of ADHD over time and prevalence studies in adulthood; (4) a discussion of factors associated with ADHD.

Methodological aspects of surveys

To generate meaningful and valid prevalence estimates, epidemiologic surveys must address a host of methodological strategies. In addition, for ADHD studies, several specific methodological choices may result in different prevalence estimates [4]. Thus, different prevalence estimates are generated depending on the specific diagnostic criteria and system applied, informant source and strategies used to collect and combine diagnostic information, and whether and how the criterion of impairment is applied to the diagnosis [4]. Therefore, these methodological aspects of any ADHD survey must be reviewed to understand the results.

One key methodological aspect of a high-quality epidemiologic study concerns who is in the sample, and how the survey sample was recruited. A survey sample's prevalence estimates can only be extrapolated to the larger population if the sample is representative of that particular community. Ideally, researchers must know and determine the probability of a given individual to be selected. Because having a complete and up-to-date list of an entire population is often virtually impossible, epidemiologic surveys often draw samples in a probabilistic fashion from birth registers [5], households [6], or schools [7], often called the *sampling frame*.

Once the sampling frame has been determined, the ascertainment strategy must not be linked to the outcome of the study (ie, the recruitment methods used for the study must not be associated with the likelihood of an ADHD diagnosis). Similarly, surveys must address the problems related to those who agree versus those who refuse to participate (volunteer bias), and those who drop out at some point in a longitudinal survey (sample attrition), potentially resulting in major problems of sample bias.

Considering that ADHD is a clinical diagnosis, the criteria adopted and validity of measures used play a major role in the results that are generated [8]. The classificatory systems (*Diagnostic and Statistical Manual of Mental Disorders* [DSM] and *International Statistical Classification of Diseases* [ICD]) have somewhat different diagnostic criteria that influence prevalence estimates. For example, the ICD-10 requires a minimum number of symptoms in all three dimensions (inattention, overactivity, and impulsivity) [9], whereas DSM-IV requires a minimum of six symptoms in one or two dimensions (inattention and hyperactivity–impulsivity) [10]. Moreover, ICD-10 specifically requires that the symptoms required for diagnosis must be identified within each of two or more settings, whereas DSM-IV does not require the full symptoms and impairment to be present in each setting, merely that sufficient symptoms be present for diagnosis across at least two settings. Not surprisingly, estimates based on ICD-10 criteria are consistently lower that those based on DSM-IV criteria [4].

Several structured and semistructured diagnostic interviews, either based on DSM or ICD criteria, have been constructed to evaluate the presence of ADHD. These can be applied by lay or clinical interviewers. Some studies have used checklists to evaluate the presence of symptoms, which commonly generate higher prevalence estimates because checklists usually do not effectively evaluate impairment nor age of onset. Studies using these less-stringent, less-precise methods tend to generate higher prevalence estimates [11].

Other points of potential controversy among investigators are how to evaluate impairment, whether impairment can be attributed to a single condition such as ADHD when most children have comorbid conditions, and what exact degree of impairment should be considered clinically significant. Given the difficulty of operationalizing these constructs, studies using different measures and approaches to assess impairment unsurprisingly provide somewhat discordant prevalence estimates [12].

Another key methodological issue in determining prevalence estimates in ADHD studies concerns the strategy adopted by investigators to collect and combine information to generate the diagnosis. Because of the structured nature of the clinical examination, children often do not exhibit ADHD symptoms during evaluation. Unfortunately, children tend to underreport externalizing behaviors, particularly ADHD and oppositional symptoms, compared with other informant sources. Thus, their reports are usually not sufficiently valid as the sole source of information for diagnosing ADHD, although older adolescents tend to better report inattentive symptoms [13]. Therefore, clinicians must rely on subjective reports of symptoms from the parents and teachers.

Interrater reliability estimates between parent and teacher reports of ADHD symptoms tend to be low [14], perhaps partly because the manifestation of symptoms is setting- and task-dependent and because parents and teachers are sensitive to different behaviors. The result of this variability among informant sources is that different prevalence rates will be generated, depending on whether the diagnosis is made based on (1) the information provided by a single informant (subject, parent, or teacher); (2) the aggregation of reports from different informants (the so-called "and rule" [ie, a symptom is considered present only if it is endorsed by two informants] or "or rule" [ie, a symptom is considered present if endorsed by one of two informants]); (3) the clinical examination, in which an experienced clinician reviews all available data, reconciles any discrepancies, and makes a diagnostic decision based on the merging of reports (best estimate procedure); or (4) direct evaluation of the individual [15].

Prevalence in childhood and adolescence

Given the growing interest and recognition of ADHD, its prevalence has been frequently studied in the past decade, with surveys conducted with different methodological approaches and in diverse cultures. Several reviews [11,15–20] have summarized this literature, including three systematic reviews that made rigorous efforts to ensure the unbiased selection of studies [4,21,22]. The most recent of these comprehensive systematic literature reviews [4] examined more than 9000 abstracts and included 102 ADHD surveys published from 1978 to 2005 and conducted worldwide. Based on a statistical computation, the pooled prevalence rate of ADHD was estimated to be 5.23%, although with significant heterogeneity among various estimates [4].

Because many additional studies have been published since that review, this article reexamines the literature, focusing only on the past decade (1997–2007) when the epidemiologic methods became more consistently rigorous. Accordingly, a systematic review of the literature published from January 1997 to June 2007 was conducted, based on search strategy used in a previous report [4]. Thus, studies were required to (1) be original surveys on ADHD/HD prevalence (point prevalence), (2) present diagnosis based either on any DSM version (III, III-R, or IV) or ICD (version 9 or 10), (3) rely on a sample ascertained from the general population (eg, households, birth registers) or from schools in a probabilistic fashion, and (4) enroll subjects aged 18 years or younger. The major methodological characteristics and results of selected studies are presented in Table 1.

The review detected 71 studies conducted in all continents. Studies showed a wide range of prevalence estimates, ranging from very low estimates of 0.2% [35], 0.4% [61], 0.7% [48], and 0.9% [33,44,59,87,88] to much higher estimates, 19.8% [39], 20.4% [31], 23.4% [54], and 27% [84]. As expected, studies using DSM-IV criteria generated higher prevalence rates than those using ICD-10. Likewise, the surveys not requiring the presence of functional impairment for diagnosis yielded higher prevalence estimates than those that did.

One might speculate that the variability of ADHD prevalence rates across the studies reported here could be a function of the geographic and cultural characteristics of study samples (ie, with higher rates of ADHD found in Western societies where cultural factors may play a role in creating or identifying cases) [89]. However, a previously reported study showed that once methodological characteristics of studies were controlled for, no differences were found between estimates from North America and Europe [4]. In contrast, differences were found between estimates from the North American and European continents compared with estimates from Middle East and Africa. Nonetheless, given the small number of studies conducted in these other countries compared with North America and Europe, firm conclusions could not be drawn about this tentative finding [4]. Until cross-national studies are performed using parallel diagnostic interview methods, identical or comparable sampling frames, and similarly defined populations, determining whether meaningful differences exist among countries will not be possible.

Prevalence in adulthood

Longitudinal studies have consistently shown that ADHD symptoms tend to decline over time, but a considerable number of affected subjects remain symptomatic and impaired in adulthood, even if the full syndrome has remitted [90,91]. Only recently has ADHD became a major focus of clinical attention [92] in studies of adults and among adult-oriented practitioners. Nevertheless, full agreement has not been reached on the phenomenology and diagnostic criteria of the disorder [93,94], which leads to ongoing uncertainty about how research findings should be interpreted. Thus, actual estimates of the proportion of children and youth who have ADHD who experience remission by adulthood depend on the conceptual definition of remission [91]. In one meta-analysis of longitudinal studies of ADHD, investigators reported a persistence rate of 15% for the full diagnosis but a rate of 40% to 60% for ADHD in partial remission [91].

In a recent reported study, investigators in the Netherlands ascertained a population-based sample of 1813 adults (aged 18–75 years) from an automated general practitioner system and evaluated them for ADHD [95]. Investigators determined that the prevalence of ADHD in adulthood was 1.0% (95% CI, 0.6–1.6) for a cutoff of six symptoms and 2.5% (95% CI, 1.9–3.4) for a cutoff of four symptoms, with the requirement of the presence of all three core symptoms during childhood. Subjects who had four or more inattentive or hyperactive–impulsive symptoms were significantly more impaired than subjects who had two or one, and those who had no symptoms [95].

Unfortunately, adult ADHD has been only rarely evaluated in epidemiologic surveys drawing on representative samples of the population and using a consistent methodology. In one of the few exceptions, a subsample of the National Comorbidity Survey Replication (a nationally representative survey of adults in the United States) was evaluated for ADHD [96]. An initial sample of 9282 individuals was screened and 5692 individuals were further selected, either because they met the required criteria for at least one disorder or because they were part of a randomly selected subsample. From these individuals, 3199 subjects (those between 18 and 44 years of age) were evaluated for ADHD. The respondents were evaluated for childhood ADHD and a single question concerning the presence or not of current ADHD symptoms was asked. Based on the results, subjects were divided into four groups: (1) absence of ADHD symptoms, (2) ADHD symptoms only during childhood, (3) diagnosis of ADHD during childhood without symptoms in adulthood, and (4) diagnosis of ADHD during childhood with symptoms in adulthood. Subsamples from each of the groups were contacted, resulting in the evaluation of 154 subjects for adult ADHD by trained clinicians. Based on the prevalence of the disorder in each of the groups and after multiple imputation to assign predicted diagnoses to respondents who did not participate in the reappraisal interviews, the

Table 1
Attention deficit hyperactivity disorder surveys in children and adolescents published from January 1997 to June 2007

Author	Country	Age (y)	Diagnostic criteria	Source of information	Requirement of impairment	Prevalence estimate (%)
Almqvist, et al [23]	Finland	8–9	DSM-III-R	Parents	Yes	7.1
Angold, et al [24]	United States	9–17	DSM-IV	Or rule	Yes	2.6
Ashenafi, et al [25]	Ethiopia	5–15	DSM-III-R	Parents	No	1.5
Bener, et al [26]	Qatar	6–12	DSM-IV	Teachers	No	9.4
Benjasuwantep, et al [27]	Thailand	6–14	DSM-IV	Best estimate	—	6.5
Breton, et al [6]	Canada	6–14	DSM-III-R	Parents	Yes	4.0
Bussing, et al [28]	United States	Kindergarten through 5th grade	DSM-IV	Parents	No	11.8
Canino, et al [12]	Puerto Rico	7–17	DSM-IV	Parents and subjects	Yes	3.7
Cardo, et al [29]	Island of Majorca	6–11	DSM-IV	Parents and teachers	No	4.6
Carlson et al [30]	United States	Grades 1–5	DSM-IV	Teachers	No	18.9
Cornejo, et al [31]	Colombia	4–17	DSM-IV	—	—	20.4
Eapen, et al [32]	United Arab Emirates	6–15	DSM-IV	Best estimate	Yes	0.5
Eapen, et al [33]	United Arab Emirates	6–18	DSM-IV	Best estimate	Yes	0.9
Ersan, et al [34]	Turkey	6–15	DSM-IV	Parents or teachers	No	8.1
Essau, et al [35]	German	12–17	DSM-IV	Subjects	Yes	0.2
Fleitlich-Bilyk and Goodman [36]	Brazil	7–14	DSM-IV	Best estimate	Yes	1.8
Fontana, et al [37]	Brazil	6–12	DSM-IV	And rule	No	13
Ford, et al [38]	Great Britain	5–15	DSM-IV	Best estimate	Yes	2.2
Gadow, et al [39]	Ukraine	10–12	DSM-IV	Parents	No	19.8
Gau, et al [40]	South Taiwan	13–15	DSM-IV	Best estimate	Yes	7.5
Gaub and Carlson [41]	United States	Grades 1–5	DSM-IV	Teachers	No	8.1
Gomez, et al [42]	Australia	5–11	DSM-IV	And rule	No	2.4
Goodman, et al [43]	England and Scotland	5–15	DSM-IV	Best estimate	Yes	2.4
Goodman, et al [44]	Brazil	5–14	DSM-IV	Best estimate	Yes	0.9
Goodman, et al [45]	Russia	7–14	ICD-10	Best estimate	Yes	1.3
Graetz, et al [46]	Australia	6–17	DSM-IV	Parents	No	7.5

Study	Country	Age	Criteria	Method	Yes/No	Prevalence
Guardiola, et al [47]	Brazil	1st grade	DSM-IV	Teachers	No	17.9
Hackett, et al [48]	South India	8–12	ICD-10	Parents	Yes	0.7
Hebrani, et al [49]	Iran	5–6	DSM-IV	Parents	Yes	12.3
Kadesjo and Gillberg [50]	Sweden	7	DSM-III-R	Best estimate	Yes	3.7
Kashala, et al [51]	Dominican Republic Congo	7–9	DSM-IV	Teachers	No	5.6
Kroes, et al [52]	The Netherlands	6–8	DSM-IV	Parents	—	3.7
Kuntsi, et al [53]	England and Wales	5	DSM-IV	Or rule	No	5.7
Kurlan, et al [54]	United States	9–17	DSM-IV	Or rule	No	23.4
Larsson, et al [55]	Sweden	8–9	DSM-III-R	Parents	No	5.4
Levy, et al [5]	Australia	4–12	DSM-III-R	Parents	No	9.9
Loeber, et al [56]	United States	7, 10, 13	DSM-III-R	Parents	No	15.7
Lynch, et al [57]	Ireland	12–15	DSM-IV	Best estimate	Yes	3.7
MacLeod, et al [58]	Canada	6–16	DSM-III	And rule	No	1.6
Malhotra, et al [59]	India	4–11	ICD-10	Best estimate	—	0.9
McArdle, et al [60]	United Kingdom	7–8	DSM-III-R	Parents	Yes	6.7
McKelvey, et al [61]	Australia	9–17	DSM-III-R	Parents	No	0.4
Merrell and Tymms [62]	England	5–6	DSM-IV	Teachers	No	11.2
Meyer [63]	South Africa	6–12	DSM-IV	Teachers	No	7.2
Meyer, et al [64]	South Africa	6–15	DSM-IV	Teachers	No	19.7
Miller, et al [65]	West Bank and Gaza	6 and older	DSM-III	Parents	No	4.6
Montiel-Nava, et al [66]	Venezuela	6–12	DSM-IV	Or rule	No	7.1
Montiel-Nava, et al [67]	Venezuela	3–13	DSM-IV	Parents	—	10.1
Mugnaini, et al [68]	Italy	6–7	DSM-IV	Teachers	Yes	7.3
Mullick and Goodman [69]	Bangladesh	5–10	ICD-10	Parents	Yes	2.0
Neuman, et al [70]	United States	7–18	DSM-IV	—	No	6.2
Owens and Hoza [71]	United States	9–13	DSM-IV	Parents	No	2.9
Pineda, et al [72]	Colombia	4–17	DSM-IV	Parents	No	16.1
Pino and Mojarro-Praxedes [73]	Spain	6–15	DSM-III-R	Parents	Yes	3.1

(continued on next page)

Table 1 (*continued*)

Author	Country	Age (y)	Diagnostic criteria	Source of information	Requirement of impairment	Prevalence estimate (%)
Puura, et al [74]	Finland	8–9	DSM-III-R	Parents	Yes	6.6
Rohde, et al [7]	Brazil	12–14	DSM-IV	Or rule	Yes	5.8
Romano, et al [75]	Canada	14–17	DSM-III-R	Parents	Yes	3.3
Rowland, et al [76]	United States	Grades 1–5	DSM-IV	Or rule	Yes	16.1
Sherman, et al [77]	United States	11–18	DSM-III-R	Parents	No	5.1
Simonoff, et al [78]	United States	8–16	DSM-III-R	Or rule	Yes	1.4
Skounti, et al [79]	Greece	7	DSM-IV			6.5
Srinath, et al [80]	India	0–16	ICD-10	Best estimate	No	1.6
Steinhausen, et al [81]	Switzerland	6–17	DSM-III-R	Parents	No	5.2
Sugawara, et al [82]	Japan	7–9	DSM-III-R	Or rule	No	10.5
Tercyak, et al [83]	United States	14–16	DSM-IV	Subjects	No	6.3
Vasconcelos, et al [84]	Brazil	6–15	DSM-IV	Teachers	No	26.8
Verhulst, et al [85]	The Netherlands	13–18	DSM-III-R	And rule	Yes	0.4
Wacharasindhu and Panyyayong [86]	Thailand	8–11	DSM-IV	—	No	5.1
West, et al [87]	Scotland	15	DSM-IV	Subjects	Yes	0.9
Yoo, et al [88]	Korea	7–12	DSM-IV	—	Yes	0.9
Zuddas, et al [14]	Italy	6–12	DSM-IV	And rule	No	1.38

Blank cells indicate that the information could not be extracted from the paper.

estimated prevalence of current adult (18–44 years of age) ADHD was 4.4% [96].

A similar approach was applied by the World Health Organization World Mental Health (WMH) Survey Initiative to assess adult ADHD in 10 countries (Belgium, Colombia, France, Germany, Italy, Lebanon, Mexico, The Netherlands, Spain, and the United States) [97]. A sample of 11,422 subjects ranging from 18 to 44 years of age was retrospectively evaluated for childhood ADHD and individuals were asked whether they continued to experience symptoms in adulthood. Based on the clinical calibration with 154 subjects in the WMH sample in the United States, multiple imputation was used to estimate the prevalence in the sample. The result for the entire sample was 3.4%, with a significantly higher estimate in France (7.3%) and significantly lower estimates in Spain (1.2%), Lebanon (1.8%), Mexico (1.9%), and Colombia (1.9%). Despite these intriguing differences, the untested assumptions implicit within the multiple imputation procedure indicate that significant questions as to whether meaningful differences would still be found across countries if more rigorous and in-depth diagnostic methods were used remains an interesting topic for future study.

Demographic and psychosocial correlates

The most consistently reported demographic factor characterizing ADHD samples across epidemiologic studies is the higher rates of ADHD among men than among women. Table 2 shows the typical higher prevalence rates for men over women, averaging 11.3% and 5.4%, respectively (approximately a 2.4:1 ratio). Replicating the overall results from Table 2, an analysis of the 2003 National Survey of Children's Health (NSCH), which screened 102,353 children, showed that the diagnosis of ADHD was 2.5 times more frequently reported for boys than girls [98]. Lastly, again consistent with this finding, the systematic review and meta-regression analysis of studies from 1978 to 2005 described earlier also found a pooled ADHD prevalence for boys that was 2.4 times higher than for girls [4]. This overall finding of an approximately 2.4:1 ratio suggests that the frequently reported 4–6:1 ratio in clinical samples may be a function of referral and treatment bias rather than true distribution in the population [11,15,99]. In adult samples, a significantly higher prevalence was also found among men compared with women [96,97].

The associations among ADHD and race, ethnicity, and socioeconomic status are not well defined and shows conflicting results [24,36,69,100]. However, access to treatment [98] and knowledge about the disorder [101] seems to be better among white, non-Hispanic, higher-educated families. Family dysfunction, parental psychopathology, poor peer relations, low self-esteem, lower academic achievement, and school failure are all correlated with ADHD, ADHD persistence, and adverse long-term outcomes in community and clinical samples [7,41,46,100,102–104].

Table 2
Attention deficit hyperactivity disorder prevalence estimates stratified by gender

Author	Male	Female
Almqvist, et al [23]	11.3	2.9
Angold, et al [24]	4.3	0.9
Ashenafi, et al [25]	1.5	1.5
Carlson, et al [30]	25.5	11.6
Essau, et al [35]	0.2	0.2
Fleitlich-Bilyk and Goodman [36]	2.7	0.7
Ford, et al [38]	3.6	0.8
Gadow, et al [39]	28.3	11.9
Gomez, et al [42]	4.2	0.8
Graetz, et al [46]	10.7	4.4
Guardiola, et al [47]	25.1	11
Kroes, et al [52]	4.3	1.4
Larsson, et al [55]	7	3.9
Merrell and Tymms [62]	15	7.1
Meyer, [63]	9.6	4.4
Meyer, et al [64]	22.6	16.5
Montiel-Nava, et al [66]	6.2	8.2
Pineda, et al [72]	19.8	12.3
Puura, et al [74]	10.8	1.4
Romano, et al [75]	5.6	0.9
Steinhausen, et al [81]	6.1	3.3
Sugawara, et al [82]	15.8	5.3
Vasconcelos, et al [84]	31.9	20.8
Wacharasindhu and Panyyayong [86]	7.8	1.6
West, et al [87]	1.3	0.7

Summary

This article reviews the major issues in the epidemiology of ADHD. ADHD surveys published in the past 10 years were selected based on a systematic search strategy. The review included 71 studies and the estimates reported showed an important variability. Findings are consistent with previous reports showing that the variability among prevalence estimates of childhood ADHD is related to methods used within specific surveys [4]. These findings indicate that the methodology of a given survey must be carefully planned and results must be understood in the context of the methodological strategies used in the surveys. Large-scale cross-national studies are needed, with common, in-depth diagnostic methods and similar sampling frames, to determine if meaningful differences exist in prevalence rates across countries.

ADHD is currently understood as a long-lasting disorder that is not restricted to childhood. Epidemiologic surveys of adult ADHD are of a paramount importance in planning of health services and must be further performed. Nevertheless, uncertainties regarding diagnostic criteria must be solved as new evidence emerges.

Although substantial progress has been made in understanding ADHD through epidemiologic and clinical treatment studies, ADHD in particular and childhood mental disorders in general are significantly undertreated worldwide, even in the United States where the most treatment resources are found [98,99,104]. Insufficient public policies and few resources exist to care for children and adolescents who have mental disorders [105]. Governments must direct their attention to childhood mental disorders to guarantee a healthy future for their countries.

Acknowledgments

The authors thank Luis Augusto Rohde for his helpful suggestions on this article.

References

[1] Costello EJ, Egger H, Angold A. 10-year research update review: the epidemiology of child and adolescent psychiatric disorders: I. Methods and public health burden. J Am Acad Child Adolesc Psychiatry 2005;44(10):972–86.

[2] Laucht M, Skowronek MH, Becker K, et al. Interacting effects of the dopamine transporter gene and psychosocial adversity on attention-deficit/hyperactivity disorder symptoms among 15-year-olds from a high-risk community sample. Arch Gen Psychiatry 2007; 64(5):585–90.

[3] Thapar A, Langley K, Fowler T, et al. Catechol O-methyltransferase gene variant and birth weight predict early-onset antisocial behavior in children with attention-deficit/hyperactivity disorder. Arch Gen Psychiatry 2005;62(11):1275–8.

[4] Polanczyk G, Lima MS, Horta BL, et al. The worldwide prevalence of ADHD: a systematic review and metaregression analysis. Am J Psychiatry 2007;164:942–8.

[5] Levy F, Hay DA, McStephen M, et al. Attention-deficit hyperactivity disorder: a category or a continuum? Genetic analysis of a large-scale twin study. J Am Acad Child Adolesc Psychiatry 1997;36(6):737–44.

[6] Breton JJ, Bergeron L, Valla JP, et al. Quebec child mental health survey: prevalence of DSM-III-R mental health disorders. J Child Psychol Psychiatry 1999;40(3):375–84.

[7] Rohde LA, Biederman J, Busnello EA, et al. ADHD in a school sample of Brazilian adolescents: a study of prevalence, comorbid conditions, and impairments. J Am Acad Child Adolesc Psychiatry 1999;38(6):716–22.

[8] Offord DR. Child psychiatric disorders: prevalence and perspectives. Psychiatr Clin North Am 1985;8(4):637–52.

[9] World Health Organization. The ICD-10 classification of mental and behavioral disorders: diagnostic criteria for research. Geneva (Switzerland): WHO; 1993.

[10] American Psychiatric Association. Diagnostic and statistical manual of mental disorders. 4th edition. Washington, DC: Washington American Psychiatric Association; 1994.

[11] Scahill L, Schwab-Stone M. Epidemiology of ADHD in school-age children. Child Adolesc Psychiatr Clin N Am 2000;9(3):541–55, vii.

[12] Canino G, Shrout PE, Rubio-Stipec M, et al. The DSM-IV rates of child and adolescent disorders in Puerto Rico: prevalence, correlates, service use, and the effects of impairment. Arch Gen Psychiatry 2004;61(1):85–93.

[13] Jensen PS, Rubio-Stipec M, Canino G, et al. Parent and child contributions to diagnosis of mental disorder: are both informants always necessary? J Am Acad Child Adolesc Psychiatry 1999;38(12):1569–79.

[14] Zuddas A, Marzocchi GM, Oosterlaan J, et al. Factor structure and cultural factors of disruptive behaviour disorders symptoms in Italian children. Eur Psychiatry 2006;21(6): 410–8.

[15] Polanczyk G, Rohde LA. Epidemiology of attention-deficit/hyperactivity disorder across the lifespan. Curr Opin Psychiatry 2007;20(4):386–92.

[16] Szatmari P. The epidemiology of attention-deficit hyperactivity disorders. Child Adolesc Psychiatr Clin N Am 1992;1(2):361–71.

[17] Biederman J, Faraone SV. Attention-deficit hyperactivity disorder. Lancet 2005;366(9481): 237–48.

[18] Staller J, Faraone SV. Attention-deficit hyperactivity disorder in girls: epidemiology and management. CNS Drugs 2006;20(2):107–23.

[19] Swanson JM, Sergeant JA, Taylor E, et al. Attention-deficit hyperactivity disorder and hyperkinetic disorder. Lancet 1998;351(9100):429–33.

[20] Rowland AS, Lesesne CA, Abramowitz AJ. The epidemiology of attention-deficit/hyperactivity disorder (ADHD): a public health view. Ment Retard Dev Disabil Res Rev 2002;8(3): 162–70.

[21] Faraone SV, Sergeant J, Gillberg C, et al. The worldwide prevalence of ADHD: is it an American condition? World Psychiatry 2003;2(2):104–13.

[22] Skounti M, Philalithis A, Galanakis E. Variations in prevalence of attention deficit hyperactivity disorder worldwide. Eur J Pediatr 2007;166(2):117–23.

[23] Almqvist F, Puura K, Kumpulainen K, et al. Psychiatric disorders in 8-9-year-old children based on a diagnostic interview with the parents. Eur Child Adolesc Psychiatry 1999; 8(Suppl 4):17–28.

[24] Angold A, Erkanli A, Farmer EM, et al. Psychiatric disorder, impairment, and service use in rural African American and white youth. Arch Gen Psychiatry 2002;59(10):893–901.

[25] Ashenafi Y, Kebede D, Desta M, et al. Prevalence of mental and behavioural disorders in Ethiopian children. East Afr Med J 2001;78(6):308–11.

[26] Bener A, Qahtani RA, Abdelaal I. The prevalence of ADHD among primary school children in an Arabian society. J Atten Disord 2006;10(1):77–82.

[27] Benjasuwantep B, Ruangdaraganon N, Visudhiphan P. Prevalence and clinical characteristics of attention deficit hyperactivity disorder among primary school students in Bangkok. J Med Assoc Thai 2002;85(Suppl 4):S1232–40.

[28] Bussing R, Zima BT, Gary FA, et al. Use of complementary and alternative medicine for symptoms of attention-deficit hyperactivity disorder. Psychiatr Serv 2002;53(9):1096–102.

[29] Cardo E, Servera M, Llobera-Canaves J. Estimation of the prevalence of attention deficit hyperactivity disorder among the standard population on the island of Majorca. Rev Neurol 2007;44(1):10–4 [Spanish].

[30] Carlson CL, Tamm L, Gaub M. Gender differences in children with ADHD, ODD, and co-occurring ADHD/ODD identified in a school population. J Am Acad Child Adolesc Psychiatry 1997;36(12):1706–14.

[31] Cornejo JW, Osio O, Sanchez Y, et al. Prevalence of attention deficit hyperactivity disorder in Colombian children and teenagers. Rev Neurol 2005;40(12):716–22 [in Spanish].

[32] Eapen V, al-Gazali L, Bin-Othman S, et al. Mental health problems among schoolchildren in United Arab Emirates: prevalence and risk factors. J Am Acad Child Adolesc Psychiatry 1998;37(8):880–6.

[33] Eapen V, Jakka ME, Abou-Saleh MT. Children with psychiatric disorders: the Al Ain Community Psychiatric Survey. Can J Psychiatry 2003;48(6):402–7.

[34] Ersan EE, Dogan O, Dogan S, et al. The distribution of symptoms of attention-deficit/hyperactivity disorder and oppositional defiant disorder in school age children in Turkey. Eur Child Adolesc Psychiatry 2004;13(6):354–61.

[35] Essau CA, Groen G, Conradt J, et al. Frequency, comorbidity and psychosocial correlates of attention-deficit/hyperactivity disorder. Results of a Bremen adolescent study. Fortschr Neurol Psychiatr 1999;67(7):296–305 [in German].

[36] Fleitlich-Bilyk B, Goodman R. Prevalence of child and adolescent psychiatric disorders in southeast Brazil. J Am Acad Child Adolesc Psychiatry 2004;43(6):727–34.

[37] Fontana RS, Vasconcelos VM, Werner J Jr, et al. ADHD prevalence in four Brazilian public schools. Arq Neuropsiquiatr 2007;65(1):134–7 [in Portuguese].

[38] Ford T, Goodman R, Meltzer H. The British Child and Adolescent Mental Health Survey 1999: the prevalence of DSM-IV disorders. J Am Acad Child Adolesc Psychiatry 2003; 42(10):1203–11.

[39] Gadow KD, Nolan EE, Litcher L, et al. Comparison of attention-deficit/hyperactivity disorder symptom subtypes in Ukrainian schoolchildren. J Am Acad Child Adolesc Psychiatry 2000;39(12):1520–7.

[40] Gau SS, Chong MY, Chen TH, et al. A 3-year panel study of mental disorders among adolescents in Taiwan. Am J Psychiatry 2005;162(7):1344–50.

[41] Gaub M, Carlson CL. Behavioral characteristics of DSM-IV ADHD subtypes in a school-based population. J Abnorm Child Psychol 1997;25(2):103–11.

[42] Gomez R, Harvey J, Quick C, et al. DSM-IV AD/HD: confirmatory factor models, prevalence, and gender and age differences based on parent and teacher ratings of Australian primary school children. J Child Psychol Psychiatry 1999;40(2):265–74.

[43] Goodman R, Ford T, Richards H, et al. The development and well-being assessment: description and initial validation of an integrated assessment of child and adolescent psychopathology. J Child Psychol Psychiatry 2000;41(5):645–55.

[44] Goodman R, Neves dos Santos D, Robatto Nunes AP, et al. The Ilha de Mare study: a survey of child mental health problems in a predominantly African-Brazilian rural community. Soc Psychiatry Psychiatr Epidemiol 2005;40(1):11–7.

[45] Goodman R, Slobodskaya H, Knyazev G. Russian child mental health—a cross-sectional study of prevalence and risk factors. Eur Child Adolesc Psychiatry 2005;14(1):28–33.

[46] Graetz BW, Sawyer MG, Hazell PL, et al. Validity of DSM-IV ADHD subtypes in a nationally representative sample of Australian children and adolescents. J Am Acad Child Adolesc Psychiatry 2001;40(12):1410–7.

[47] Guardiola A, Fuchs FD, Rotta NT. Prevalence of attention-deficit hyperactivity disorders in students. Comparison between DSM-IV and neuropsychological criteria. Arq Neuropsiquiatr 2000;58(2B):401–7.

[48] Hackett R, Hackett L, Bhakta P, et al. The prevalence and associations of psychiatric disorder in children in Kerala, South India. J Child Psychol Psychiatry 1999;40(5):801–7.

[49] Hebrani P, Abdolahian E, Behdani F, et al. The prevalence of attention deficit hyperactivity disorder in preschool-age children in Mashhad, north-East of Iran. Arch Iran Med 2007; 10(2):147–51.

[50] Kadesjo B, Gillberg C. The comorbidity of ADHD in the general population of Swedish school-age children. J Child Psychol Psychiatry 2001;42(4):487–92.

[51] Kashala E, Tylleskar T, Elgen I, et al. Attention deficit and hyperactivity disorder among school children in Kinshasa, Democratic Republic of Congo. Afr Health Sci 2005;5(3): 172–81.

[52] Kroes M, Kalff AC, Kessels AG, et al. Child psychiatric diagnoses in a population of Dutch schoolchildren aged 6 to 8 years. J Am Acad Child Adolesc Psychiatry 2001; 40(12):1401–9.

[53] Kuntsi J, Eley TC, Taylor A, et al. Co-occurrence of ADHD and low IQ has genetic origins. Am J Med Genet B Neuropsychiatr Genet 2004;124(1):41–7.

[54] Kurlan R, Como PG, Miller B, et al. The behavioral spectrum of tic disorders: a community-based study. Neurology 2002;59(3):414–20.

[55] Larsson JO, Lichtenstein P, Fried I, et al. Parents' perception of mental development and behavioural problems in 8 to 9-year-old children. Acta Paediatr 2000;89(12):1469–73.

[56] Loeber R, Farrington DP, Stouthamer-Loeber M, et al. Male mental health problems, psychopathy, and personality traits: key findings from the first 14 years of the Pittsburgh Youth Study. Clin Child Fam Psychol Rev 2001;4(4):273–97.

[57] Lynch F, Mills C, Daly I, et al. Challenging times: prevalence of psychiatric disorders and suicidal behaviours in Irish adolescents. J Adolesc 2006;29(4):555–73.

[58] MacLeod RJ, McNamee JE, Boyle MH, et al. Identification of childhood psychiatric disorder by informant: comparisons of clinic and community samples. Can J Psychiatry 1999;44(2):144–50.

[59] Malhotra S, Kohli A, Arun P. Prevalence of psychiatric disorders in school children in Chandigarh, India. Indian J Med Res 2002;116:21–8.

[60] McArdle P, Prosser J, Kolvin I. Prevalence of psychiatric disorder: with and without psychosocial impairment. Eur Child Adolesc Psychiatry 2004;13(6):347–53.

[61] McKelvey RS, Sang DL, Baldassar L, et al. The prevalence of psychiatric disorders among Vietnamese children and adolescents. Med J Aust 2002;177(8):413–7.

[62] Merrell C, Tymms PB. Inattention, hyperactivity and impulsiveness: their impact on academic achievement and progress. Br J Educ Psychol 2001;71(Pt 1):43–56.

[63] Meyer A. Attention deficit/hyperactivity disorder among North Sotho speaking primary school children in South Africa: prevalence and sex ratios. Journal of Psychology in Africa 1998;8(2):186–95.

[64] Meyer A, Ellertsen DR, Sundet JM, et al. Cross-cultural similarities in ADHD-like behaviour amongst South African primary school children. S Afr J Psychol 2004;34(1):122–38.

[65] Miller T, el-Masri M, Allodi F, et al. Emotional and behavioural problems and trauma exposure of school-age Palestinian children in Gaza: some preliminary findings. Med Confl Surviv 1999;15(4):368–78.

[66] Montiel-Nava C, Pena JA, Lopez M, et al. Estimations of the prevalence of attention deficit hyperactivity disorder in Marabino children. Rev Neurol 2002;35(11):1019–24 [in Spanish].

[67] Montiel-Nava C, Pena JA, Montiel-Barbero I. Epidemiological data about attention deficit hyperactivity disorder in a sample of Marabino children. Rev Neurol 2003;37(9):815–9 [in Spanish].

[68] Mugnaini D, Masi G, Brovedani P, et al. Teacher reports of ADHD symptoms in Italian children at the end of first grade. Eur Psychiatry 2006;21(6):419–26.

[69] Mullick MS, Goodman R. The prevalence of psychiatric disorders among 5-10 year olds in rural, urban and slum areas in Bangladesh: an exploratory study. Soc Psychiatry Psychiatr Epidemiol 2005;40(8):663–71.

[70] Neuman RJ, Sitdhiraksa N, Reich W, et al. Estimation of prevalence of DSM-IV and latent class-defined ADHD subtypes in a population-based sample of child and adolescent twins. Twin Res Hum Genet 2005;8(4):392–401.

[71] Owens J, Hoza B. Diagnostic utility of DSM-IV-TR symptoms in the prediction of DSM-IV-TR ADHD subtypes and ODD. J Atten Disord 2003;7(1):11–27.

[72] Pineda D, Ardila A, Rosselli M, et al. Prevalence of attention-deficit/hyperactivity disorder symptoms in 4- to 17-year-old children in the general population. J Abnorm Child Psychol 1999;27(6):455–62.

[73] Pino P, Mojarro-Praxedes M. Hyperkinetic D disorders: double-phase epidemiological study of a population from Sevilla. An Psiquiatria 2001;17(6):265–70 [in Spanish].

[74] Puura K, Almqvist F, Tamminen T, et al. Psychiatric disturbances among prepubertal children in southern Finland. Soc Psychiatry Psychiatr Epidemiol 1998;33(7):310–8.

[75] Romano E, Tremblay RE, Vitaro F, et al. Prevalence of psychiatric diagnoses and the role of perceived impairment: findings from an adolescent community sample. J Child Psychol Psychiatry 2001;42(4):451–61.

[76] Rowland AS, Umbach DM, Catoe KE, et al. Studying the epidemiology of attention-deficit hyperactivity disorder: screening method and pilot results. Can J Psychiatry 2001;46(10): 931–40.

[77] Sherman DK, McGue MK, Iacono WG. Twin concordance for attention deficit hyperactivity disorder: a comparison of teachers' and mothers' reports. Am J Psychiatry 1997; 154(4):532–5.

[78] Simonoff E, Pickles A, Meyer JM, et al. The Virginia twin study of adolescent behavioral development. Influences of age, sex, and impairment on rates of disorder. Arch Gen Psychiatry 1997;54(9):801–8.

[79] Skounti M, Philalithis A, Mpitzaraki K, et al. Attention-deficit/hyperactivity disorder in schoolchildren in Crete. Acta Paediatr 2006;95(6):658–63.

[80] Srinath S, Girimaji SC, Gururaj G, et al. Epidemiological study of child & adolescent psychiatric disorders in urban & rural areas of Bangalore, India. Indian J Med Res 2005; 122(1):67–79.

[81] Steinhausen HC, Metzke CW, Meier M, et al. Prevalence of child and adolescent psychiatric disorders: the Zurich epidemiological study. Acta Psychiatr Scand 1998;98(4):262–71.

[82] Sugawara M, Mukai T, Kitamura T, et al. Psychiatric disorders among Japanese children. J Am Acad Child Adolesc Psychiatry 1999;38(4):444–52.

[83] Tercyak KP, Lerman C, Audrain J. Association of attention-deficit/hyperactivity disorder symptoms with levels of cigarette smoking in a community sample of adolescents. J Am Acad Child Adolesc Psychiatry 2002;41(7):799–805.

[84] Vasconcelos MM, Werner J Jr, Malheiros AF, et al. Attention deficit/hyperactivity disorder prevalence in an inner city elementary school. Arq Neuropsiquiatr 2003;61(1): 67–73 [in Portuguese].

[85] Verhulst FC, van der Ende J, Ferdinand RF, et al. The prevalence of DSM-III-R diagnoses in a national sample of Dutch adolescents. Arch Gen Psychiatry 1997;54(4):329–36.

[86] Wacharasindhu A, Panyyayong B. Psychiatric disorders in Thai school-aged children: I prevalence. J Med Assoc Thai 2002;85(Suppl 1):S125–36.

[87] West P, Sweeting H, Der G, et al. Voice-DISC identified DSM-IV disorders among 15-year-olds in the west of Scotland. J Am Acad Child Adolesc Psychiatry 2003;42(8):941–9.

[88] Yoo HI, Cho SC, Kim BN, et al. Psychiatric morbidity of second and third grade primary school children in Korea. Child Psychiatry Hum Dev 2005;36(2):215–25.

[89] Timimi S. Effect of globalisation on children's mental health. BMJ 2005;331(7507):37–9.

[90] Biederman J, Mick E, Faraone SV. Age-dependent decline of symptoms of attention deficit hyperactivity disorder: impact of remission definition and symptom type. Am J Psychiatry 2000;157(5):816–8.

[91] Faraone SV, Biederman J, Mick E. The age-dependent decline of attention deficit hyperactivity disorder: a meta-analysis of follow-up studies. Psychol Med 2006;36(2):159–65.

[92] Wilens TE, Faraone SV, Biederman J. Attention-deficit/hyperactivity disorder in adults. JAMA 2004;292(5):619–23.

[93] McGough JJ, Barkley RA. Diagnostic controversies in adult attention deficit hyperactivity disorder. Am J Psychiatry 2004;161(11):1948–56.

[94] Faraone SV, Biederman J, Spencer T, et al. Diagnosing adult attention deficit hyperactivity disorder: are late onset and subthreshold diagnoses valid? Am J Psychiatry 2006;163(10): 1720–9.

[95] Kooij JJ, Buitelaar JK, van den Oord EJ, et al. Internal and external validity of attention-deficit hyperactivity disorder in a population-based sample of adults. Psychol Med 2005; 35(6):817–27.

[96] Kessler RC, Adler L, Barkley R, et al. The prevalence and correlates of adult ADHD in the United States: results from the National Comorbidity Survey Replication. Am J Psychiatry 2006;163(4):716–23.

[97] Fayyad J, De Graaf R, Kessler R, et al. Cross-national prevalence and correlates of adult attention-deficit hyperactivity disorder. Br J Psychiatry 2007;190:402–9.

[98] Mental health in the United States. Prevalence of diagnosis and medication treatment for attention-deficit/hyperactivity disorder—United States, 2003. MMWR Morb Mortal Wkly Rep 2005;54(34):842–7.

[99] A 14-month randomized clinical trial of treatment strategies for attention-deficit/hyperactivity disorder. The MTA Cooperative Group. Multimodal Treatment Study of Children with ADHD. Arch Gen Psychiatry 1999;56(12):1073–86.

[100] Scahill L, Schwab-Stone M, Merikangas KR, et al. Psychosocial and clinical correlates of ADHD in a community sample of school-age children. J Am Acad Child Adolesc Psychiatry 1999;38(8):976–84.
[101] McLeod JD, Fettes DL, Jensen PS, et al. Public knowledge, beliefs, and treatment preferences concerning attention-deficit hyperactivity disorder. Psychiatr Serv 2007;58(5): 626–31.
[102] Jensen PS, Arnold LE, Swanson JM, et al. 3-year follow-up of the NIMH MTA study. J Am Acad Child Adolesc Psychiatry 2007;46(8):989–1002.
[103] Owens EB, Hinshaw SP, Kraemer HC, et al. Which treatment for whom for ADHD? Moderators of treatment response in the MTA. J Consult Clin Psychol 2003;71(3):540–52.
[104] Swanson JM, Hinshaw SP, Arnold LE, et al. Secondary evaluations of MTA 36-month outcomes: propensity score and growth mixture model analyses. J Am Acad Child Adolesc Psychiatry 2007;46(8):1003–14.
[105] Belfer ML, Saxena S. WHO Child Atlas project. Lancet 2006;367(9510):551–2.

ELSEVIER
SAUNDERS

Child Adolesc Psychiatric Clin N Am
17 (2008) 261–284

CHILD AND
ADOLESCENT
PSYCHIATRIC CLINICS
OF NORTH AMERICA

Genetics of Attention Deficit Hyperactivity Disorder

Eric Mick, ScD[a], Stephen V. Faraone, PhD[b],*

[a]Department of Psychiatry, Massachusetts General Hospital and Harvard Medical School,
Warren 705, 55 Fruit Street, Boston, MA 02114-2622, USA
[b]Departments of Psychiatry and Neuroscience and Physiology, SUNY Upstate Medical
University, 750 East Adams Street, Syracuse, NY 13210-2375, USA

Attention deficit hyperactivity disorder (ADHD) is among the most common childhood onset psychiatric disorders. The worldwide prevalence of ADHD in children is 8% to 12% [1], and the prevalence of ADHD in adults in the United States was estimated to be 4% in the National Comorbidity Survey [2]. Early studies found the risk of ADHD among parents of children with ADHD to be increased by between twofold and eightfold, with similarly elevated risk among the siblings of ADHD subjects (for a review of this literature see [3]). Faraone and colleagues [4] recently extended these findings to families ascertained via adult probands meeting criteria for either full ADHD, as defined by the *Diagnostic and Statistical Manual of Mental Disorders, Fourth Edition* (DSM-IV), or late-onset ADHD.

However, adoption and twin studies are necessary to disentangle genetic from environmental sources of transmission observed in family studies. Three studies found that biologic relatives of ADHD [5] or hyperactive children [6,7] were more likely to have hyperactivity than adoptive relatives. A more direct method of examining the heritability of ADHD is to study twins: the extent to which monozygotic twins are more concordant for ADHD than dizygotic twins can be used to compute the degree to which

Dr. Eric Mick receives or has received grant support from, is or has been a speaker for, or is or has been on the advisory board for the following sources: McNeil Pediatrics and Janssen Pharmaceuticals, Pfizer, Shire, and the National Institute of Mental Health (NIMH). Dr. Stephen V. Faraone receives or has received grant support from, is or has been a speaker for, or is or has been on the advisory board for the following sources: McNeil Pediatrics, Eli Lilly & Company, the NIMH, the National Institute of Child Health and Development, and the National Institute of Neurological Diseases and Stroke.
    * Corresponding author.
    E-mail address: faraones@upstate.edu (S.V. Faraone).

variability in ADHD in the population can be accounted for by genes (ie, heritability). Faraone and colleagues [4] reviewed 20 twin studies from the United States, Australia, Scandinavia, and the European Union and reported a mean heritability estimate of 76%, demonstrating that ADHD is among the most heritable of psychiatric disorders.

In an attempt to find regions of chromosomes that might harbor genes for ADHD, three groups have conducted genome-wide linkage scans. This approach examines many DNA markers across the genome to determine whether any chromosomal regions are shared more often than expected among ADHD family members. A study of 126 American-affected sib-pairs found three regions showing some evidence of linkage (limit of detection [LOD] scores > 1.5): 5p12, 10q26, 12q23, and 16p13 [8]. An expanded sample of 203 families found stronger evidence for the 16p13 region, previously implicated in autism, with a maximum LOD score of 4 [9]. A study of 164 Dutch-affected sib-pairs also identified a peak previously noted in autism, at 15q15, with a peak LOD score of 3.5 [10]. Two other peaks, at 7p13 and 9q33, yielded LOD scores of 3.0 and 2.1, respectively. A genome-wide scan of families from a genetically isolated community in Colombia implicated 8q12, 11q23, 4q13, 17p11, 12q23, and 8p23 [11]. Although pooled analyses of [9,10] suggest that the genetic background in the differing populations is quite distinct and that the lack of consistent findings is a reflection of this variance between population heterogeneity [12], they did identify an area of linkage (5p13) that may reflect a common risk locus. A study of 155 sib-pairs from Germany reported a maximum LOD score of 2.59 for chromosome 5p at 17cM. The study also reported nominal evidence for linkage to chromosomes 6q, 7p, 9q, 11q, 12q, and 17p, which had also been identified in previous scans [13].

Although there is some overlap in nominally significant linkage peaks, there is no evidence for the replication of a genome-wide significant finding that uses strict criteria [14]. Nevertheless, given that these studies show some overlap for peaks at lower LOD scores and that each, individually, had low power to detect linkage to genes of small effect, these regions remain of interest for replication studies and for fine-mapping efforts. For ADHD, the lack of replication across the available studies completed so far suggests that genes of moderately large effect are unlikely to exist and that the method of association will be more fruitful in the search for ADHD-susceptibility genes.

In contrast to the scarcity of linkage studies, many candidate gene association studies have been conducted. Several recent meta-analyses suggest strong association with ADHD and the dopamine D4 receptor gene (DRD4, 48-bp variable number of tandem repeat [VNTR]; [15]), the dopamine D5 receptor gene (DRD5, 148-bp microsatellite marker; [15]), the dopamine beta-hydroxylase gene (DBH, 5′ taq1 A allele; [4]), the synaptosomal-associated protein 25 gene (SNAP-25, T1065G single-nucleotide polymorphism [SNP], [4]), the serotonin transporter gene (SLC6A4, 44-bp insertion/deletion in the promoter region [5-HTTLPR]; [4]), and the seroto-nin 1B receptor gene (HTR1B, G861C SNP; [4]). Conversely, meta-analysis has suggested a weak association with ADHD and the dopamine trans-porter gene (SLC6A3, 480-bp VNTR in the 3' untranslated region [UTR]; [15–17]) and no association with the catechol-O-methyltransferase gene (COMT, Val108Met polymorphism; [18]).

A major recent advance in the molecular genetics of ADHD was the pub-lication of the International Multisite ADHD Gene (IMAGE) project in which 51 genes were analyzed for association with ADHD. Families were recruited via an ADHD combined-type child proband (N = 674) who had at least one full sibling (N = 808) and one biological parent (N = 1227 par-ents) available for study. A high-density SNP map was constructed for genes involved in the regulation of neurotransmitter pathways implicated in ADHD (dopamine, norepinephrine, and serotonin) based on tagging SNPs and SNPs within known functional regions. This study—the most in-depth genetic association study performed in the largest set of ADHD pa-tients to date—found evidence of association with ADHD and 18 genes.

Taken together, this literature strongly suggests a contribution of genetic factors in the etiology of ADHD. This article provides an update on the progress of molecular genetic studies published since the completion of these meta-analyses. Results from the IMAGE projects are discussed separately for each gene.

Catecholaminergic genes

The dopamine D4 receptor

Both noradrenaline and dopamine are potent agonists of DRD4 [19], and the D4 receptor is prevalent in frontal-subcortical networks implicated in the pathophysiology of ADHD by neuroimaging and neuropsychologic studies [20]. Researchers have predominantly focused on a tandem repeat polymorphism in exon III of DRD4 because in vitro studies have shown that one variant (the 7-repeat allele) produces a blunted response to dopa-mine [21,22]. Faraone and colleagues [4] conducted a meta-analysis of the 7-repeat allele of the exon III polymorphism and found statistically signifi-cant association with ADHD in both case-control (odds ratio [OR] = 1.45; 95% CI, 1.27–1.65) and family-based (OR = 1.16; 95% CI, 1.03–1.31) stud-ies. Most recently, Li and colleagues [15] reported a pooled OR of 1.34 (1.23–1.45) in 33 studies.

Not included in these meta-analyses of the exon III DRD4 48-bp VNTR were a prospective follow-up study of German children in which the 7-re-peat DRD4 allele was associated with increased incidence and persistence of ADHD in boys up to 11 years of age [23], a positive association with the 6- and 7-repeat alleles in a sample of 44 Indian ADHD trios (relative risk [RR] = 1.81; P = .03) [24], and a negative association in 126 Korean

ADHD families ($P = .67$) [25]. Carrasco and colleagues [26] also failed to document an association with the 7-repeat allele in a small case-control study of 26 Chilean children with ADHD, but found a significant interaction with this DRD4 marker and the dopamine transporter gene, suggesting that children with the risk alleles at both loci are at greater risk of ADHD. In the large and comprehensive IMAGE project, the association with this VNTR and ADHD was not statistically significant ($P<.09$), but the OR (1.18) was very close to that observed in meta-analyses.

A small number of studies have assessed other DRD4 polymorphisms; however, these data have not been conclusive. McCracken and colleagues [27,28] found an association between ADHD and a 5' 120-bp repeat 1.2 kb upstream of the initiation codon. However, Barr and colleagues [29], Todd and colleagues [30], Brookes and colleagues [31], and Bhaduri and colleagues [32] found no association between ADHD and this marker. Significant evidence of association was found by Arcos-Burgos and colleagues [11], but only with the 5' 120-bp marker included with exon III 48-bp 7-repeat allele in haplotype analysis.

Barr and colleagues [29] found no association between ADHD and two SNPs in the promoter region (rs747302 and rs1800955), but Lowe and colleagues [33] observed a significant overtransmission of the rs1800955-A allele and a trend toward association with the rs747302-C allele. Brookes and colleagues [34] did not genotype these SNPS in the IMAGE project, but observed nominal association with SNP (rs9195457) for which the linkage disequilibrium structure with previously associated SNPs could not be determined.

Although it has been suggested that the DRD4 gene may be particularly relevant to symptoms of inattention, the recent literature suggests that this may not be so. Rowe and colleagues [35] found that fathers of ADHD children with the 7-repeat allele had higher levels of retrospectively reported inattention symptoms, and Levitan and colleagues [36] found an association between this allele and greater self-reported childhood inattention in women with seasonal affective disorder. However, Todd and colleagues [37] found no association with the exon III 48-bp VNTR and any ADHD symptom profiles or DSM-IV subtypes in pooled analysis of 2090 children. Similarly, Mill and colleagues [38] found no association with the 7-repeat allele and a quantitative measure of ADHD symptom profiles in 329 pairs of male twins ascertained in England and Wales. Although the 7-repeat allele was not present in a sample of Korean ADHD children, Kim and colleagues [25] reported no variation of inattentive symptoms with the number of repeats, but rather observed a greater severity of hyperactive/impulsive symptoms in subjects with a 5-repeat allele.

The literature is similarly inconclusive when examining neuropsychologic measures of attention. Kieling and colleagues [39] found increased errors of omission and commission in ADHD subjects with the 7-repeat allele, whereas others have found that subjects possessing the 7-repeat allele demonstrated significantly better attention than subjects with fewer repeats [40–42] or demonstrated no difference on similar measures of attention [43]. However, Bellgrove and colleagues [42] found that the rs747302-A allele was associated with sustained attention deficits, whereas the 7-repeat allele of the exon III VNTR was associated with improved performance. Thus, they conclude that such risk alleles have dissociable effects on cognition in ADHD children [42].

Two studies have provided evidence documenting strength of a DRD4–ADHD relationship relative to other phenotypes hypothesized to also be associated with DRD4: autism [44] and a novelty-seeking temperament [45]. Grady and colleagues [44] found no evidence of an overrepresentation of rare DRD4 variants in a sample of children with autism relative to geographically matched controls, whereas a sample of ADHD children had a fourfold increase in novel alleles compared with geographically matched controls. Furthermore, Lynn and colleagues [45] examined the relationship between ADHD/novelty-seeking and the exon III DRD4 48-bp VNTR and found independent associations with ADHD/novelty seeking and ADHD/DRD4, but not between DRD4/novelty seeking. Although not conclusive, these studies suggest that the association between ADHD and DRD4 is relatively specific (ie, relative to autism) and not confounded by common comorbid behaviors (ie, increased novelty seeking).

The dopamine 5 receptor

The most widely studied polymorphism for DRD5 has been a dinucleotide repeat that maps approximately 18.5 kb 5′ to the transcription start site [46]. Meta-analysis of 14 independent family-based studies suggested a significant association of the 148-bp allele with ADHD (OR = 1.2; 95% CI, 1.1–1.4) [47] that was confirmed in updated analyses recently conducted by Li and colleagues [15] (OR = 1.3; 95% CI, 1.2–1.5). Not included in these meta-analyses is a study by Mill and colleagues [38] examining quantitative measures of ADHD symptoms in 329 pairs of male twins ascertained in England and Wales. Again, the 148-bp allele was statistically significantly associated with ADHD, but unfortunately the direction of effect was in the opposite direction: the risk allele was associated with lower hyperactivity scores [38].

Other markers within DRD5 have also been found to be associated with ADHD. Hawi and colleagues [46] studied two additional 5′ microsatellite markers and an SNP in the 3′ UTR. The 3′ SNP was associated with ADHD (RR = 1.6), and haplotype analyses showed an association with ADHD and a two-marker haplotype of one of the 5′ microsatellite markers (D4S1582) and the dinucleotide repeat (DRD5-PCR1) (P = .000107), a two-marker haplotype comprising DRD5-PCR1 and the 3′ SNP (P = .0099), and a haplotype comprising all three of these markers (P = .0013).

The dopamine transporter gene

There are several reasons that the dopamine transporter gene (SLC6A3) has been considered a suitable candidate for ADHD. Stimulant medications, which are efficacious in treating ADHD, block the dopamine transporter as one mechanism of action for achieving their therapeutic effects [48]. In mice, eliminating SLC6A3 gene function leads to two features suggestive of ADHD: hyperactivity and deficits in inhibitory behavior. Treating these "knockout" mice with stimulants reduces their hyperactivity [49,50].

Using a family-based association study, Cook and colleagues [51] first reported an association between ADHD and the 10-repeat allele of 3' UTR VNTR. The present authors' previous meta-analysis of family-based studies resulted in a small but significant OR (1.13; 95% CI, 1.03–1.24), but Li and colleagues [15] updated this work and found no evidence of association with ADHD and the 10-repeat allele in family-based studies (OR = 1.04; 95% CI, 0.99–1.14) and considerable evidence of heterogeneity between studies (p(Q) = 0.000001). The most recent meta-analysis of this gene found small but significant association with ADHD for family-based transmission disequilibrium test (TDT) studies (OR = 1.17; 95% CI, 1.05–1.30) [16]. The OR for seven family-based haplotype-based haplotype relative risk (HHRR) studies was 1.5, but it was not significant, perhaps owing to the small number of studies. Although there were only six case-control studies, their combined OR of 0.95 would seem to disconfirm the family-based studies [16].

Thus, the lack of consistent association with the 3' UTR VNTR suggests that this marker itself is not directly involved in the etiology of ADHD, but that may be tagging a proximate functional polymorphism in partial linkage disequilibrium with the 10-repeat allele. For example, Genro and colleagues [52] found an association with rs2652511, and Brookes and colleagues [34] found an association with rs40184 in samples for which there was no evidence of association with the 3' UTR VNTR. In an attempt to further refine the SLC6A3 risk variant for ADHD, Brookes and colleagues [53] reported that association with a haplotype comprised the 10-repeat allele in the 3' UTR and the 6-repeat allele of a 30-bp VNTR in intron 8. Of the four possible haplotype combinations of the two markers, only the 10-6 haplotype was associated with increased risk for ADHD in both populations. This finding was replicated by Brookes and colleagues [34] (OR = 1.19, $P < .06$) and Asherson and colleagues [54] in the second set of 383 ADHD probands from the IMAGE sample (OR = 1.27, $P = .002$). Bakker and colleagues [55], however, failed to identify an overall association with this haplotype ($P = .2$) or preferential overtransmission of the 10-6 variant in 198 Dutch probands with ADHD.

However, evidence is emerging that environmental risk factors for ADHD are important mediators of the risk for ADHD associated with

SLC6A3. Brookes and colleagues [53] also reported a gene–environment interaction that suggests that the risk for ADHD was increased only in the presence of 10-6 SLC6A3 haplotype when also exposed to maternal alcohol use during pregnancy. Although the 9-repeat allele was significantly overtransmitted in the sample [56] used by Neuman and colleagues [57], they documented an increased risk for the severe combined ADHD profile with both SLC6A3 and the DRD4 7-repeat allele only in children also exposed to maternal cigarette smoking during pregnancy. Similarly, Laucht and colleagues [58] found that the 3' UTR 10-repeat allele, the intron 8 6-repeat allele, and the 10-6 haplotype were associated with ADHD symptoms only in families exposed to higher psychosocial adversity.

Dopamine beta-hydroxylase

DBH is the primary enzyme responsible for conversion of dopamine to norepinephrine. Comings and colleagues [59,60] examined a Taq1 restriction-site polymorphism in intron 5 and found a significant association with the A1 allele and ADHD symptom scores in children with Tourette's syndrome (TS) [60]. Smith and colleagues [61] subsequently replicated this association (OR = 1.96; 95% CI, 1.01–3.79) in ADHD subjects, but Daly and colleagues [62] and Roman and colleagues [63] found overtransmission of the A2 allele. Both also found that the association was stronger in combined-type ADHD cases, but Daly and colleagues [62] found that parental history of ADHD strengthened the association, whereas Roman and colleagues [63] found stronger evidence of association in those with no parental history of ADHD. In a Canadian study of 117 families with children with ADHD, Wigg and colleagues [64] reported a nonsignificant excess transmission of the A2 allele. Subsequently, a case-control study of Indian ADHD children [65] and both case-control and family-based analyses of persistent ADHD cases in Canada [66] have failed to document a significant association with this marker of DBH.

Other markers of DBH have also failed to identify significant association with ADHD. Wigg and colleagues [64] observed no evidence of linkage or association for the dinucleotide repeat polymorphism and an insertion/deletion polymorphism in the region 5' to the transcription start site (both of which had been associated with serum DBH levels). A G/T SNP in exon 5 of DBH was examined in 104 trios from the United Kingdom (Payton and colleagues [67]) and in 86 trios from Ireland (Hawi and colleagues [46]); no evidence of association was found in either study. Hawi and colleagues [68] also examined an EcoN1 restriction-site polymorphism in exon 2 and an MspI polymorphism in intron 9 and found association for only a haplotype composed of allele 1 of the exon 2 polymorphism and A2 of the Taq1 polymorphism. A -1021C > T polymorphism in the 5' flanking region of DBH has been shown to account for as much as 50% of plasma DBH activity and was associated with ADHD in the Han Chinese

[69] but not in a sample of Indian ADHD children [65]. Finally, 33 SNPs were tagged for this gene in the IMAGE project, but no nominally significant associations with ADHD were found [34].

Monoamine oxidase A

The monoamine oxidase A (MAO-A) enzyme moderates levels of norepinephrine, dopamine, and serotonin, and MAO-A knockout mice display numerous abnormalities in these neurotransmitter systems [70]. A case-control study of a 30-bp pair tandem repeat in the promoter region in 129 Israeli ADHD suggested association with ADHD and a particularly large effect was noted in subset of female cases (N = 19) [71]. The 4- and 5-repeat alleles of this promoter-region VNTR were also significantly associated with ADHD in a sample of 133 Israeli families [71] but not in a similarly sized family-based study by Lawson and colleagues [72]. In contrast, Das and colleagues [73] found overtransmission of the shorter repeats (ie, 3.5 repeats, or 324 bp) in a sample of 21 Indian male ADHD probands and their mothers. A CA-repeat microsatellite in intron 2 was associated with ADHD [74] in 82 Chinese, but this was not replicated in samples of white subjects [67,75].

Domschke and colleagues [75] also examined an SNP in exon 8 (941G > T) and found association with the high-activity G941T allele and with a haplotype containing the G941T allele, the 3-repeat allele of 30-bp VNTR, and the 6-repeat of the CA microsatellite described above. Xu and colleagues [76] replicated the association with G941T allele and the overtransmission of a haplotype containing the G941T allele and the shorter 3-repeat allele of the promoter VNTR in a Taiwanese sample. Five tagged SNPs for MAO-A were statistically significantly associated with ADHD in the IMAGE sample [34]. The 941G > T SNP was not included in that analysis, but the region covered by the widow of significant SNPs incorporated the location of this SNP.

The dopamine D2 receptor

DRD2 has been less extensively studied in ADHD than have DRD4 and DRD5. Comings and colleagues [77] compared 104 ADHD subjects (nearly all with comorbid TS) with controls and found a significant association with the TaqIA1 allele of DRD2, which they subsequently replicated [59]. More recently, this finding was replicated in a case-control sample of Czech boys with ADHD [78], but not in a sample of Korean alcoholics with and without ADHD [79].

Family-based studies of DRD2 have been uniformly negative, however. Rowe and colleagues [80] examined 164 ADHD children from 125 families and found no excess transmission of the Taq1A1 allele. A subsequent study of Taiwanese families likewise found no association [81]. Kirley and colleagues [82] examined two polymorphisms in 118 ADHD children and their families. No significant associations were identified, though they reported a trend toward significance ($P = .07$) for the Ser311 polymorphism when paternally transmitted. Finally, the IMAGE project examined 23 tag SNPs and found no nominally significant association with ADHD.

The dopamine D3 receptor

Barr and colleagues [83] examined a Ser9Gly exon 1 polymorphism and an intron 5 MspI restriction-site polymorphism in 100 Canadian families, but neither the individual loci nor haplotypes of the two were associated with ADHD. Negative results for the Ser9Gly polymorphism were also reported in a family-based study of 105 families in the United Kingdom [67] and a study of 39 families of ADHD adults [84]. Comings and colleagues [85] also found no evidence for association with ADHD and comorbid TS. In a sample of 146 German patients referred for forensic evaluation [86], heterozygosity at this polymorphism was associated with higher impulsivity scores, although this effect was only seen among those with a history of violence. Similarly, none of the 28 dopamine D3 receptor (DRD3) SNPs tagged for the IMAGE project were nominally significant [34].

Catechol-O-methyltransferase

COMT catalyzes a major step in the degradation of dopamine, norepinephrine, and epinephrine. The most extensively studied marker for the COMT gene is the Val108Met polymorphism, which yields either a high- or low-activity form of COMT [87]. Cheuk and Wong [18] conducted a meta-analysis of this marker and found no evidence of association with ADHD in case-control studies (OR = 0.95; CI, 0.75–1.2, $P = .7$) or family-based studies using the TDT (OR = 0.95; CI, 0.84–1.09, $P = .5$) or the HHRR (OR = 1.02; CI, 0.78–1.34, $P = .9$). Reuter and colleagues [88] found that higher symptom scores were associated with the MET/MET genotype in German adults who were healthy or diagnosed with eating or substance use disorders. Gothelf and colleagues [89] documented a fivefold increased risk for the MET allele in 55 subjects with velocardiofacial syndrome and comorbid ADHD relative to those without comorbid ADHD. The lack of significant results from the IMAGE project [90] is consistent with the negative meta-analysis conducted by Cheuk and colleagues [18].

The noradrenergic system

Noradrenergic receptors: alpha-2A adrenergic receptor, 2C, and 1C

Three adrenergic receptors have been examined in ADHD. The alpha-2A adrenergic receptor (ADRA2A) has a promoter-region SNP (-1291

C > G) that has been examined in both case-control and family-based studies. Comings and colleagues [91] reported an association between genotypes at this SNP and ADHD symptom scores and that the G-1291C allele was associated with ADHD and oppositional defiant or conduct disorder symptoms, whereas the C-1291G allele was associated with a spectrum of other conditions, including panic attacks, obsessive-compulsive disorder, addictions, and affective and schizoid symptoms. However, family-based studies failed to detect association with -1291C > G polymorphism and the diagnosis of ADHD [92–98]. The G-1291C allele of this marker has been shown to be associated with ADHD symptom scores, but the direction of effect has been inconsistent—some studies found association with only inattentive symptoms [99], whereas others found association with both inattentive and hyperactive symptoms [93,94]. In contrast, Wang and colleagues [97] found no association with ADHD in a sample of Han Chinese but a trend toward lower ADHD symptom scores in subjects homozygous for the G-1291C allele. Examination of other markers have been similarly inconsistent, with the G-1291C allele being included in a significantly overtransmitted haplotype in a sample of 51 trios [94], whereas the C-1291G allele was included in a significant haplotype in sib-pair linkage study of 93 ADHD probands and 50 of their unaffected siblings [98].

Although these results suggest either a weak or no association with ADHD and polymorphism -1291G > C polymorphism, they do not take heterogeneity in the presentation of ADHD into account. Schmitz and colleagues [95] conducted a unique study of exclusively inattentive-type ADHD children and found a significant association with the G-1291C allele in case-control but not family-based analyses. Waldman and colleagues [100] evaluated the moderating and mediating effects of executive function deficits on the association of ADRA2A and ADHD and found that association with ADHD was more robust in children with poorer cognitive performance. Although Stevenson and colleagues [96] reported no overall association with ADRA2A, there was a significant overtransmission of the G-1291C allele in the subsample with a reading disability.

A dinucleotide-repeat polymorphism located approximately 6 kb from the gene that codes for the ADRA2C has also been examined in both case-control and family-based analyses. Comings and colleagues [101] found an association between this polymorphism and ADHD symptom scores (it was, however, not significant after Bonferroni correction), but two subsequent family-based analyses showed no evidence of association [102,103]. The former study also examined a C-to-T SNP in codon 492 of the 1C receptor (ADRA1C) that changes cysteine to arginine; no evidence of linkage was found [102]. In the IMAGE project, there was no nominally significant association with any of SNPs tagged for ADRA2A or ADRA2C [34].

The norepinephrine transporter (SLC6A2)

SLC6A2 has been examined in ADHD because drugs that block the nor-epinephrine transporter are efficacious in treating ADHD [104]. Comings and colleagues [85] found evidence for association of an SNP in SLC6A2 with ADHD symptoms. Subsequently, Barr and colleagues [105] examined three SNPs in SLC6A2 (one each in exon 9, intron 9, and intron 13) in 122 ADHD families and found no evidence of association for these loci or haplotypes comprising them. Others have found no association with SNPs in intron 7 or 9 [106] or with a restriction fragment-length polymorphism in ADHD adults [103]. However, Xu and colleagues [107] investigated 21 SNPs spanning the norepinephrine transporter region in 180 cases and 334 controls and reported nominally significant association with rs3785157 that was later replicated by Bobb and colleagues [108] with the additional significant association with rs998424. Although these SNPs were not found to be associated with ADHD in the IMAGE study [34], 2 of the 43 tagged SNPs (rs3785143 and rs11568324) for SLC6A2 did reach nominal statistical significance. Finally, a novel promoter SNP has recently been shown to be possibly associated with ADHD in a sample of association in a set of 94 ADHD cases and 60 controls [109].

The serotonergic system

Serotonin receptors: HTR1B and HTR2A

Of the family-based association studies of a silent SNP (861G > C) in the gene coding for the serotonin HTR1B receptor [108,110–114], only the multi-site study by Hawi and colleagues [110] reached statistical significance, sug-gesting overtransmission of the G861C allele. Smoller and colleagues pooled data from [110–112] and identified statistically significant overtrans-mission of this allele (OR = 1.35; CI, 1.13–1.62, $P = .009$) that strongly sug-gested paternal ($P = .00005$) rather than maternal transmission ($P = .2$) [112]. There was a weak trend suggesting overtransmission of the G681 allele in Li and colleagues [114] when examining primarily inattentive ADHD subjects separately. Smoller and colleagues [112] also identified association with this ADHD subtype and a 6-SNP haplotype, including the G681C allele and two promoter SNPs with functional effects on HTR1B expression. Heiser and colleagues [113] identified no association with the G681C allele, but exam-ined only the combined ADHD subtype and did not assess for paternal trans-mission separately. The analysis of combined-type ADHD in the IMAGE project did not identify association with any of the tag SNPs selected [34].

The T102C, G1438A, and His452Tyr polymorphisms of the serotonin HTR2A receptor gene have also been examined for association with ADHD [110,113,115–119]. No association has been reported for the T102C and the G1438A SNPs for ADHD in [113,116,117,119]. Likewise, Bobb and colleagues [108] found no evidence of association with ADHD and any of the SNPs of the HTR2A gene examined in either case-control or family-based analyses. However, Levitan and colleagues [120] found an association with C102T allele and greater scores on a self-report measure of childhood ADHD in a sample of women with seasonal affective disorder. Li and colleagues [118] found that the A1438G allele was associated with functional remission from ADHD in Han Chinese adolescents. A coding polymorphism in the HTR2A receptor gene (His452Tyr) was associated with ADHD in [115,119] but not in [110,113].

Li and colleagues [121] found significant overtransmission of the C-759T/ G-697C haplotype within the HTR2C gene, but no association was observed in Bobb and colleagues [108] or in the IMAGE project [34]. Li and colleagues have also reported significant undertransmission of the C83097T/G83198A haplotype in the HTR4 gene [122], but no association with markers in HTR5A and HTR6 [117] or HTR1D [123]. Genes for additional serotonin receptors (HTR1E and HTR3B) evaluated in the IMAGE project [34] have also failed to yield any significant association with ADHD.

Serotonin transporter (HTT, SLC6A4)

A 44-base pair insertion/deletion polymorphism (HTTLPR) in the promoter region of SLC6A4 may be the most studied genetic marker in psychiatric genetics, with associations reported for a broad range of diagnoses and traits [124,125]. When the HTTLPR studies published by 2005 were combined [4], the pooled ORs for the long allele was 1.31 (95%; CI, 1.09– 1.59). Curran and colleagues [126] found nominal evidence of overtransmission of the long allele and strong evidence of association with a 4 SNP haplotype upstream that included the 5-HTTPR insertion/deletion polymorphism. However, subsequent studies of this marker in 126 Korean ADHD families [127], 197 ADHD families from the United Kingdom [128], 196 Taiwanese ADHD families [128,129], 56 Indian ADHD families [130], 209 Canadian ADHD families [131], and 102 German ADHD families [113] have failed to identify an association with the HTTLPR. Li and colleagues [132] found statistically significant overtransmission of the short (rather than the long) allele in 279 Han Chinese ADHD families.

A 17-bp VNTR in intron 2 of SLC6A4 (STint2) was first associated with ADHD in a case-control study conducted by [116], with the 12-12 genotype being underrepresented in cases than in controls. Banerjee and colleagues [130] found significant overtransmission of the 12 allele, but Heiser and colleagues [113], Xu and colleagues [128], and Kim and colleagues [127] found no association, and Li and colleagues [132] found evidence of undertransmission of a haplotype with the HTTLPR long allele and the STint2 12 allele. The IMAGE project found no association for the tag SNPs examined [34], and Wigg and colleagues [131] found no association with two functional SLC6A4 polymorphisms— rs3813034 (T/G) and Ile425Val (A/G)—and ADHD.

Tryptophan hydroxylase

Tryptophan hydroxylase (TPH) is the rate-limiting enzyme in the synthesis of serotonin, and TPH polymorphisms have been associated with aggression and impulsivity [133]. Two family-based studies examined the TPH gene in ADHD. One study of 69 Han Chinese trios found no association with an SNP (A218C) in intron 7 [134]. A second study examined two SNPs among more than 350 Han Chinese youth with ADHD, with and without learning disability, and their families [135,136]. Although neither SNP showed biased transmission individually, a haplotype composed of the A218 and G-6526 alleles appeared to be undertransmitted ($P = .03$).

The gene for a second form of TPH (TPH-2), located on chromosome 12q15, has received more attention because it has been found to specifically synthesize serotonin in the mouse brain [137]. Walitza and colleagues examined two SNPs located in the transcriptional control region of TPH-2 (rs4570625 and rs11178997) and a third located in intron 2 (rs4565946). Tests of the transcriptional SNPs individually and in a two-SNP haplotype were modestly associated with ADHD in the 225 affected children (103 families), but the intron 2 SNP was not associated. Sheehan and colleagues [138] studied eight additional SNPs in 179 ADHD families and found statistically significant evidence of association with the rs1843809-T allele ($P = .0006$) and the rs1386497-A allele ($P = .048$) as well as a trend suggesting association with the rs1386493-C allele ($P = .09$). In the IMAGE project, rs1843809 and rs1386497 were also significantly associated with ADHD, but the direction of effect observed in Sheehan and colleagues [138] was not [34]. Brookes and colleagues [34] also reported an association with rs1007023, which was in perfect linkage disequilibrium with rs1386497 from Sheehan and colleagues. However, Brookes and colleagues did not replicate the finding reported by Walitza and colleagues [139], and Sheehan and colleagues [140] was not able to replicate their earlier findings in a smaller sample of 63 ADHD trios.

Other candidate genes

Synaptasomal-associated protein of 25kD

SNAP25 is a 206 amino acid protein found on chromosome 20p12. The gene product is a presynaptic plasma membrane protein involved in the regulation of neurotransmitter release. Its relevance to ADHD was motivated by the coloboma mouse, which has a hemizygous two centimorgan deletion of a segment on chromosome 2q, including the gene-encoding SNAP25. The coloboma mutation leads to spontaneous hyperactivity, delays in achieving complex neonatal motor abilities, deficits in hippocampal physiology (which may contribute to learning deficiencies), and deficits in Ca2+-dependent dopamine release in dorsal striatum [141]. Four family-based studies of SNAP25 examined two biallelic SNPs (1069T > C and 1065T > G) separated by four base pairs at the 3′ end of the gene [142–146]. Meta-analysis of these studies showed significant evidence for an association with ADHD and T1065G (OR = 1.19; 95% CI, 1.03–1.38). Feng and colleagues [147] examined 12 SNPs in two independent samples of ADHD families and found significant overtransmission of the rs66039806-C, rs362549-A, rs362987-A, and the rs362998-C alleles in families from Toronto but not California. The IMAGE analysis of pooled data did not test these specific markers, but did demonstrate nominally statistically significant association with SNAP-25 and other markers (rs363020 and rs362567) [34] the 5′ UTR. Kim and colleagues [148] examined the previously implicated SNPs and 5 additional SNPs (rs6077699, rs363006, rs362549, rs362987, rs362998), but found no evidence of association with ADHD in tests of individual markers or haplotypes. However, a combined TDT analysis of pooled data was modestly significant for rs3746544-T ($P = .048$) and rs6077690-T ($P = .031$). Stratification by psychiatric comorbidity further suggested that subjects with ADHD and comorbid depression may demonstrate stronger association with SNPs in SNAP-25 [148].

Acetylcholine receptors: cholinergic receptor, nicotinic, alpha 4

The nicotinic acetylcholine receptors are ligand-gated ion channels composed of five subunits, one of which is the alpha-4 subunit (cholinergic receptor, nicotinic, alpha 4 [CHRNA4]), which has been examined in several studies in ADHD. Comings and colleagues [149] found evidence of association with an intron 1 dinucleotide repeat polymorphism of the CHRNA4 gene and ADHD symptoms in a case-control study of children with TS, but Kent and colleagues [150] found no significant evidence of association with a Cfo1 restriction-site polymorphism in exon 5 in a study of 68 trios. Todd and colleagues [151] examined seven SNPs encompassing exons 2 and 5 as well as haplotypes of these markers and found significant association for inattentive ADHD with an intronic SNP (G/A) near the exon/intron boundary at the 3′ end of exon 2. Subsequent examination of CHRNA4 in samples of combined-type ADHD cases has not replicated this association [34,108], although the IMAGE project did report association with an SNP in the 5′ flanking region. Lee and colleagues [152] failed to replicate the association with SNPs from Todd and colleagues [151] or the IMAGE study [34] for either categorical ADHD diagnosis or symptom profile scores. In contrast to Todd and colleagues [151], Lee and colleagues [152] found overtransmission of the rs2273505-G and rs3787141-T alleles with the combined ADHD subtype and hyperactivity–impulsivity scores.

Glutamate receptors

The glutamate receptor, ionotropic, N-methyl D-aspartate 2A (GRIN2A) gene, which codes a subunit of the N-methyl D-aspartate receptor, has been examined in family-based studies of ADHD. Glutamate and the N-methyl D-aspartate receptor have been implicated in cognition in both animal and human studies; the GRIN2A gene is an appealing positional candidate gene as well, located under a linkage peak at 16p13 previously associated with ADHD [9]. In a family-based analysis of 238 families, an SNP in exon 5 (Grin2a_5) was significantly associated with ADHD ($P = .01$); haplotypes, including additional SNPs, were more weakly associated [153]. However, among 183 families, no evidence for association was identified for this SNP ($P = .74$) or three others [154].

Brain-derived neurotrophic factor

Brain-derived neurotrophic factor (BDNF) is a protein that supports survival of central nervous system neurons and stimulates growth and differentiation of developing neurons. A polymorphism producing an amino acid substitution (valine to methionine) at codon 66 of the BDNF may impact intracellular trafficking and activity-dependent secretion of BDNF [155]. Kent and colleagues [156] found overtransmission of the Val66 allele and that this was accounted for by paternal ($P = .0005$) rather than maternal ($P = 1.0$) transmission in 341 white ADHD probands and their family members. However, Xu and colleagues [157] failed to replicate these associations with Val66 in samples from the United Kingdom or Taiwan. Xu and colleagues also examined the 270C > T SNP in the 5'-noncoding region of intron 1 and found significant overtransmission of the C720T allele in Taiwanese ADHD families but not in those from the United Kingdom [157]. Twenty SNPs in the BDNF gene were tagged for the IMAGE project, but none were statistically significantly associated with ADHD [34].

Summary

Although twin studies demonstrate that ADHD is a highly heritable condition, molecular genetic studies suggest that the genetic architecture of ADHD is complex. The handful of genome-wide scans that have been conducted thus far show divergent findings and are, therefore, not conclusive. Similarly, many of the candidate genes reviewed here (ie, DBH, MAO-A, SLC6A2, TPH-2, SLC6A4, CHRNA4, GRIN2A) are theoretically compelling from a neurobiologic systems perspective, but available data are sparse and inconsistent. However, candidate gene studies of ADHD have produced substantial evidence implicating several genes in the etiology of the disorder. The literature published since recent meta-analyses is particularly supportive of a role of the genes coding for DRD4, DRD5, SLC6A3, SNAP-25, and HTR1B in the etiology of ADHD.

Yet, even these associations are small and consistent with the idea that the genetic vulnerability to ADHD is mediated by many genes of small effects. These small effects emphasize the need for future candidate gene studies to implement strategies that will provide enough statistical power to detect such small effects. One such strategy, examination of refined phenotypes that may reduce heterogeneity, is beginning to bear fruit, but more research is needed to extend the work focused on ADHD subtypes (eg, inattentive subtype and HTR1B); comorbid psychopathology or cognitive impairment (eg, depression and SNAP-25, reading disability, and ADRA2A), and gene-environment interactions (eg, prenatal or psychosocial risk factors for ADHD and SLC6A3). The ongoing efforts to develop larger collaborative studies with adequate sizes for genome-wide association studies will also be critical in understanding the molecular genetics of ADHD.

References

[1] Faraone SV, Sergeant J, Gillberg C, et al. The worldwide prevalence of ADHD: is it an American condition? World Psychiatry 2003;2(2):104–13.

[2] Kessler RC, Adler L, Barkley R, et al. The prevalence and correlates of adult ADHD in the United States: results from the national comorbidity survey replication. Am J Psychiatry 2006;163(4):716–23.

[3] Faraone SV, Biederman J. Nature, nurture, and attention deficit hyperactivity disorder. Dev Rev 2000;20:568–81.

[4] Faraone SV, Perlis RH, Doyle AE, et al. Molecular genetics of attention deficit hyperactivity disorder. Biol Psychiatry 2005;57(11):1313–23.

[5] Sprich S, Biederman J, Crawford MH, et al. Adoptive and biological families of children and adolescents with ADHD. J Am Acad Child Adolesc Psychiatry 2000;39(11): 1432–7.

[6] Cantwell DP. Genetics of hyperactivity. J Child Psychol Psychiatry 1975;16:261–4.

[7] Morrison JR, Stewart MA. The psychiatric status of the legal families of adopted hyperactive children. Arch Gen Psychiatry 1973;28(June):888–91.

[8] Fisher SE, Francks C, McCracken JT, et al. A genomewide scan for loci involved in attention-deficit/hyperactivity disorder. Am J Hum Genet 2002;70(5):1183–96.

[9] Smalley SL, Kustanovich V, Minassian SL, et al. Genetic linkage of attention-deficit/hyperactivity disorder on chromosome 16p13, in a region implicated in autism. Am J Hum Genet 2002;71(4):959–63.

[10] Bakker SC, van der Meulen EM, Buitelaar JK, et al. A whole-genome scan in 164 Dutch sib pairs with attention-deficit/hyperactivity disorder: suggestive evidence for linkage on chromosomes 7p and 15q. Am J Hum Genet 2003;72(5):1251–60.

[11] Arcos-Burgos M, Castellanos FX, Konecki D, et al. Pedigree disequilibrium test (PDT) replicates association and linkage between DRD4 and ADHD in multigenerational and extended pedigrees from a genetic isolate. Mol Psychiatry 2004;9(3):252–9.

[12] Ogdie MN, Bakker SC, Fisher SE, et al. Pooled genome-wide linkage data on 424 ADHD ASPs suggests genetic heterogeneity and a common risk locus at 5p13. Mol Psychiatry 2006; 11(1):5–8.

[13] Hebebrand J, Dempfle A, Saar K, et al. A genome-wide scan for attention-deficit/hyperactivity disorder in 155 german sib-pairs. Mol Psychiatry 2006;11(2):196–205.

[14] Lander E, Kruglyak L. Genetic dissection of complex traits: guidelines for interpreting and reporting linkage results. Nat Genet 1995;11:241–7.

[15] Li D, Sham PC, Owen MJ, et al. Meta-analysis shows significant association between dopamine system genes and attention deficit hyperactivity disorder (ADHD). Hum Mol Genet 2006;15(4):2276–84.

[16] Yang B, Chan RC, Jing J, et al. A meta-analysis of association studies between the 10-repeat allele of a VNTR polymorphism in the 3'-UTR of dopamine transporter gene and attention deficit hyperactivity disorder. Am J Med Genet B Neuropsychiatr Genet 2007;144B(4): 541–50.

[17] Purper-Ouakil D, Wohl M, Mouren MC, et al. Meta-analysis of family-based association studies between the dopamine transporter gene and attention deficit hyperactivity disorder. Psychiatr Genet 2005;15(1):53–9.

[18] Cheuk DK, Wong V. Meta-analysis of association between a Catechol-O-Methyltransferase gene polymorphism and attention deficit hyperactivity disorder. Behav Genet 2006;36: 651–9.

[19] Lanau F, Zenner M, Civelli O, et al. Epinephrine and norepinephrine act as potent agonists at the recombinant human dopamine D4 receptor. J Neurochem 1997;68(2): 804–12.

[20] Faraone SV, Biederman J. Neurobiology of attention-deficit hyperactivity disorder. Biol Psychiatry 1998;44(10):951–8.

[21] Van Tol HH, Wu CM, Guan HC, et al. Multiple dopamine D4 receptor variants in the human population. Nature 1992;358(6382):149–52.

[22] Asghari V, Sanyal S, Buchwaldt S, et al. Modulation of intracellular cyclic AMP levels by different human dopamine D4 receptor variants. J Neurochem 1995;65(3):1157–65.

[23] El-Faddagh M, Laucht M, Maras A, et al. Association of dopamine D4 receptor (DRD4) gene with attention-deficit/hyperactivity disorder (ADHD) in a high-risk community sample: a longitudinal study from birth to 11 years of age. J Neural Transm 2004;111(7):883–9.

[24] Bhaduri N, Sinha S, Chattopadhyay A, et al. Analysis of polymorphisms in the dopamine Beta hydroxylase gene: association with attention deficit hyperactivity disorder in Indian children. Indian Pediatr 2005;42(2):123–9.

[25] Kim YS, Leventhal BL, Kim SJ, et al. Family-based association study of DAT1 and DRD4 polymorphism in Korean children with ADHD. Neurosci Lett 2005;390(3):176–81.

[26] Carrasco X, Rothhammer P, Moraga M, et al. Genotypic interaction between DRD4 and DAT1 loci is a high risk factor for attention-deficit/hyperactivity disorder in Chilean families. Am J Med Genet B Neuropsychiatr Genet 2006;141(1):51–4.

[27] McCracken JT, Smalley SL, McGough JJ, et al. Evidence for linkage of a tandem duplication polymorphism upstream of the dopamine D4 receptor gene (DRD4) with attention deficit hyperactivity disorder (ADHD). Mol Psychiatry 2000;5(5):531–6.

[28] Kustanovich V, Ishii J, Crawford L, et al. Transmission disequilibrium testing of dopamine-related candidate gene polymorphisms in ADHD: confirmation of association of ADHD with DRD4 and DRD5. Mol Psychiatry 2004;9:711–7.

[29] Barr CL, Feng Y, Wigg KG, et al. 5'-untranslated region of the dopamine D4 receptor gene and attention-deficit hyperactivity disorder. Am J Med Genet 2001;105(1):84–90.

[30] Todd RD, Neuman RJ, Lobos EA, et al. Lack of association of dopamine D4 receptor gene polymorphisms with ADHD subtypes in a population sample of twins. Am J Med Genet 2001;105(5):432–8.

[31] Brookes KJ, Xu X, Chen CK, et al. No evidence for the association of DRD4 with ADHD in a Taiwanese population within-family study. BMC Med Genet 2005;6:31.

[32] Bhaduri N, Das M, Sinha S, et al. Association of dopamine D4 receptor (DRD4) polymorphisms with attention deficit hyperactivity disorder in Indian population. Am J Med Genet B Neuropsychiatr Genet 2006;141B(1):61–6.

[33] Lowe N, Kirley A, Mullins C, et al. Multiple marker analysis at the promoter region of the DRD4 gene and ADHD: evidence of linkage and association with the SNP-616. Am J Med Genet 2004;131B(1):33–7.

[34] Brookes K, Xu X, Chen W, et al. The analysis of 51 genes in DSM-IV combined type attention deficit hyperactivity disorder: association signals in DRD4, DAT1 and 16 other genes. Mol Psychiatry; 2006;11:934–53.

[35] Rowe DC, Stever C, Chase D, et al. Two dopamine genes related to reports of childhood retrospective inattention and conduct disorder symptoms. Mol Psychiatry 2001;6(4): 429–33.

[36] Levitan RD, Masellis M, Lam RW, et al. Childhood inattention and dysphoria and adult obesity associated with the dopamine D4 receptor gene in overeating women with seasonal affective disorder. Neuropsychopharmacology 2004;29(1):179–86.

[37] Todd RD, Huang H, Smalley SL, et al. Collaborative analysis of DRD4 and DAT genotypes in population-defined ADHD subtypes. J Child Psychol Psychiatry 2005;46(10): 1067–73.

[38] Mill J, Xu X, Ronald A, et al. Quantitative trait locus analysis of candidate gene alleles associated with attention deficit hyperactivity disorder (ADHD) in five genes: DRD4, DAT1, DRD5, SNAP-25, and 5HT1B. Am J Med Genet B Neuropsychiatr Genet 2005;133B(1): 68–73.

[39] Kieling C, Roman T, Doyle AE, et al. Association between DRD4 gene and performance of children with ADHD in a test of sustained attention. Biol Psychiatry 2006;60:1163–5.

[40] Swanson J, Oosterlaan J, Murias M, et al. Attention deficit/hyperactivity disorder children with a 7-repeat allele of the dopamine receptor D4 gene have extreme behavior but normal performance on critical neuropsychological tests of attention. Proc Natl Acad Sci USA 2000;97(9):4754–9.

[41] Manor I, Tyano S, Eisenberg J, et al. The short DRD4 repeats confer risk to attention deficit hyperactivity disorder in a family-based design and impair performance on a continuous performance test (TOVA). Mol Psychiatry 2002;7(7):790–4.

[42] Bellgrove MA, Hawi Z, Lowe N, et al. DRD4 gene variants and sustained attention in attention deficit hyperactivity disorder (ADHD): effects of associated alleles at the VNTR and -521 SNP. Am J Med Genet B Neuropsychiatr Genet 2005;136(1):81–6.

[43] Langley K, Marshall L, van den Bree M, et al. Association of the dopamine D4 receptor gene 7-repeat allele with neuropsychological test performance of children with ADHD. Am J Psychiatry 2004;161(1):133–8.

[44] Grady DL, Harxhi A, Smith M, et al. Sequence variants of the DRD4 gene in autism: further evidence that rare DRD4 7R haplotypes are ADHD specific. Am J Med Genet B Neuropsychiatr Genet 2005;136(1):33–5.

[45] Lynn DE, Lubke G, Yang M, et al. Temperament and character profiles and the dopamine D4 receptor gene in ADHD. Am J Psychiatry 2005;162(5):906–13.

[46] Hawi Z, Lowe N, Kirley A, et al. Linkage disequilibrium mapping at DAT1, DRD5 and DBH narrows the search for ADHD susceptibility alleles at these loci. Mol Psychiatry 2003;8(3):299–308.

[47] Lowe N, Kirley A, Hawi Z, et al. Joint analysis of DRD5 marker concludes association with ADHD confined to the predominantly inattentive and combined subtypes. Am J Hum Genet 2004;74(2):348–56.

[48] Spencer T, Biederman J, Wilens T. Pharmacotherapy of attention deficit hyperactivity disorder. Child Adolesc Psychiatr Clin N Am 2000;9(1):77–97.

[49] Giros B, Jaber M, Jones SR, et al. Hyperlocomotion and indifference to cocaine and amphetamine in mice lacking the dopamine transporter. Nature 1996;379(6566):606–12.

[50] Gainetdinov RR, Wetsel WC, Jones SR, et al. Role of serotonin in the paradoxical calming effect of psychostimulants on hyperactivity. Science 1999;283:397–402.

[51] Cook EH, Stein MA, Krasowski MD, et al. Association of attention deficit disorder and the dopamine transporter gene. Am J Hum Genet 1995;56:993–8.

[52] Genro JP, Zeni C, Polanczyk GV, et al. A promoter polymorphism (-839 C > T) at the dopamine transporter gene is associated with attention deficit/hyperactivity disorder in Brazilian children. Am J Med Genet B Neuropsychiatr Genet 2006;11(12):1066–7.

[53] Brookes KJ, Mill J, Guindalini C, et al. A common haplotype of the dopamine transporter gene associated with attention-deficit/hyperactivity disorder and interacting with maternal use of alcohol during pregnancy. Arch Gen Psychiatry 2006;63(1):74–81.

[54] Asherson P, Brookes K, Franke B, et al. Confirmation that a specific haplotype of the dopamine transporter gene is associated with combined-type ADHD. Am J Psychiatry 2007; 164(4):674–7.

[55] Bakker SC, van der Meulen EM, Oteman N, et al. DAT1, DRD4, and DRD5 polymorphisms are not associated with ADHD in Dutch families. Am J Med Genet B Neuropsychiatr Genet 2005;132(1):50–2.

[56] Todd RD. Neural development is regulated by classical neurotransmitters: dopamine D2 receptor stimulation enhances neurite outgrowth. Biol Psychiatry 1992;31:794–807.

[57] Neuman RJ, Lobos E, Reich W, et al. Prenatal smoking exposure and dopaminergic genotypes interact to cause a severe ADHD subtype. Biol Psychiatry 2007;61(12): 1320–8.

[58] Laucht M, Skowronek MH, Becker K, et al. Interacting effects of the dopamine transporter gene and psychosocial adversity on attention-deficit/hyperactivity disorder symptoms among 15-year-olds from a high-risk community sample. Arch Gen Psychiatry 2007; 64(5):585–90.

[59] Comings DE, Muhleman D, Gysin R. Dopamine D2 receptors (DRD2) gene and susceptibility to posttraumatic stress disorder: a study and replication. Biol Psychiatry 1996;40: 368–72.

[60] Comings DE, Wu H, Chiu C, et al. Polygenic inheritance of Tourette syndrome, stuttering, attention deficit hyperactivity, conduct and oppositional defiant disorder: the additive and subtractive effect of the three dopaminergic genes—DRD2, DBH and DAT1. Am J Med Genet 1996;67:264–88.

[61] Smith KM, Daly M, Fischer M, et al. Association of the dopamine beta hydroxylase gene with attention deficit hyperactivity disorder: genetic analysis of the Milwaukee longitudinal study. Am J Med Genet 2003;119B(1):77–85.

[62] Daly G, Hawi Z, Fitzgerald M, et al. Mapping susceptibility loci in attention deficit hyperactivity disorder: preferential transmission of parental alleles at DAT1, DBH and DRD5 to affected children. Mol Psychiatry 1999;4:192–6.

[63] Roman T, Schmitz M, Polanczyk GV, et al. Further evidence for the association between attention- deficit/hyperactivity disorder and the dopamine-beta-hydroxylase gene. Am J Med Genet 2002;114(2):154–8.

[64] Wigg K, Zai G, Schachar R, et al. Attention deficit hyperactivity disorder and the gene for dopamine Beta-hydroxylase. Am J Psychiatry 2002;159(6):1046–8.

[65] Bhaduri N, Mukhopadhyay K. Lack of significant association between -1021C–>T polymorphism in the dopamine beta hydroxylase gene and attention deficit hyperactivity disorder. Neurosci Lett 2006;402(1–2):12–6.

[66] Inkster B, Muglia P, Jain U, et al. Linkage disequilibrium analysis of the dopamine beta-hydroxylase gene in persistent attention deficit hyperactivity disorder. Psychiatr Genet 2004;14(2):117–20.

[67] Payton A, Holmes J, Barrett JH, et al. Examining for association between candidate gene polymorphisms in the dopamine pathway and attention-deficit hyperactivity disorder: a family-based study. Am J Med Genet 2001;105(5):464–70.

[68] Hawi Z, Foley D, Kirley A, et al. Dopa decarboxylase gene polymorphisms and attention deficit hyperactivity disorder (ADHD): no evidence for association in the Irish population. Mol Psychiatry 2001;6(4):420–4.

[69] Zhang HB, Wang YF, Li J, et al. [Association between dopamine beta hydroxylase gene and attention deficit hyperactivity disorder complicated with disruptive behavior disorder] [Chinese]. Zhonghua Er Ke Za Zhi 2005;43(1):26–30.

[70] Cases O, Lebrand C, Giros B, et al. Plasma membrane transporters of serotonin, dopamine, and norepinephrine mediate serotonin accumulation in atypical locations in the developing brain of monoamine oxidase A knock-outs. J Neurosci 1998;18(17):6914–27.

[71] Manor I, Tyano S, Mel E, et al. Family-based and association studies of monoamine oxidase A and attention deficit hyperactivity disorder (ADHD): preferential transmission of

the long promoter-region repeat and its association with impaired performance on a continuous performance test (TOVA). Mol Psychiatry 2002;7(6):626–32.

[72] Lawson DC, Turic D, Langley K, et al. Association analysis of monoamine oxidase A and
attention deficit hyperactivity disorder. Am J Med Genet 2003;116B(1):84–9.

[73] Das M, Das Bhowmik A, Sinha S, et al. MAOA promoter polymorphism and attention deficit hyperactivity disorder (ADHD) in Indian children. Am J Med Genet B Neuropsychiatr
Genet 2006;141B(6):637–42.

[74] Jiang S, Xin R, Lin S, et al. Linkage studies between attention-deficit hyperactivity disorder
and the monoamine oxidase genes. Am J Med Genet 2001;105(8):783–8.

[75] Domschke K, Sheehan K, Lowe N, et al. Association analysis of the monoamine oxidase A
and B genes with attention deficit hyperactivity disorder (ADHD) in an Irish sample: preferential transmission of the MAO-A 941G allele to affected children. Am J Med Genet B
Neuropsychiatr Genet 2005;134B(1):110–4.

[76] Xu X, Brookes K, Chen CK, et al. Association study between the monoamine oxidase A
gene and attention deficit hyperactivity disorder in Taiwanese samples. BMC Psychiatry
2007;7(1):10.

[77] Comings DE, Comings BG, Muhleman D, et al. The dopamine D2 receptor locus as a mod-
ifying gene in neuropsychiatric disorders. J Am Med Assoc 1991;266(13):1793–800.

[78] Sery O, Drtilkova I, Theiner P, et al. Polymorphism of DRD2 gene and ADHD. Neuro
Endocrinol Lett 2006;27(1–2):236–40.

[79] Kim JW, Park CS, Hwang JW, et al. Clinical and genetic characteristics of Korean male
alcoholics with and without attention deficit hyperactivity disorder. Alcohol Alcohol
2006;41(4):407–11.

[80] Rowe DC, den Oord EJ, Stever C, et al. The DRD2 TaqI polymorphism and symptoms of
attention deficit hyperactivity disorder. Mol Psychiatry 1999;4(6):580–6.

[81] Huang YS, Lin SK, Wu YY, et al. A family-based association study of attention-deficit hyperactivity disorder and dopamine D2 receptor TaqI A alleles. Chang Gung Med J 2003;
26(12):897–903.

[82] Kirley A, Hawi Z, Daly G, et al. Dopaminergic system genes in ADHD: toward a biological
hypothesis. Neuropsychopharmacology 2002;27(4):607–19.

[83] Barr CL, Wigg KG, Wu J, et al. Linkage study of two polymorphisms at the dopamine D3
receptor gene and attention-deficit hyperactivity disorder. Am J Med Genet 2000;96(1):
114–7.

[84] Muglia P, Jain U, Kennedy JL. A transmission disequilibrium test of the Ser9/Gly dopamine D3 receptor gene polymorphism in adult attention-deficit hyperactivity disorder.
Behav Brain Res 2002;130(1–2):91–5.

[85] Comings DE, Gade-Andavolu R, Gonzalez N, et al. Comparison of the role of dopamine,
serotonin, and noradrenaline genes in ADHD, ODD and conduct disorder: multivariate re-
gression analysis of 20 genes. Clin Genet 2000;57(3):178–96.

[86] Retz W, Rosler M, Supprian T, et al. Dopamine D3 receptor gene polymorphism and vio-
lent behavior: relation to impulsiveness and ADHD-related psychopathology. J Neural
Transm 2003;110(5):561–72.

[87] Syvanen AC, Tilgmann C, Rinne J, et al. Genetic polymorphism of catechol-O-methyltransferase (COMT): correlation of genotype with individual variation of S-COMT activity
and comparison of the allele frequencies in the normal population and Parkinsonian patients in Finland. Pharmacogenetics 1997;7(1):65–71.

[88] Reuter M, Kirsch P, Hennig J. Inferring candidate genes for attention deficit hyperactivity
disorder (ADHD) assessed by the World Health Organization Adult ADHD Self-Report
Scale (ASRS). J Neural Transm 2006;113(7):929–38.

[89] Gothelf D, Michaelovsky E, Frisch A, et al. Association of the low-activity COMT 158 Met
allele with ADHD and OCD in subjects with velocardiofacial syndrome. Int J Neuropsychopharmacol 2007;10(3):301–8.

[90] Brookes KJ, Knight J, Xu X, et al. DNA pooling analysis of ADHD and genes regulating vesicle release of neurotransmitters. Am J Med Genet B Neuropsychiatr Genet 2005;139:33–7.

[91] Comings DE, Gonzalez NS, Cheng Li SC, et al. A "line item" approach to the identification of genes involved in polygenic behavioral disorders: the adrenergic alpha2A (ADRA2A) gene. Am J Med Genet 2003;118B(1):110–4.

[92] Xu C, Schachar R, Tannock R, et al. Linkage study of the alpha2A adrenergic receptor in attention-deficit hyperactivity disorder families. Am J Med Genet 2001;105(2):159–62.

[93] Roman T, Schmitz M, Polanczyk GV, et al. Is the alpha-2A adrenergic receptor gene (ADRA2A) associated with attention-deficit/hyperactivity disorder? Am J Med Genet 2003;120B(1):116–20.

[94] Park L, Nigg JT, Waldman ID, et al. Association and linkage of alpha-2A adrenergic receptor gene polymorphisms with childhood ADHD. Mol Psychiatry 2005;10(6): 572–80.

[95] Schmitz M, Denardin D, Silva TL, et al. Association between Alpha-2a-adrenergic receptor gene and ADHD inattentive type. Biol Psychiatry 2006;60(10):1028–33.

[96] Stevenson J, Langley K, Pay H, et al. Attention deficit hyperactivity disorder with reading disabilities: preliminary genetic findings on the involvement of the ADRA2A gene. J Child Psychol Psychiatry 2005;46(10):1081–8.

[97] Wang B, Wang Y, Zhou R, et al. Possible association of the alpha-2A adrenergic receptor gene (ADRA2A) with symptoms of attention-deficit/hyperactivity disorder. Am J Med Genet B Neuropsychiatr Genet 2006;141B(2):130–4.

[98] Deupree JD, Smith SD, Kratochvil CJ, et al. Possible involvement of alpha-2A adrenergic receptors in attention deficit hyperactivity disorder: radioligand binding and polymorphism studies. Am J Med Genet B Neuropsychiatr Genet 2006;141(8):877–84.

[99] Roman T, Polanczyk GV, Zeni C, et al. Further evidence of the involvement of alpha-2A-adrenergic receptor gene (ADRA2A) in inattentive dimensional scores of attention-deficit/hyperactivity disorder. Mol Psychiatry 2006;11(1):8–10.

[100] Waldman ID, Nigg JT, Gizer IR, et al. The adrenergic receptor alpha-2A gene (ADRA2A) and neuropsychological executive functions as putative endophenotypes for childhood ADHD. Cogn Affect Behav Neurosci 2006;6(1):18–30.

[101] Comings D, Gade-Andavolu R, Gonzalez N, et al. Additive effect of three noradenergic genes (ADRA2A, ADRA2C, DBH) on attention-deficit hyperactivity disorder and learning disabilities an Tourette syndrome subjects. Clin Genet 1999;55(3):160–72.

[102] Barr CL, Wigg K, Zai G, et al. Attention-deficit hyperactivity disorder and the adrenergic receptors alpha1C and alpha2C. Mol Psychiatry 2001;6(3):334–7.

[103] De Luca V, Muglia P, Vincent JB, et al. Adrenergic alpha 2C receptor genomic organization: association study in adult ADHD. Am J Med Genet B Neuropsychiatr Genet 2004; 127B(1):65–7.

[104] Biederman J, Spencer T. Non-stimulant treatments for ADHD. Eur Child Adolesc Psychiatry 2000;9(Suppl 1):I51–9.

[105] Barr CL, Kroft J, Feng Y, et al. The norepinephrine transporter gene and attention-deficit hyperactivity disorder. Am J Med Genet 2002;114(3):255–9.

[106] McEvoy B, Hawi Z, Fitzgerald M, et al. No evidence of linkage or association between the norepinephrine transporter (NET) gene polymorphisms and ADHD in the Irish population. Am J Med Genet 2002;114(6):665–6.

[107] Xu X, Knight J, Brookes K, et al. DNA pooling analysis of 21 norepinephrine transporter gene SNPs with attention deficit hyperactivity disorder: no evidence for association. Am J Med Genet B Neuropsychiatr Genet 2005;134B(1):115–8.

[108] Bobb AJ, Addington AM, Sidransky E, et al. Support for association between ADHD and two candidate genes: NET1 and DRD1. Am J Med Genet B Neuropsychiatr Genet 2005; 134B(1):67–72.

[109] Kim CH, Hahn MK, Joung Y, et al. A polymorphism in the norepinephrine transporter gene alters promoter activity and is associated with attention-deficit hyperactivity disorder. Proc Natl Acad Sci USA 2006;103(50):19164–9.

[110] Hawi Z, Dring M, Kirley A, et al. Serotonergic system and attention deficit hyperactivity disorder (ADHD): a potential susceptibility locus at the 5-HT(1B) receptor gene in 273 nuclear families from a multi-centre sample. Mol Psychiatry 2002;7(7):718–25.

[111] Quist JF, Barr CL, Schachar R, et al. The serotonin 5-HT1B receptor gene and attention deficit hyperactivity disorder. Mol Psychiatry 2003;8(1):98–102.

[112] Smoller JW, Biederman J, Arbeitman L, et al. Association between the 5HT1B Receptor Gene (HTR1B) and the Inattentive Subtype of ADHD. Biol Psychiatry 2006;59(5):460–7.

[113] Heiser P, Dempfle A, Friedel S, et al. Family-based association study of serotonergic candidate genes and attention-deficit/hyperactivity disorder in a German sample. J Neural Transm 2007;114(4):513–21.

[114] Li J, Wang Y, Zhou R, et al. Serotonin 5-HT1B receptor gene and attention deficit hyperactivity disorder in Chinese Han subjects. Am J Med Genet B Neuropsychiatr Genet 2005; 132B(1):59–63.

[115] Quist JF, Barr CL, Schachar R, et al. Evidence for the serotonin HTR2A receptor gene as a susceptibility factor in attention deficit hyperactivity disorder (ADHD). Mol Psychiatry 2000;5(5):537–41.

[116] Zoroglu SS, Erdal ME, Alasehirli B, et al. Significance of serotonin transporter gene 5-HTTLPR and variable number of tandem repeat polymorphism in attention deficit hyperactivity disorder. Neuropsychobiology 2002;45(4):176–81.

[117] Li J, Wang Y, Zhou R, et al. No association of attention-deficit/hyperactivity disorder with genes of the serotonergic pathway in Han Chinese subjects. Neurosci Lett 2006;403:172–5.

[118] Li J, Kang C, Wang Y, et al. Contribution of 5-HT2A receptor gene -1438A > G polymorphism to outcome of attention-deficit/hyperactivity disorder in adolescents. Am J Med Genet B Neuropsychiatr Genet 2006;141B:473–6.

[119] Guimaraes AP, Zeni C, Polanczyk GV, et al. Serotonin genes and attention deficit/hyperactivity disorder in a Brazilian sample: preferential transmission of the HTR2A 452His allele to affected boys. Am J Med Genet B Neuropsychiatr Genet 2007;144(1):69–73.

[120] Levitan R, Masellis M, Basile V, et al. Polymorphism of the serotonin-2A receptor gene (HTR2A) associated with childhood attention deficit hyperactivity disorder (ADHD) in adult women with seasonal affective disorder. J Affect Disord 2002;71(1–3):229–33.

[121] Li J, Wang Y, Zhou R, et al. Association between polymorphisms in serotonin 2C receptor gene and attention-deficit/hyperactivity disorder in Han Chinese subjects. Neurosci Lett 2006;407:107–11.

[122] Li J, Wang Y, Zhou R, et al. Association of attention-deficit/hyperactivity disorder with serotonin 4 receptor gene polymorphisms in Han Chinese subjects. Neurosci Lett 2006; 401:6–9.

[123] Li J, Zhang X, Wang Y, et al. The serotonin 5-HT1D receptor gene and attention-deficit hyperactivity disorder in Chinese Han subjects. Am J Med Genet B Neuropsychiatr Genet 2006;141B(8):874–6.

[124] Anguelova M, Benkelfat C, Turecki G. A systematic review of association studies investigating genes coding for serotonin receptors and the serotonin transporter: I. Affective disorders. Mol Psychiatry 2003;8(6):574–91.

[125] Anguelova M, Benkelfat C, Turecki G. A systematic review of association studies investigating genes coding for serotonin receptors and the serotonin transporter: II. Suicidal behavior. Mol Psychiatry 2003;8(7):646–53.

[126] Curran S, Purcell S, Craig I, et al. The serotonin transporter gene as a QTL for ADHD. Am J Med Genet B Neuropsychiatr Genet 2005;134B(1):42–7.

[127] Kim SJ, Badner J, Cheon KA, et al. Family-based association study of the serotonin transporter gene polymorphisms in Korean ADHD trios. Am J Med Genet B Neuropsychiatr Genet 2005;139(1):14–8.

[128] Xu X, Mill J, Chen CK, et al. Family-based association study of serotonin transporter gene polymorphisms in attention deficit hyperactivity disorder: no evidence for association in UK and Taiwanese samples. Am J Med Genet B Neuropsychiatr Genet 2005;139(1):11–3.

[129] Xu M, Hu XT, Cooper DC, et al. Elimination of cocaine-induced hyperactivity and dopamine-mediated neurophysiological effects in dopamine D1 receptor mutant mice [see comments]. Cell 1994;79(6):945–55.

[130] Banerjee E, Sinha S, Chatterjee A, et al. A family-based study of Indian subjects from Kolkata reveals allelic association of the serotonin transporter intron-2 (STin2) polymorphism and attention-deficit-hyperactivity disorder (ADHD). Am J Med Genet B Neuropsychiatr Genet 2006;141(4):361–6.

[131] Wigg KG, Takhar A, Ickowicz A, et al. Gene for the serotonin transporter and ADHD: no association with two functional polymorphisms. Am J Med Genet B Neuropsychiatr Genet 2006;141B(6):566–70.

[132] Li J, Wang Y, Zhou R, et al. Association between polymorphisms in serotonin transporter gene and attention deficit hyperactivity disorder in Chinese Han subjects. Am J Med Genet B Neuropsychiatr Genet 2007;144(1):14–9.

[133] Manuck SB, Flory JD, Ferrell RE, et al. Aggression and anger-related traits associated with a polymorphism of the tryptophan hydroxylase gene. Biol Psychiatry 1999;45(5): 603–14.

[134] Tang G, Ren D, Xin R, et al. Lack of association between the tryptophan hydroxylase gene A218C polymorphism and attention-deficit hyperactivity disorder in Chinese Han population. Am J Med Genet 2001;105(6):485–8.

[135] Li J, Wang YF, Zhou RL, et al. [Association between tryptophan hydroxylase gene polymorphisms and attention deficit hyperactivity disorder with or without learning disorder]. Zhonghua Yi Xue Za Zhi 2003;83(24):2114–8.

[136] Li J, Wang Y, Zhou R, et al. Association between tryptophan hydroxylase gene polymorphisms and attention deficit hyperactivity disorder in Chinese Han population. Am J Med Genet B Neuropsychiatr Genet 2006;141B:126–9.

[137] Walther DJ, Peter JU, Bashammakh S, et al. Synthesis of serotonin by a second tryptophan hydroxylase isoform. Science 2003;299(5603):76.

[138] Sheehan K, Lowe N, Kirley A, et al. Tryptophan hydroxylase 2 (TPH2) gene variants associated with ADHD. Mol Psychiatry 2005;10(10):944–9.

[139] Walitza S, Renner TJ, Dempfle A, et al. Transmission disequilibrium of polymorphic variants in the tryptophan hydroxylase-2 gene in attention-deficit/hyperactivity disorder. Mol Psychiatry 2005;10(12):1126–32.

[140] Sheehan K, Hawi Z, Gill M, et al. No association between TPH2 gene polymorphisms and ADHD in a UK sample. Neurosci Lett 2007;412(2):105–7.

[141] Wilson MC. Coloboma mouse mutant as an animal model of hyperkinesis and attention deficit hyperactivity disorder. Neurosci Biobehav Rev 2000;24(1):51–7.

[142] Barr CL, Feng Y, Wigg K, et al. Identification of DNA variants in the SNAP-25 gene and linkage study of these polymorphisms and attention-deficit hyperactivity disorder. Mol Psychiatry 2000;5(4):405–9.

[143] Brophy K, Hawi Z, Kirley A, et al. Synaptosomal-associated protein 25 (SNAP-25) and attention deficit hyperactivity disorder (ADHD): evidence of linkage and association in the Irish population. Mol Psychiatry 2002;7(8):913–7.

[144] Kustanovich V, Merriman B, McGough J, et al. Biased paternal transmission of SNAP-25 risk alleles in attention-deficit hyperactivity disorder. Mol Psychiatry 2003;8(3):309–15.

[145] Mill J, Curran S, Kent L, et al. Association study of a SNAP-25 microsatellite and attention deficit hyperactivity disorder. Am J Med Genet 2002;114(3):269–71.

[146] Mill J, Richards S, Knight J, et al. Haplotype analysis of SNAP-25 suggests a role in the aetiology of ADHD. Mol Psychiatry 2004;9:801–10.

[147] Feng Y, Crosbie J, Wigg K, et al. The SNAP25 gene as a susceptibility gene contributing to attention-deficit hyperactivity disorder. Mol Psychiatry 2005;10(11):998–1005, 973.

[148] Kim JW, Biederman J, Arbeitman L, et al. Investigation of variation in SNAP-25 and ADHD and relationship to co-morbid major depressive disorder. Am J Med Genet B Neuropsychiatr Genet 2007;144:781–90.

[149] Comings DE, Gade-Andavolu R, Gonzalez N, et al. Multivariate analysis of associations of 42 genes in ADHD, ODD and conduct disorder. Clin Genet 2000;58(1):31–40.

[150] Kent L, Middle F, Hawi Z, et al. Nicotinic acetylcholine receptor alpha4 subunit gene polymorphism and attention deficit hyperactivity disorder. Psychiatr Genet 2001;11(1):37–40.

[151] Todd RD, Lobos EA, Sun LW, et al. Mutational analysis of the nicotinic acetylcholine receptor alpha 4 subunit gene in attention deficit/hyperactivity disorder: evidence for association of an intronic polymorphism with attention problems. Mol Psychiatry 2003;8(1):103–8.

[152] Lee J, Laurin N, Crosbie J, et al. Association study of the nicotinic acetylcholine receptor alpha4 subunit gene, CHRNA4, in attention-deficit hyperactivity disorder. Genes Brain Behav; 2007.

[153] Turic D, Langley K, Mills S, et al. Follow-up of genetic linkage findings on chromosome 16p13: evidence of association of N-methyl-D aspartate glutamate receptor 2A gene polymorphism with ADHD. Mol Psychiatry 2004;9(2):169–73.

[154] Adams J, Crosbie J, Wigg K, et al. Glutamate receptor, ionotropic, N-methyl D-aspartate 2A (GRIN2A) gene as a positional candidate for attention-deficit/hyperactivity disorder in the 16p13 region. Mol Psychiatry 2004;9(5):494–9.

[155] Egan MF, Kojima M, Callicott JH, et al. The BDNF val66met polymorphism affects activity-dependent secretion of BDNF and human memory and hippocampal function. Cell 2003;112(2):257–69.

[156] Kent L, Green E, Hawi Z, et al. Association of the paternally transmitted copy of common Valine allele of the Val66Met polymorphism of the brain-derived neurotrophic factor (BDNF) gene with susceptibility to ADHD. Mol Psychiatry 2005;10:939–43.

[157] Xu X, Mill J, Zhou K, et al. Family-based association study between brain-derived neurotrophic factor gene polymorphisms and attention deficit hyperactivity disorder in UK and Taiwanese samples. Am J Med Genet B Neuropsychiatr Genet 2007;144(1):83–6.

ELSEVIER
SAUNDERS

Child Adolesc Psychiatric Clin N Am
17 (2008) 285–307

CHILD AND
ADOLESCENT
PSYCHIATRIC CLINICS
OF NORTH AMERICA

Neurobiology of Attention Deficit Hyperactivity Disorder

Christian Kieling, MD[a,*],
Renata R.F. Goncalves, MA[a],
Rosemary Tannock, PhD[b],
Francisco X. Castellanos, MD[c,d]

[a]Department of Psychiatry, Federal University of Rio Grande do Sul, Rua Ramiro Barcelos,
2350 - 2201A 90035-903, Porto Alegre, RS, Brazil
[b]Neuroscience and Mental Health Research Program, The Hospital for Sick Children, 555
University Avenue, Toronto, Ontario M5G 1X8, Canada
[c]New York University Child Study Center, 215 Lexington Avenue, 14th Floor,
New York, NY 10016, USA
[d]Nathan S. Kline Institute for Psychiatric Research, 140 Old Orangeburg Road,
Orangeburg, NY 10962, USA

Uncovering the neurobiological bases of mental disorders is a core enterprise in the contemporary psychiatric research agenda [1]. As revisions to the diagnostic system are being debated, the transition from a phenomenologically based classification system toward an etiologic and neurodevelopmentally oriented framework will require a substantial body of evidence to be accumulated and synthesized. For the development of this novel nosologic paradigm in the field of psychiatry, it is not enough to have all the puzzle pieces, it is also important to begin to understand how they fit together.

The investigation of the origins, nature, and course of psychopathology across childhood and adolescence and into adulthood is important for scientific and clinical purposes. Identifying etiologic factors, characterizing the developmental course of symptom expression, and understanding the

R. Tannock has received research funds from Eli Lilly and Shire, currently, sits on the Advisory Boards of Eli Lilly and Pfizer, acts as a consultant to Eli Lilly, and has received honoraria from Eli Lilly, Shire, Janssen-Ortho, McNeil, and Pfizer. All such funding is donated to The Hospital for Sick Children Foundation for attention deficit hyperactivity disorder research.

* Corresponding author. Hospital de Clínicas de Porto Alegre, Rua Ramiro Barcelos, 2350 - 2201A 90035-903, Porto Alegre, RS, Brazil.
    E-mail address: ckieling@ufrgs.br (C. Kieling).

1056-4993/08/$ - see front matter © 2008 Elsevier Inc. All rights reserved.
doi:10.1016/j.chc.2007.11.012
childpsych.theclinics.com

mechanisms underlying continuity long have been major goals in the study of child and adolescent psychiatry. More recently, these theoretic goals have become practical challenges, as a growing body of research suggests that continuing along a maladaptive pathway increases the individual risk for psychopathology and diminishes the chance of reclaiming a typical developmental trajectory [2,3].

The first phase of the process of developing the psychiatric nosology began in 1980 with the publication of *Diagnostic and Statistical Manual of Mental Disorders, Revised Third Edition (DSM-III)*, which eschewed etiologic models in favor of a focus restricted to the description of clusters of symptoms and characteristics of clinical course [1]. Since then, advances in psychopharmacology and in molecular and imaging methods have raised hopes that neurobiological factors soon will be included in the etiologic models of mental disorders. Direct linkages between genes or brain morphology and diagnoses, however, so far have been mostly disappointing [4].

Attention deficit hyperactivity disorder (ADHD) is one of the most extensively investigated psychiatric disorders of childhood and adolescence [5]. Notwithstanding the empiric research on the identification of etiologic factors and the achievement of some remarkably well-replicated findings, comprehensive testable theories remain underspecified [6,7]. As evidence accumulates that ADHD is a highly heterogeneous disorder, not only in terms of clinical presentation but also in terms of etiologic bases [8], the ADHD construct continues to be reevaluated at the phenotypic level [9].

Over a decade ago, family studies indicated that ADHD runs in families [10], and subsequent twin studies consistently have demonstrated heritability estimates of approximately 0.80, suggesting that the etiology of ADHD is largely attributable to genetic factors. Nonetheless, environmental factors that increase the risk for ADHD also have been identified [11], such as exposure to nicotine during pregnancy [12] or to lead during early childhood [13]. Moreover, recent studies suggest that causal pathways are likely to involve complex interactions between genetic and environmental factors, which are associated with developmentally dependent (and perhaps gender-specific) variation in brain structure and function and phenotypic expression.

Few attempts have been made so far to work across different levels of analysis in an attempt to integrate genetic, environmental, cognitive, and behavioral mechanisms underlying ADHD. Moreover, to link these data and provide a full account of ADHD, it is necessary to evaluate the phenotype as it evolves over time in males and females. Longitudinal studies will need to examine the very early periods of child development and look at the interplay between risks in pregnancy, infancy, and preschool years if more is to be learned about the developmental pathways from early predisposing risk factors to the development of full-blown chronic ADHD, as it is expressed throughout the lifespan [14,15].

This article reviews studies on ADHD in an attempt to place biological findings in the context of a complex brain disorder. An exhaustive review of neurobiological findings on ADHD is beyond the scope of this article. Aiming at an integrative developmental model for the neurobiology of ADHD, this article focuses on empiric research supporting a pathway that links genetic and environmental variations to structural and functional brain abnormalities that ultimately will lead to a set of age-dependent behavioral manifestations. Integrating biological findings of ADHD studies into a developmental perspective, however, remains hampered by limitations in research design and methodology. This review therefore divided this article in three sections. The first presents evidence of risk factors for ADHD, emphasizing gene–environment interactions; the second examines neural structures and circuits involved in ADHD and how neuroimaging studies may help further the understanding of the pathophysiological bases of the disorder. Finally, the third section highlights the clinical expression of ADHD as it develops across childhood and adolescence and into adulthood.

Risk factors: genetic and environmental

Given the high heritability estimates, varying between 60% and 91% in twin studies [16], current trends in the investigation of the etiology of ADHD emphasize the role of genetic factors (for a comprehensive review on genetic studies of ADHD, see the article by Faraone in this issue). Although ADHD is a highly heritable condition, none of the investigated genes has proven to be sufficient or necessary for causing the disorder. As for all complex traits, the etiology of ADHD is thought to involve a combination of multiple genes of moderate effect [16,17] interacting with environmental factors. The possible roles of pre- and perinatal exposures are the main focus of research on environmental risk factors for ADHD, as current approaches to the analysis of gene–environment interactions seek to answer not only the question of which environmental factors are the most important in this interplay, but also how the pathologic process develops from pregnancy through school years.

Perinatal exposure

Despite a general worldwide trend toward decreased cigarette smoking (eg, reviews by US Centers for Disease Control and Prevention) [18], the rate of smoking and other substance abuse among pregnant women remains high (eg, approximately 25% of all pregnancies in Finland) [19,20]. Moreover, even among nonsmoking mothers, a substantial number of infants (around 14%) experience daily prenatal environmental tobacco exposure (ETS) from paternal and other nonmaternal sources, according to a recent epidemiologic study in China, where maternal smoking during pregnancy is much lower (4.6%) than in the United States [21].

Maternal smoking during pregnancy has been found to be associated with ADHD or the symptom dimensions of ADHD in the offspring in several clinical [22,23] and population-based studies [24–27]. Converging evidence is provided by studies in various countries (eg, Netherlands, Finland, United Kingdom, New Zealand, Australia, United States, Canada, Brazil), using different experimental designs (eg, retrospective clinical case–control, community cohort, population-based prospective follow-up, and twin studies) and methodologies (eg, self-reported smoking in pregnancy, bioassay, child behavior ratings, clinical diagnostic interviews) [12,24,25,28–31]. For example, a recent review showed a pooled odds ratio derived from case–control studies indicating a more than twofold increase in the risk for ADHD diagnosis in those individuals whose mothers smoked during pregnancy [30]. Confounding risk factors such as parental psychopathology, parent ADHD, alcohol and drug use, birth weight, IQ, and psychosocial adversity do not appear to account fully for this association [24,31,32] but do contribute [20,33,34].

Preclinical work indicates that nicotine binds to nicotinic acetylcholine receptors (nACHRs), which play a key role in brain development (eg, cell replication and differentiation, synaptic development) when stimulated by endogenous acetylcholine [35]. In rodent studies, prenatal exposure to nicotine stimulates nACHRs and produces persistent cholinergic and serotonergic hypoactivity [35] and disrupts auditory processing and learning [36]. Moreover, exposure to nicotine during adolescent development of rodents has similar effects on brain development to prenatal exposure, although smaller in magnitude [35]. Collectively, findings from these animal studies suggest that initial changes in neuronal maturation and brain structure elicited by prenatal nicotine exposure and/or ETS profoundly influence the development of cells that emerge later during postnatal life. Thus, prenatal exposure to nicotine may lead to far-reaching disturbances in central nervous system (CNS) function that are not detectable at birth, but which manifest as adverse neurobehavioral outcomes later in development and may predispose the offspring to early initiation of smoking and/or nicotine dependence [37–40].

As in the animal studies, maternal smoking during pregnancy and ETS also have been associated with small but persistent deficits in intellectual function and auditory processing [41–43]. ETS has been associated with poor academic outcomes in the offspring [44,45]. Furthermore, although paternal smoking was not found to add to the effects of maternal smoking during pregnancy, parental smoking after the child's birth (ie, ETS) increases the risk of academic underachievement, particularly in arithmetic and spelling [29]. Notably, academic problems have been found to be associated closely with ADHD [46,47]. A recurrent observation is that pre- and postnatal nicotine exposure by means of maternal smoking during pregnancy and/or ETS is associated with fetal growth restriction, prematurity, and low birth weight (LBW, less than 2500 g) [48–50], which in turn may lead to developmental disorders in the child [51]. For instance, several studies have investigated the association between LBW or extremely low birth weight (ELBW, 1000 g) and subsequent manifestation of psychiatric symptoms or disorders. Overall, they have suggested that LBW is a risk factor for several behavioral outcomes, including emotional, behavioral, social, and academic problems [52]. Evidence, however, suggests a specific link between LBW and subsequent development of ADHD. When 137 LBW children were compared at 12 years with a sample of matched peers on several psychiatric symptoms, the main psychiatric risk was for manifesting ADHD, with 23% ELBW children meeting clinical criteria, compared with 6% of their peers [53]. ELBW has been suggested as a specific risk factor for ADHD [54], and small body size at birth has been shown to predict behavioral symptoms of ADHD [55]. Preterm birth (less than 37 weeks) also carries more than twice the relative risk for developing ADHD [56].

Women at risk for preterm delivery (ie, LBW and ELBW offspring) typically are treated with synthetic glucocorticoids, which, according to animal studies, cross the fetoplacental barrier and affect the development and function of fetal hypothalamic-pituitary-adrenal (HPA) axis and cognitive function in ways that persist into adult life and possibly into the next generation (an epigenetic mechanism) [15,57,58]. Thus it is unclear whether the link between ELBW/LBW and ADHD is mediated at least in part by treatment-induced effects of synthetic glucocorticoids on fetal pathophysiology, which in turn appears to be linked with subsequent cardiovascular, metabolic, neuroendocrine, neurocognitive, and psychiatric disorders [58].

Interestingly, this chain of risks goes further, as LBW and prematurity are associated with prenatal nicotine exposure, which, in turn, is associated with alcohol use during pregnancy. Addressing the association between ADHD and prenatal exposure to maternal cigarette smoking and alcohol, Mick and colleagues [31] found that ADHD cases were 2.1 times more likely to have been exposed to cigarettes and 2.5 times more likely to have been exposed to alcohol in utero than were the non-ADHD control subjects, evidencing that the disorder is associated with prenatal exposure to alcohol independently of the association between ADHD and nicotine. Significant associations also have been found between child ADHD and maternal and paternal alcohol dependence. Mothers who had alcohol abuse or dependence were more likely to drink during pregnancy and were also more likely to smoke beyond the first trimester [59].

These studies have contributed to the notion that the risk effect of environmental factors for ADHD arise from a combination of multiple factors rather than a single variable. The neurobiology of psychiatric disorders is not about inevitability but is instead about vulnerability and propensity; it is only in certain environments that the disease is likely to emerge [60]. Nevertheless, the study of genetically mediated child psychopathology outside twin/adoption studies or molecular genetic paradigms makes it difficult to separate the effect of environmental factors from the genetic liability imparted by parents [61]. That is, as mothers and offspring share on average half of their genes, and both the outcome (ADHD) and the study variables (smoking or alcohol) are highly heritable conditions, shared genetic vulnerability between smoking and ADHD is an alternative explanation for the increased rate of ADHD among the offspring of smokers or drinkers.

This seems to be the case at least for nicotine exposure. In a population-based sample of twins, Thapar and colleagues [24] showed that smoking during pregnancy accounted for only a small proportion of the total variance in ADHD symptom scores, rated by parents and teachers. Genetic influences accounted for most of the variance in offspring ADHD, although maternal smoking during pregnancy still was found to show a significant environmentally mediated association. Another important consideration in the analysis of these presumed risk factors is that they may be acting as a proxy for other factors related to the outcome. Thus, parental alcoholism may predict increased risk of offspring ADHD, but children of alcoholics are also significantly more likely to experience other high-risk environmental exposures [62].

Gene-environment interactions

The effect of a single variable—whether genetic or environmental—on a complex disorder is expected to explain only a small proportion of the phenotypic variance. There are certainly several reasons for the difficulties in replicating findings of genetic studies of psychiatric disorders, but one is of particular importance in this context. One of the explanations why results of genetic studies of ADHD have been contradictory is that not all individuals carrying a vulnerable genotype develop the disorder as the genetic effect may only become apparent among the subgroup of individuals exposed to a certain environmental risk. Thus, the importance of studying gene–environment interactions in behavioral disorders lies in the hypothesis that some genes show effects only in groups of individuals subjected to specific environmental stressors [63]. Based on findings from animal studies, suggesting that perinatal tobacco exposure interacts with the dopamine transporter (DAT1) gene products to yield a selective up-regulation of nicotine receptors [64], Kahn and colleagues [65] examined the independent and joint association of a DAT1 polymorphism and maternal prenatal smoking on hyperactive-impulsive, inattentive, and oppositional behaviors among 5-year-old children, using a prospective longitudinal cohort followed from age 6 months to 60 months. They found that children who were both exposed to prenatal smoking and homozygous for the DAT1 10-repeat allele were at significantly increased risk of hyperactivity–impulsivity and oppositional symptoms, and that neither prenatal smoke exposure alone nor DAT1 10/10 genotype alone was associated significantly with increased scores of disruptive behavior. The DAT1 gene again was linked to an increased risk for ADHD in both British and Taiwanese samples of children prenatally exposed to alcohol [66]. The authors suggested that the risk conferred by a DAT1 haplotype moderates the environmental risk associated with mothers' use of alcohol during pregnancy.

A twin study confirmed the role of gene–environment interactions in modulating the risk for ADHD, as the strength of the associations between ADHD and polymorphisms of the DAT1 or dopamine-4 receptor (DRD4) genes were increased if mothers reported smoking during pregnancy. For twins who were exposed in utero to tobacco, the odds of a *DSM-IV* diagnosis of ADHD combined subtype was 2.9 times greater if they had inherited the DAT1 10-repeat allele and 2.8 times greater if they carried the DRD4 7-repeat allele, compared with unexposed twins without the risk alleles [67]. Furthermore, a recent study extended these findings to the neural nicotinic acetylcholine receptor alpha 4 subunit gene (CHRNA4), which is located on presynaptic dopaminergic neurons [68]. Specifically, not only was a significant interaction found between prenatal exposure to nicotine and CHRNA4 for severe combined type of ADHD (defined by latent class analysis), but it also was found that prenatal nicotine exposure interacted with genotypes at three loci (CHRNA4, DAT1 and DRD4) in modulating the risk for severe combined-type ADHD [68].

The moderating effects of environmental exposures on the associations of genes with psychopathology are not limited to the pre- and perinatal period. Laucht and colleagues [69] recently reported that psychosocial adversity moderates the effect of DAT1 genotype on ADHD symptoms in adolescents from a high-risk community sample. Psychosocial adversity is characterized by adverse family environments, including marital discord, parental psychopathology, low maternal education, and single parenthood. Adolescents homozygous for the DAT1 10-repeat allele polymorphism who grew up in greater psychosocial adversity exhibited significantly more inattention and hyperactivity–impulsivity than adolescents with other genotypes or who lived in less adverse family conditions.

In the future, genetic information may be incorporated into psychiatric nosology, helping to diminish clinical heterogeneity and thus refining psychiatric diagnoses. Data from two independent birth cohorts, from Britain and New Zealand, showed that both the 7-repeat of DRD4 and the 10-repeat allele of DAT1 were associated with variation in intellectual functioning among children diagnosed as having ADHD, independent of the severity of their symptoms. As one of the cohorts was followed up to the age of 26 years, the study was also able to show a significant association between number of genotypic risks (no, one, or two risks) and adult outcomes. Interestingly, this association became nonsignificant after controlling for IQ, indicating that the effect of dopaminergic risk genotypes on adult psychosocial adjustment is mediated partly by IQ deficits [70].

Another promising strategy is the evaluation of the functional role of candidate genes in subgroups of patients with ADHD. The refinement of the ADHD phenotype by means of the concept of endophenotypes might enhance sensitivity to specific dimensions of the syndrome, thus allowing for the identification of individual pathways contributing to the clinical expression of the disorder [71]. Among studies that adopted neuropsychological variables as outcome measures, the DRD4 7-repeat allele is one of the most investigated polymorphisms. Results have been variable, with two studies evidencing associations between the DRD4 7-repeat allele and an error-prone response style [72,73] and three studies demonstrating greater inattention, impulsivity, and reaction time anomalies in patients lacking the 7-repeat allele [74–76]. Although these apparently conflicting results could be understood as reflecting the effect of a genetic variant of ADHD expressed by behavioral excesses without deficits in speed and variability on reaction times [77], methodological differences still limit comparison among results. Of major interest are the effects of potential confounding variables such as severity of ADHD symptoms, IQ, environmental factors, and especially age, as both gene expression and cognitive performance are believed to change over time.

Pathophysiological processes: brain imaging

The complex pathophysiology of psychiatric disorders is reflected in microscopic and quantitative, rather than macroscopic and qualitative, differences in brain development [78]. The overt behavioral signs of ADHD (ie, excessive inattention, hyperactivity, and impulsivity) are thought to result from underlying deficits in response inhibition, delay aversion, and executive functioning. In turn, these neuropsychological deficits are presumed to be linked to structural and functional brain abnormalities in frontal-striatal-cerebellar circuits [79]. The mapping of attentional functions onto different brain regions may help elucidate the underlying neurophysiology of ADHD, with the ultimate goal of determining how different phenotypes relate to specific alterations in brain structure and function.

Brain volume

Early brain imaging studies with ADHD children suggested a smaller than normal size for several brain regions, including corpus callosum, caudate nucleus, and right frontal cortex [80–82]. Overall, the last two decades of extensive investigation have confirmed these original findings, and it now is accepted that the brains of children who have ADHD are significantly smaller, on average, than the brains of healthy comparison children throughout childhood and adolescence [83–85].

The brain volume reduction observed in ADHD is widespread, affecting the cerebrum and cerebellum. The largest study performed to date compared regional brain volumes of 152 children and adolescents who had ADHD and 139 controls collected at the National Institute of Mental Health (NIMH) in Bethesda, Md, between 1992 and 2000. Children who had ADHD showed overall cerebral volumes that were 3.2% smaller than controls, affecting all four major lobes (frontal, parietal, temporal, and occipital) [83]. Durston and colleagues [84] found a similar volumetric reduction (4%) when comparing 30 boys who had ADHD with 30 matched controls. In a sample of 12 boys who had ADHD and 12 age-matched controls, those who had ADHD had on average 8.3% smaller total cerebral volumes, and the decreased size of the frontal lobe was shown to account for 48% of the reduction in total brain volume [85]. Swanson and colleagues [86] summarized effect size differences for regional brain volumes in ADHD. In addition to an overall reduction in size, four other major findings were notable. Relative to controls, individuals who had ADHD showed (1) smaller MRI-based volumes of the caudate nucleus and globus pallidus, (2) larger posterior regions and smaller anterior brain regions, (3) smaller cerebellar vermis, and (4) smaller white matter tracts. A recent meta-analysis of structural imaging findings confirmed a global brain reduction for ADHD subjects compared with control subjects, with the largest differences observed in cerebellar vermis, corpus callosum, total and right cerebral volume, and right caudate [87]. A volumetric MRI study with 50 boys found that total brain volume was 5% smaller than matched comparison subjects, and this effect was not accounted for by age, height, weight, or IQ; a subsequent study showed that total brain size correlated significantly with the vocabulary subtest score of the Wechsler Intelligence Scale for Children-Revised (WISC-R) in a sample of boys who had ADHD [88]. In a group of 50 girls who had ADHD, total brain volume correlated with the scores of full-scale IQ and attention problems as measured by the Child Behavior Checklist [89].

Beyond differences in brain volume, there is more conflicting evidence than certainties. Although converging findings from studies on the neuropharmacology, genetics, neuropsychology, and neuroimaging of ADHD attribute a central role to frontostriatal pathway disruption in ADHD [90], current theories suggest that the disorder may result from a disruption in a more distributed circuitry, including the frontal brain regions, as well as the basal ganglia, the cerebellar hemispheres, and the cerebellar vermis [79]. Moreover, additional structures and networks are hypothesized to be involved in the pathophysiology of ADHD. A recent resting-state functional MRI report demonstrated that adults who have ADHD exhibit decreased functional connectivity in long-range connections linking the anterior cingulate region and two posterior components of the so-called default-mode network (precuneus and posterior cingulate) [91].

Nevertheless, the most significant findings on structural and functional neuroimaging studies of ADHD delineate three anatomic regions: the frontal cortex, particularly the prefrontal cortex, the basal ganglia, and the cerebellum. Neuroimaging studies have assumed a central role in the definition of an accurate model for the pathophysiology of ADHD. Methodological limitations, however—such as small sample sizes, moderate effect sizes, lack of consistency in MRI methodology, the nonspecificity of deficits to ADHD, the variation of symptoms according to subtype, age, sex, and clinical setting, and a lack of replication studies—prevent more definitive conclusions.

Frontal cortex

A similar pattern of deficits observed in patients presenting with ADHD and with frontal lobe lesions first implicated the prefrontal cortex in the pathophysiology of ADHD. As catecholaminergic agents were found to have a primary role in the treatment of ADHD, this association was reinforced further by the fact that the prefrontal region is highly influenced by catecholaminergic nuclei [92]. Numerous structural neuroimaging studies have reported significantly smaller volumes of the frontal cortex in children who have ADHD compared with healthy controls [88,93–95]. This volume decrease appears to be particularly significant in the right prefrontal cortex, reducing the typical right greater than left (R > L) asymmetry of the prefrontal cortex in children who have ADHD [80,88].

Right frontal volume reductions were reported to correlate significantly with impaired performance on tasks indexing response inhibition [96] and rapid color naming [97], both of which are known to be impaired in ADHD [98–100]. Moreover, functional imaging studies have shown that an expected increase in prefrontal metabolism during response inhibition tasks is reduced markedly in ADHD subjects [101,102]. In fact, a recent meta-analysis of 16 published functional neuroimaging studies of ADHD revealed that significant patterns of frontal hypoactivity are detected across studies in patients who have ADHD, affecting anterior cingulate, dorsolateral prefrontal, and inferior prefrontal cortices [103].

More recently, innovative analytic methods have allowed the assessment of other cortical regions in patients who have ADHD. A detailed spatial mapping of cortical morphology and gray matter density described by Sowell and colleagues [104] revealed significant differences in the morphology of frontal cortices in patients who had ADHD, with size reductions noted bilaterally in the inferior dorsolateral aspects of this region, but also in the lateral aspects of anterior and midtemporal cortices. This study supports the hypothesis that attention and behavioral inhibition deficits are associated with anatomic abnormalities of a distributed neural system including the prefrontal cortex and other heteromodal association cortices.

Using automated computational techniques, Shaw and colleagues [105] examined the relationships among cortical thickness measures, baseline diagnosis, and clinical outcome in the NIMH cohort of children and adolescents who had ADHD. Results confirmed previous findings of cortical abnormalities, prominently in medial and superior prefrontal and precentral regions, which are important for attentional control and motor output. A thinner medial prefrontal cortex in baseline discriminated poor from good outcome in patients who had ADHD, as a fixed thinning of this area was observed in children who had a worse outcome, whether this outcome was defined on the basis of overall functioning or persistence of *DSM-IV*-defined ADHD. The developmental trajectory of cortical thickness also differed between outcome groups; only the good outcome group showed normalization of right parietal cortical thickness, a region speculated to support compensatory changes in posterior attentional systems through adolescence.

A subsequent innovative study integrating genetic, neuroimaging and clinical data [106] identified that distinct trajectories in cortical development were associated with ADHD diagnosis and DRD4 gene polymorphisms. There was a stepwise increment in thickness in the right orbitofrontal and posterior parieto-occipital cortices according to diagnostic and genotypic statuses: subjects who had ADHD and a DRD4 7-repeat allele presented the thinnest cortex, followed by those with ADHD but without the 7-repeat allele, healthy 7-repeat carriers, and finally by healthy noncarriers. Interestingly, the presence of a 7-repeat allele was also associated with cortical normalization and a better clinical outcome over time. In a recent study [107], the NIMH group also reported a longitudinal comparison of cortical thickness between 223 patients who had ADHD and 223 healthy controls. They showed that rather than a deviation from typical development, ADHD exhibited a marked delay in reaching peak thickness in most cortical regions (median age 10.5 and 7.5 years for the ADHD and control groups, respectively).

Basal ganglia

As the caudate nuclei and associated subcortical circuits receive inputs from cortical regions implicated in executive functioning and attentional processes, research also has focused on the role of the basal ganglia on the pathophysiology of ADHD. The basal ganglia are neural structures within the motor and cognitive control circuits in the mammalian forebrain, which are organized into multiple parallel processing loops that project mainly toward motor and prefrontal areas of the frontal lobes. Their largest input station, the striatum, collects inputs from the entire neocortex and sends processed information to areas of the frontal cortex that have been implicated in motor planning, sequencing, learning, and execution. Anatomical studies indicate that the putamen is involved most directly in regulation of motor activity and movement, whereas the anterior caudate subserves higher cognitive functions [108]. Abnormalities of the caudate nucleus, the putamen, and the globus pallidus have been reported in children and adolescents who have ADHD, but findings have been inconsistent across studies [79].

One of the earliest findings of caudate differences in ADHD was based on studies using regional cerebral blood flow, which found decreased metabolism in the striatal region, particularly the right caudate [109,110]. Later studies have shown size reductions of the right globus pallidus [88] and smaller volumes of left [82,93,97] and right caudate [111]. Indices of asymmetry are intrinsically less reliable [111]; accordingly right greater than left (R>L) [82,112] and left greater than right (R<L) [113,114] asymmetries and symmetric caudate volumes [88,93] have all been reported to be associated with ADHD.

A study by Castellanos and colleagues in 2002 [83], however, found that such volumetric differences may be transient and possibly related to developmental changes in symptoms of ADHD with increasing age.

Decreased volumes of total caudate in ADHD subjects were found up to the age of 16, but not beyond that age; around age 16, caudate volumes appeared to converge, as a decrease was seen in caudate volumes of normal controls, but not in the ADHD group.

Anatomical abnormalities typically are reflected by atypical brain activation patterns. Comparison of neuropsychological and basal ganglia measures in ADHD showed that performance on response inhibition tasks correlated with the volume of the caudate and globus pallidus, but not the putamen. The significant correlations between task performance and anatomic measures of the caudate nuclei were predominantly in the right hemisphere, supporting the role of right frontostriatal circuitry in response to inhibition and ADHD [96]. A significant relationship has been described between reversed caudate asymmetry and measures of inhibition and externalizing behavior, as children who had reversed caudate asymmetry performed more poorly on measures of inhibition regardless of group membership [97]. A study exclusively with girls demonstrated that the pallidum and caudate volumes correlated significantly with ratings of ADHD severity and cognitive performance [89]. Further support for striatal models of ADHD comes from a brain–behavior study in monozygotic twins discordant for ADHD, which showed that affected twins had significantly smaller caudate volumes than their unaffected cotwins [115].

Cerebellum

The role played by cerebellar structures in circuitries involved in cognitive and affective processes, beyond its traditional involvement in motor coordination [116], has led to its investigation as an area possibly implicated in pathophysiological processes underlying ADHD. In particular, the smaller posterior inferior lobe (lobules VIII-X) of the vermis consistently has been replicated in ADHD. In a recent longitudinal study, the global nonprogressive reduction in total volume [83] was shown to be more specific to the superior cerebellar vermis, a region that exhibited a volumetric developmental trajectory associated with better or worse clinical outcomes [117].

Behavioral manifestations: clinical expression

Although ADHD increasingly is conceptualized as a neurodevelopmental disorder, several issues remain unresolved regarding the nature of biological and psychological processes underlying symptom expression throughout childhood. Once considered as a disorder affecting primarily males in middle childhood, recent research has led to a reconceptualization of ADHD as a chronic disorder affecting both sexes [118]. The persistence of the disorder, which previously was thought to remit largely in adolescence, has been shown to carry substantial risk for additional morbidity and disability [119].

Because ADHD is conceptualized as a neurodevelopmental disorder, precursor problems would be expected in infancy. The Ben-Gurion Infant Development Study (BIDS) provides an innovative approach to this issue; this is a prospective longitudinal investigation of infants at high familial risk for ADHD, who are thus classified on the basis of paternal symptoms of ADHD [120]. Differences in activity level between the ADHD high- and low-risk groups were evident in the neonatal period, with the ADHD risk group having marginally higher activity levels than the comparison group as measured by the Neonatal Behavioral Assessment Scales [121]. Moreover, differences in attention were also evident in the high-risk group in infancy. The ADHD risk group showed less interest in a block play task at 7 months and less vigilance in a puppet paradigm at 12 months in laboratory assessments [120,122]. Moreover, the ADHD risk group also received higher parent ratings for activity level and anger as well as lower ratings on a composite measure of effortful control at 7, 12, and 25 months of age [121]. It remains to be seen what proportion of these high-risk infants subsequently meet diagnostic criteria for ADHD.

Typically, ADHD is not diagnosed before the age of 3 years, as the diagnosis is particularly challenging in preschool-aged children, for which the normative ranges of levels of activity, impulsivity, and attention span are much broader than at older ages [118,123]. Diagnosis of preschool-aged children thus requires the identification of excessive levels of such characteristics for that age, leading to substantial impairment in terms of socialization, learning, or parent–child interaction. Nevertheless, it is estimated that roughly 2% of preschool-aged children meet criteria for ADHD [124] and all three subtypes of the disorder (predominantly inattentive, predominantly hyperactive/impulsive, and combined subtype) have been validly identified in four-to-six-year-old children. Symptoms and associated impairments observed in these children include social and academic difficulties, more placements in special education, and more unintentional injuries than non-ADHD children [125]. Lahey and colleagues [126] demonstrated that the great majority of children who meet full diagnostic criteria for ADHD at 4 to 6 years of age continue to exhibit ADHD symptoms well into elementary school, with enduring impairments reported across different sources, including parent, teacher, interviewer, and child reports.

It is indisputable that ADHD is a disorder that typically has its onset of symptoms during childhood. Current diagnostic criteria for ADHD, however, based on *DSM-IV*, requires that the beginning of some symptoms of inattention or hyperactivity/impulsivity causing impairment occurs before the age of 7 years. Contrary to this explicit age-of-onset requirement, researchers have argued that the selection of a specific cutoff at age 7 for the onset of the disorder is too restrictive, based only in a committee decision, and not empirically validated [127]. Studies that examined the diagnostic validity of this requirement in different cultures have not found support for an age-of-onset cutoff for ADHD [128,129], as subjects with late-onset and full ADHD diagnostic criteria had similar patterns of psychiatric comorbidity, functional impairment and familial transmission [130], neuropsychological dysfunction [131], and response to medication [132].

Although a specific age-of-onset cutoff has not been validated, evidence of a childhood history of ADHD symptoms remains essential to an accurate diagnosis. First evidence of ADHD symptoms in adolescence, even in the presence of the full clinical syndrome, should prompt consideration of other diagnoses. The possibility that these are only ADHD-like symptoms and that the current complaints can be explained best by another axis 1 disorder must be considered [133].

Prospective, longitudinal studies with follow-up periods from 4 to 12 years provide compelling evidence of the continuation of ADHD. Persistence rates for the diagnosis of ADHD vary widely [134–137], but a recent review found a persistence rate of 74% [138]. These studies, however, should be interpreted cautiously, as most were based on clinical samples and included patients who varied substantially in age. This is particularly important, as it has been suggested that persistence rates for ADHD decrease substantially every 5 years beginning at the age of 9 [139]. Additionally, remission rates have been shown to vary considerably according with the definition used [138,140,141]. A recent meta-analysis demonstrated that when only patients meeting full *DSM-IV* criteria for ADHD are classified as having persistent ADHD, the proportion of persistence is not very high, approximately 15% at age 25 years. On the other hand, when cases in partial remission are included, the rate of persistence reaches approximately 65% [142].

Independent of specific remission or retention rates, ADHD symptoms lessen with age. An earlier age-of-onset is seen for the combined and hyperactive subtypes compared with the inattentive type of ADHD [143]. Hyperactivity and impulsivity symptoms tend to decline with age more rapidly than symptoms of inattention [137,140], which become increasingly more evident during secondary school years [144]. Accordingly, children rarely remain in the hyperactive/impulsive classification over time; rather, they mostly shift to the combined subtype in later years [145]. Again, the interpretation of such findings must take into account the fact that the set of hyperactive behaviors investigated in these longitudinal studies may not have been adequate to identify adolescent and/or adult hyperactivity, as the original constructs were developed for males in midchildhood.

Although ADHD behaviors decline over time, this developmental trajectory does not result in normalization necessarily. The persistence of ADHD is associated with a range of educational and social adjustment outcomes [146], including less formal schooling and lower-ranking occupational positions [147]. At least two factors have been identified as predicting the persistence of ADHD into adulthood—familiality with ADHD and psychiatric comorbidity [137].

The development of aggression or delinquency problems in children with ADHD is also of particular concern. ADHD has been found to co-occur with oppositional defiant disorder (ODD) and/or conduct disorder (CD) in 30% to 50% of cases both in epidemiologic and clinical samples [148,149], often leading to a diagnosis of antisocial disorder in adulthood [150,151]. Youth who have ADHD are at increased risk for cigarette smoking and substance abuse during adolescence [150–153] and tend to show a longer course of addiction compared with non-ADHD peers [154–157]. ADHD has also a significant overlap with learning disorders, especially reading disability. Further longitudinal studies are required to confirm the causality of these associations, establishing whether continued ADHD behaviors mediate the risk for negative outcomes in adolescence or are a proxy for other processes that result in negative outcomes [118].

Summary

Key elements of the neurobiological bases of ADHD are starting to be uncovered, as new neuroimaging and molecular techniques allow research to aim at increasingly sophisticated goals. Studies have identified relevant genetic and environmental risk factors for ADHD, making genes, like DRD4 and DAT1, and exposures to substances, such as nicotine and alcohol, necessary study variables for subsequent etiologic research. Brain studies are proving to be an essential transitional point of analysis, building the necessary link between disease susceptibility and clinical expression, as it is discovered how specific combinations of genes relate to various abnormalities in brain-based functions.

The validation of initial theories regarding neurobiological underpinnings of ADHD was accomplished by the replication of findings across cultures and ethnicities. As research advanced, additional elements were found to be part of the pathophysiology of ADHD, leading to the refinement of theories and to the development of new hypotheses. Although catecholaminergic imbalance is still central in ADHD theory, genes coding for other neurotransmitter systems have been found to be also associated with the disorder. The cardinal role attributed to the prefrontal cortex as key structure in cognitive and affective processes also is being discussed as functional circuits involving basal ganglia and cerebellum are depicted. All these findings corroborate the complex nature of the disorder, evidencing the heterogeneity of ADHD at both etiologic and phenomenological levels.

A translational approach to ADHD decipherment is essential for putting together neuroscience and nosology. The recognition of biological bases of behavioral processes might reduce the stigma associated with mental disorders [158]. Most importantly, insights from the neurobiology of ADHD may strengthen its validity as a clinical syndrome, and improve diagnosis and treatment. A promising strategy for future research is to integrate information from multiple levels of analysis, by studying genetic, neurophysiological, and clinical processes across the developmental continuum.

References

[1] Kupfer DJ, First MB, Regier DA. A research agenda for DSM-V. 1st edition. Washington, DC: American Psychiatric Association; 2002.

[2] Caspi A, Moffitt TE, Newman DL, et al. Behavioral observations at age 3 years predict adult psychiatric disorders. Longitudinal evidence from a birth cohort. Arch Gen Psychiatry 1996;53(11):1033–9.

[3] Lynam DR, Caspi A, Moffitt TE, et al. Longitudinal evidence that psychopathy scores in early adolescence predict adult psychopathy. J Abnorm Psychol 2007;116(1):155–65.

[4] Porges SW. Asserting the role of biobehavioral sciences in translational research: the behavioral neurobiology revolution. Dev Psychopathol 2006;18(3):923–33.

[5] Goldman LS, Genel M, Bezman RJ, et al. Diagnosis and treatment of attention-deficit/hyperactivity disorder in children and adolescents. Council on Scientific Affairs, American Medical Association. JAMA 1998;279(14):1100–7.

[6] Sonuga-Barke EJ, Sergeant J. The neuroscience of ADHD: multidisciplinary perspectives on a complex developmental disorder. Dev Sci 2005;8(2):103–4.

[7] Coghill D, Nigg J, Rothenberger A, et al. Whither causal models in the neuroscience of ADHD? Dev Sci 2005;8(2):105–14.

[8] Volkmar F. Toward understanding the basis of ADHD. Am J Psychiatry 2005;162(6): 1043–4.

[9] Spencer TJ, Biederman J, Wilens TE, et al. Overview and neurobiology of attention-deficit/ hyperactivity disorder. J Clin Psychiatry 2002;63(Suppl 12):3–9.

[10] Biederman J, Faraone SV, Keenan K, et al. Family-genetic and psychosocial risk factors in DSM-III attention deficit disorder. J Am Acad Child Adolesc Psychiatry 1990;29(4): 526–33.

[11] Banerjee TD, Middleton F, Faraone SV. Environmental risk factors for attention-deficit hyperactivity disorder. Acta Paediatr 2007;96(9):1269–74.

[12] Linnet KM, Dalsgaard S, Obel C, et al. Maternal lifestyle factors in pregnancy risk of attention deficit hyperactivity disorder and associated behaviors: review of the current evidence. Am J Psychiatry 2003;160(6):1028–40.

[13] Braun JM, Kahn RS, Froehlich T, et al. Exposures to environmental toxicants and attention deficit hyperactivity disorder in US children. Environ Health Perspect 2006;114(12): 1904–9.

[14] Dopfner M, Rothenberger A, Sonuga-Barke E. Areas for future investment in the field of ADHD: preschoolers and clinical networks. Eur Child Adolesc Psychiatry 2004;13(Suppl 1):I130–5.

[15] Kapoor A, Petropoulos S, Matthews SG. Fetal programming of hypothalamic-pituitary-adrenal (HPA) axis function and behavior by synthetic glucocorticoids. Brain Res Rev 2007, in press.

[16] Thapar A, Holmes J, Poulton K, et al. Genetic basis of attention deficit and hyperactivity. Br J Psychiatry 1999;174:105–11.

[17] Smalley SL. Genetic influences in childhood-onset psychiatric disorders: autism and attention-deficit/hyperactivity disorder. Am J Hum Genet 1997;60(6):1276–82.

[18] Centers for Disease Control and Prevention (CDC). Cigarette smoking among adults— United States, 2006. MMWR Morb Mortal Wkly Rep 2007;56(44):1157–61.

[19] Bardy AH, Seppala T, Lillsunde P, et al. Objectively measured tobacco exposure during pregnancy: neonatal effects and relation to maternal smoking. Br J Obstet Gynaecol 1993;100(8):721–6.

[20] Kuczkowski KM. The effects of drug abuse on pregnancy. Curr Opin Obstet Gynecol 2007; 19:578–85.

[21] Leung GM, Ho LM, Lam TH. The economic burden of environmental tobacco smoke in the first year of life. Arch Dis Child 2003;88:767–71.

[22] Milberger S, Biederman J, Faraone SV, et al. Is maternal smoking during pregnancy a risk factor for attention deficit hyperactivity disorder in children? Am J Psychiatry 1996;153(9): 1138–42.

[23] Milberger S, Biederman J, Faraone SV, et al. Further evidence of an association between maternal smoking during pregnancy and attention-deficit hyperactivity disorder: findings from a high-risk sample of siblings. J Clin Child Psychol 1998;27(3):352–8.

[24] Thapar A, Fowler T, Rice F, et al. Maternal smoking during pregnancy and attention-deficit hyperactivity disorder symptoms in offspring. Am J Psychiatry 2003;160(11):1985–9.

[25] Kotimaa AJ, Moilanen I, Taanila A, et al. Maternal smoking and hyperactivity in 8-year-old children. J Am Acad Child Adolesc Psychiatry 2003;42(7):826–33.

[26] Rodriguez A, Bohlin G. Are maternal smoking and stress during pregnancy related to ADHD symptoms in children? J Child Psychol Psychiatry 2005;46(3):246–54.

[27] Schmitz M, Denardin D, Laufer Silva T, et al. Smoking during pregnancy and attention-deficit/hyperactivity disorder, predominantly inattentive type: a case-control study. J Am Acad Child Adolesc Psychiatry 2006;45(11):1338–45.

[28] Ernst M, Heishman SJ, Spurgeon L, et al. Smoking history and nicotine effects on cognitive performance. Neuropsychopharmacology 2001;25:313–9.

[29] Batstra L, Hadders-ALgra M, Neeleman J. Effect of antenatal exposure to maternal smoking on behavioural problems and academic achievement in childhood: prospective evidence from a Dutch birth cohort. Early Hum Dev 2003;75(1–2):21–33.

[30] Langley K, Rice F, van den Bree MB, et al. Maternal smoking during pregnancy as an environmental risk factor for attention-deficit hyperactivity disorder behaviour. A review. Minerva Pediatr 2005;57(6):359–71.

[31] Mick E, Biederman J, Faraone SV, et al. Case–control study of attention-deficit hyperactivity disorder and maternal smoking, alcohol use, and drug use during pregnancy. J Am Acad Child Adolesc Psychiatry 2002;41(4):378–85.

[32] Weissman MM, Warner V, Wickramaratne PJ, et al. Maternal smoking during pregnancy and psychopathology in offspring followed to adulthood. J Am Acad Child Adolesc Psychiatry 1999;38:892–9.

[33] Goodwin RD, Keyes K, Simuro N. Mental disorders and nicotine dependence among pregnant women in the United States. Obstet Gynecol 2007;109(4):875–83.

[34] Williams JH, Ross L. Consequences of prenatal toxin exposure for mental health in children and adolescents: a systematic review. Eur Child Adolesc Psychiatry 2007;16:243–53.

[35] Slotkin TA, MacKillop EA, Rudder CL, et al. Permanent, sex-selective effects of prenatal or adolescent nicotine exposure, separately or sequentially, in rat brain regions: indices of cholinergic and serotonergic synaptic function, cell signaling, and neural cell number and size at 6 months of age. Neuropsychopharmacology 2007;32:1082–97.

[36] Liang K, Poytress BS, Chen Y, et al. Neonatal nicotine exposure impairs nicotinic enhancement of central auditory processing and auditory learning in adult rats. Eur J Neurosci 2006;24(3):857–66.

[37] Roy TS, Seidler FJ, Slotkin TA. Prenatal nicotine exposure evokes alterations of cell structure in hippocampus and somatosensory cortex. J Pharmacol Exp Ther 2002;300:124–33.

[38] Slawecki CJ, Thomas JD, Riley EP, et al. Neonatal nicotine exposure alters hippocampal EEG and event-related potentials (ERPs) in rats. Pharmacol Biochem Behav 2000;65:711–8.

[39] Slawecki CJ, Thorsell A, Ehlers CL. Long-term neurobehavioral effects of alcohol or nicotine exposure in adolescent animal models. Ann N Y Acad Sci 2004;1021:448–52.

[40] Vaglenova J, Birru S, Pandiella NM, et al. An assessment of the long-term developmental and behavioral teratogenicity of prenatal nicotine exposure. Behav Brain Res 2004; 150(1–2):159–70.

[41] Fried PA, Watkinson B, Siegel LS. Reading and language in 9- to 12-year olds prenatally exposed to cigarettes and marijuana. Neurotoxicol Teratol 1997;19(3):171–83.

[42] Fried PA, Watkinson B, Gray R. Differential effects on cognitive functioning in 13- to 16-year-olds prenatally exposed to cigarettes and marihuana. Neurotoxicol Teratol 2003; 25(4):427–36.

[43] Jacobsen LK, Slotkin TA, Mencl WE, et al. Gender-specific effects of prenatal and adolescent exposure to tobacco smoke on auditory and visual attention. Neuropsychopharmacology 2007;32(12):2453–64.

[44] Collins BN, Wileyto EP, Murphy MF, et al. Adolescent environmental tobacco smoke exposure predicts academic achievement test failure. J Adolesc Health 2007;41(4):363–70.

[45] Yolton K, Dietrich K, Auinger P, et al. Exposure to environmental tobacco smoke and cognitive abilities among US children and adolescents. Environ Health Perspect 2005;113(1): 98–103.

[46] Currie J, Stabile M. Child mental health and human capital accumulation: the case of ADHD. J Health Econ 2006;25(6):1094–118.

[47] Frazier TW, Youngstrom EA, Glutting JJ, et al. ADHD and achievement: meta-analysis of the child, adolescent, and adult literatures and a concomitant study with college students. J Learn Disabil 2007;40(1):49–65.

[48] Kharrazi M, DeLorenze GN, Kaufman FL, et al. Environmental tobacco smoke and pregnancy outcome. Epidemiology 2004;15(6):660–70.

[49] Delpisheh A, Kelly Y, Rizwan S, et al. Population attributable risk for adverse pregnancy outcomes related to smoking in adolescents and adults. Public Health 2007;121(11):861–8.

[50] Ward C, Lewis S, Coleman T. Prevalence of maternal smoking and environmental tobacco smoke exposure during pregnancy and impact on birth weight: retrospective study using Millennium Cohort. BMC Public Health 2007;7:81.

[51] Mikkola K, Ritari N, Tommiska V, et al. Neurodevelopmental outcome at 5 years of age of a national cohort of extremely low birth weight infants who were born in 1996–1997. Pediatrics 2005;116(6):1391–400.

[52] Indredavik MS, Vik T, Heyerdahl S, et al. Psychiatric symptoms in low birth weight adolescents, assessed by screening questionnaires. Eur Child Adolesc Psychiatry 2005; 14(4):226–36.

[53] Botting N, Powls A, Cooke RW, et al. Attention-deficit hyperactivity disorders and other psychiatric outcomes in very low birth weight children at 12 years. J Child Psychol Psychiatry 1997;38(8):931–41.

[54] Szatmari P, Saigal S, Rosenbaum P, et al. Psychiatric disorders at five years among children with birth weights less than 1000 g: a regional perspective. Dev Med Child Neurol 1990; 32(11):954–62.

[55] Lahti J, Raikkonen K, Kajantie E, et al. Small body size at birth and behavioural symptoms of ADHD in children aged five to six years. J Child Psychol Psychiatry 2006;47(11): 1167–74.

[56] Bhutta AT, Cleves MA, Casey PH, et al. Cognitive and behavioral outcomes of school-aged children who were born preterm: a meta-analysis. JAMA 2002;288(6):728–37.

[57] Emgard M, Paradisi M, Pirondi S, et al. Prenatal glucocorticoid exposure affects learning and vulnerability of cholinergic neurons. Neurobiol Aging 2007;28(1):112–21.

[58] Seckl JR, Holmes MC. Mechanisms of disease: glucocorticoids, their placental metabolism, and fetal programming of adult pathophysiology. Nat Clin Pract Endocrinol Metab 2007; 3(6):479–88.

[59] Knopik VS, Sparrow EP, Madden PA, et al. Contributions of parental alcoholism, prenatal substance exposure, and genetic transmission to child ADHD risk: a female twin study. Psychol Med 2005;35(5):625–35.

[60] Sapolsky RM. Gene therapy for psychiatric disorders. Am J Psychiatry 2003;160(2): 208–20.

[61] Biederman J, Faraone SV, Monuteaux MC. Differential effect of environmental adversity by gender: Rutter's index of adversity in a group of boys and girls with and without ADHD. Am J Psychiatry 2002;159(9):1556–62.

[62] Knopik VS, Heath AC, Jacob T, et al. Maternal alcohol use disorder and offspring ADHD: disentangling genetic and environmental effects using a children-of-twins design. Psychol Med 2006;36(10):1461–71.

[63] Caspi A, McClay J, Moffitt TE, et al. Role of genotype in the cycle of violence in maltreated children. Science 2002;297(5582):851–4.

[64] Slotkin TA, Pinkerton KE, Auman JT, et al. Perinatal exposure to environmental tobacco smoke up-regulates nicotinic cholinergic receptors in monkey brain. Brain Res Dev Brain Res 2002;133(2):175–9.

[65] Kahn RS, Khoury J, Nichols WC, et al. Role of dopamine transporter genotype and maternal prenatal smoking in childhood hyperactive–impulsive, inattentive, and oppositional behaviors. J Pediatr 2003;143(1):104–10.

[66] Brookes KJ, Mill J, Guindalini C, et al. A common haplotype of the dopamine transporter gene associated with attention-deficit/hyperactivity disorder and interacting with maternal use of alcohol during pregnancy. Arch Gen Psychiatry 2006;63(1):74–81.

[67] Neuman RJ, Lobos E, Reich W, et al. Prenatal smoking exposure and dopaminergic genotypes interact to cause a severe ADHD subtype. Biol Psychiatry 2007;61(12):1320–8.

[68] Todd RD, Neuman RJ. Gene–environment interactions in the development of combined type ADHD: evidence for a synapse-based model. Am J Med Genet B Neuropsychiatr Genet 2007;144B(8):971–5.

[69] Laucht M, Skowronek MH, Becker K, et al. Interacting effects of the dopamine transporter gene and psychosocial adversity on attention-deficit/hyperactivity disorder symptoms among 15-year-olds from a high-risk community sample. Arch Gen Psychiatry 2007; 64(5):585–90.

[70] Mill J, Caspi A, Williams BS, et al. Prediction of heterogeneity in intelligence and adult prognosis by genetic polymorphisms in the dopamine system among children with attention-deficit/hyperactivity disorder: evidence from 2 birth cohorts. Arch Gen Psychiatry 2006;63(4):462–9.

[71] Castellanos FX, Tannock R. Neuroscience of attention-deficit/hyperactivity disorder: the search for endophenotypes. Nat Rev Neurosci 2002;3(8):617–28.

[72] Langley K, Marshall L, van den Bree M, et al. Association of the dopamine D4 receptor gene 7-repeat allele with neuropsychological test performance of children with ADHD. Am J Psychiatry 2004;161(1):133–8.

[73] Kieling C, Roman T, Doyle AE, et al. Association between DRD4 gene and performance of children with ADHD in a test of sustained attention. Biol Psychiatry 2006;60(10):1163–5.

[74] Swanson J, Oosterlaan J, Murias M, et al. Attention-deficit/hyperactivity disorder children with a 7-repeat allele of the dopamine receptor D4 gene have extreme behavior but normal performance on critical neuropsychological tests of attention. Proc Natl Acad Sci U S A 2000;97(9):4754–9.

[75] Manor I, Tyano S, Eisenberg J, et al. The short DRD4 repeats confer risk to attention-deficit hyperactivity disorder in a family-based design and impair performance on a continuous performance test (TOVA). Mol Psychiatry 2002;7(7):790–4.

[76] Bellgrove MA, Hawi Z, Lowe N, et al. DRD4 gene variants and sustained attention in attention-deficit hyperactivity disorder (ADHD): effects of associated alleles at the VNTR and -521 SNP. Am J Med Genet B Neuropsychiatr Genet 2005;136(1):81–6.

[77] Swanson JM, Kinsbourne M, Nigg J, et al. Etiologic subtypes of attention-deficit/hyperactivity disorder: brain imaging, molecular genetic and environmental factors, and the dopamine hypothesis. Neuropsychol Rev 2007;17(1):39–59.

[78] Levitt P. Developmental neurobiology and clinical disorders: lost in translation? Neuron 2005;46(3):407–12.

[79] Krain AL, Castellanos FX. Brain development and ADHD. Clin Psychol Rev 2006;26(4): 433–44.

[80] Hynd GW, Semrud-Clikeman M, Lorys AR, et al. Brain morphology in developmental dyslexia and attention-deficit disorder/hyperactivity. Arch Neurol 1990;47(8):919–26.

[81] Hynd GW, Semrud-Clikeman M, Lorys AR, et al. Corpus callosum morphology in attention-deficit hyperactivity disorder: morphometric analysis of MRI. J Learn Disabil 1991; 24(3):141–6.

[82] Hynd GW, Hern KL, Novey ES, et al. Attention-deficit hyperactivity disorder and asymmetry of the caudate nucleus. J Child Neurol 1993;8(4):339–47.

[83] Castellanos FX, Lee PP, Sharp W, et al. Developmental trajectories of brain volume abnormalities in children and adolescents with attention-deficit/hyperactivity disorder. JAMA 2002;288(14):1740–8.

[84] Durston S, Hulshoff Pol HE, Schnack HG, et al. Magnetic resonance imaging of boys with attention-deficit/hyperactivity disorder and their unaffected siblings. J Am Acad Child Adolesc Psychiatry 2004;43(3):332–40.

[85] Mostofsky SH, Cooper KL, Kates WR, et al. Smaller prefrontal and premotor volumes in boys with attention-deficit/hyperactivity disorder. Biol Psychiatry 2002;52(8):785–94.

[86] Swanson JM, Hinshaw SP, Arnold LE, et al. Clinical and cognitive definitions of attention deficits in children with attention-deficit/hyperactivity disorder. In: Posner MI, editor. Cognitive neuroscience of attention. New York: Guilford; 2004. p. 430–45.

[87] Valera EM, Faraone SV, Murray KE, et al. Meta-analysis of structural imaging findings in attention-deficit/hyperactivity disorder. Biol Psychiatry 2007;61(12):1361–9.

[88] Castellanos FX, Giedd JN, Marsh WL, et al. Quantitative brain magnetic resonance imaging in attention-deficit hyperactivity disorder. Arch Gen Psychiatry 1996;53(7):607–16.

[89] Castellanos FX, Giedd JN, Berquin PC, et al. Quantitative brain magnetic resonance imaging in girls with attention-deficit/hyperactivity disorder. Arch Gen Psychiatry 2001; 58(3):289–95.

[90] Durston S. A review of the biological bases of ADHD: what have we learned from imaging studies? Ment Retard Dev Disabil Res Rev 2003;9(3):184–95.

[91] Castellanos FX, Margulies DS, Clare Kelly AM, et al. Cingulate precuneus interactions: a new locus of dysfunction in adult attention-deficit/hyperactivity disorder. Biological Psychiatry, in press.

[92] Halperin JM, Schulz KP. Revisiting the role of the prefrontal cortex in the pathophysiology of attention-deficit/hyperactivity disorder. Psychol Bull 2006;132(4):560–81.

[93] Filipek PA, Semrud-Clikeman M, Steingard RJ, et al. Volumetric MRI analysis comparing subjects having attention-deficit hyperactivity disorder with normal controls. Neurology 1997;48(3):589–601.

[94] Kates WR, Frederikse M, Mostofsky SH, et al. MRI parcellation of the frontal lobe in boys with attention-deficit hyperactivity disorder or Tourette syndrome. Psychiatry Res 2002; 116(1–2):63–81.

[95] Hill DE, Yeo RA, Campbell RA, et al. Magnetic resonance imaging correlates of attention-deficit/hyperactivity disorder in children. Neuropsychology 2003;17(3):496–506.

[96] Casey BJ, Castellanos FX, Giedd JN, et al. Implication of right frontostriatal circuitry in response inhibition and attention-deficit/hyperactivity disorder. J Am Acad Child Adolesc Psychiatry 1997;36(3):374–83.

[97] Semrud-Clikeman M, Steingard RJ, Filipek P, et al. Using MRI to examine brain–behavior relationships in males with attention-deficit disorder with hyperactivity. J Am Acad Child Adolesc Psychiatry 2000;39(4):477–84.

[98] Willcutt EG, Doyle AE, Nigg JT, et al. Validity of the executive function theory of attention-deficit/hyperactivity disorder: a meta-analytic review. Biol Psychiatry 2005;57(11):1336–46.

[99] Tannock R, Martinussen R, Frijters J. Naming speed performance and stimulant effects indicate effortful, semantic processing deficits in attention-deficit/hyperactivity disorder. J Abnorm Child Psychol 2000;28(3):237–52.

[100] Tannock R, Banaschewski T, Gold D. Color naming deficits and attention-deficit/hyperactivity disorder: a retinal dopaminergic hypothesis. Behav Brain Funct 2006;2:4.
[101] Rubia K, Overmeyer S, Taylor E, et al. Hypofrontality in attention-deficit hyperactivity disorder during higher-order motor control: a study with functional MRI. Am J Psychiatry 1999;156(6):891–6.
[102] Rubia K, Smith AB, Brammer MJ, et al. Abnormal brain activation during inhibition and error detection in medication-naive adolescents with ADHD. Am J Psychiatry 2005;162(6):1067–75.
[103] Dickstein SG, Bannon K, Xavier Castellanos F, et al. The neural correlates of attention-deficit hyperactivity disorder: an ALE meta-analysis. J Child Psychol Psychiatry 2006;47(10):1051–62.
[104] Sowell ER, Thompson PM, Welcome SE, et al. Cortical abnormalities in children and adolescents with attention-deficit hyperactivity disorder. Lancet 2003;362(9397):1699–707.
[105] Shaw P, Lerch J, Greenstein D, et al. Longitudinal mapping of cortical thickness and clinical outcome in children and adolescents with attention-deficit/hyperactivity disorder. Arch Gen Psychiatry 2006;63(5):540–9.
[106] Shaw P, Gornick M, Lerch J, et al. Polymorphism of the dopamina D4 receptor, clinical outcome, and cortical structure in attention-deficit/hyperactivity disorder. Arch Gen Psychiatry 2007;64(8):921–31.
[107] Shaw P, Eckstrand K, Sharp W, et al. Attention-deficit/hyperactivity disorder is characterized by a delay in cortical maturation. PNAS 2007;104(49):19649–54.
[108] Graybiel AM, Aosaki T, Flaherty AW, et al. The basal ganglia and adaptive motor control. Science 1994;265(5180):1826–31.
[109] Lou HC, Henriksen L, Bruhn P. Focal cerebral hypoperfusion in children with dysphasia and/or attention-deficit disorder. Arch Neurol 1984;41(8):825–9.
[110] Lou HC, Henriksen L, Bruhn P, et al. Striatal dysfunction in attention-deficit and hyperkinetic disorder. Arch Neurol 1989;46(1):48–52.
[111] Castellanos FX, Giedd JN, Eckburg P, et al. Quantitative morphology of the caudate nucleus in attention-deficit/hyperactivity disorder. Am J Psychiatry 1994;151(12):1791–6.
[112] Mataro M, Garcia-Sanchez C, Junque C, et al. Magnetic resonance imaging measurement of the caudate nucleus in adolescents with attention-deficit/hyperactivity disorder and its relationship with neuropsychological and behavioral measures. Arch Neurol 1997;54(8):963–8.
[113] Giedd JN, Castellanos FX, Casey BJ, et al. Quantitative morphology of the corpus callosum in attention-deficit/hyperactivity disorder. Am J Psychiatry 1994;151(5):665–9.
[114] Pineda DA, Restrepo MA, Sarmiento RJ, et al. Statistical analyses of structural magnetic resonance imaging of the head of the caudate nucleus in Colombian children with attention-deficit/hyperactivity disorder. J Child Neurol 2002;17(2):97–105.
[115] Castellanos FX, Sharp WS, Gottesman RF, et al. Anatomic brain abnormalities in monozygotic twins discordant for attention-deficit/hyperactivity disorder. Am J Psychiatry 2003;160(9):1693–6.
[116] Allen G, Buxton RB, Wong EC, et al. Attentional activation of the cerebellum independent of motor involvement. Science 1997;275(5308):1940–3.
[117] Mackie S, Shaw P, Lenroot R, et al. Cerebellar development and clinical outcome in attention- deficit/hyperactivity disorder. Am J Psychiatry 2007;164(4):647–55.
[118] Willoughby MT. Developmental course of ADHD symptomatology during the transition from childhood to adolescence: a review with recommendations. J Child Psychol Psychiatry 2003;44(1):88–106.
[119] Wilens TE, Biederman J, Spencer TJ. Attention-deficit/hyperactivity disorder across the lifespan. Annu Rev Med 2002;53:113–31.
[120] Auerbach JG, Atzaba-Poria N, Berger A, et al. Emerging developmental pathways to ADHD: possible path markers in early infancy. Neural Plast 2004;11(1–2):29–43.
[121] Auerbach JG, Landau R, Berger A, et al. Neonatal behavior of infants at familial risk for ADHD. Infant Behav Dev 2005;28:220–4.

[122] Berger A, Neuman K, Sagi-Shmueli A, et al. Vigilance in 1-year-old infants at familial risk for attention-deficit/hyperactivity disorder, submitted for publication.

[123] Blackman JA. Attention-deficit/hyperactivity disorder in preschoolers. Does it exist, and should we treat it? Pediatr Clin North Am 1999;46(5):1011–25.

[124] Lavigne JV, Gibbons RD, Christoffel KK, et al. Prevalence rates and correlates of psychiatric disorders among preschool children. J Am Acad Child Adolesc Psychiatry 1996;35(2): 204–14.

[125] Lahey BB, Pelham WE, Stein MA, et al. Validity of DSM-IV attention-deficit/hyperactivity disorder for younger children. J Am Acad Child Adolesc Psychiatry 1998;37(7):695–702.

[126] Lahey BB, Pelham WE, Loney J, et al. Three-year predictive validity of DSM-IV attention-deficit/ hyperactivity disorder in children diagnosed at 4–6 years of age. Am J Psychiatry 2004;161(11):2014–20.

[127] Barkley RA, Biederman J. Toward a broader definition of the age-of-onset criterion for attention-deficit/hyperactivity disorder. J Am Acad Child Adolesc Psychiatry 1997;36(9): 1204–10.

[128] Applegate B, Lahey BB, Hart EL, et al. Validity of the age-of-onset criterion for ADHD: a report from the DSM-IV field trials. J Am Acad Child Adolesc Psychiatry 1997;36(9): 1211–21.

[129] Rohde LA, Biederman J, Zimmermann H, et al. Exploring ADHD age-of-onset criterion in Brazilian adolescents. Eur Child Adolesc Psychiatry 2000;9(3):212–8.

[130] Faraone SV, Biederman J, Spencer T, et al. Diagnosing adult attention-deficit/hyperactivity disorder: are late-onset and subthreshold diagnoses valid? Am J Psychiatry 2006; 163(10):1720–9, quiz 1859.

[131] Faraone SV, Biederman J, Doyle A, et al. Neuropsychological studies of late-onset and subthreshold diagnoses of adult attention-deficit/hyperactivity disorder. Biol Psychiatry 2006;60(10):1081–7.

[132] Reinhardt MC, Benetti L, Victor MM, et al. Is age-at-onset criterion relevant for the response to methylphenidate in attention-deficit/hyperactivity disorder? J Clin Psychiatry 2007;68(7):1109–16.

[133] Rucklidge J, Tannock R. Apparent adolescent onset of ADHD—beware! J Am Acad Child Adolesc Psychiatry 2000;39(9):1075–6.

[134] August GJ, Stewart MA, Holmes CS. A four-year follow-up of hyperactive boys with and without conduct disorder. Br J Psychiatry 1983;143:192–8.

[135] Biederman J, Faraone SV, Milberger S, et al. Is childhood oppositional–defiant disorder a precursor to adolescent conduct disorder? Findings from a four-year follow-up study of children with ADHD. J Am Acad Child Adolesc Psychiatry 1996;35(9):1193–204.

[136] Cantwell DP, Baker L. Stability and natural history of DSM-III childhood diagnoses. J Am Acad Child Adolesc Psychiatry 1989;28(5):691–700.

[137] Hart EL, Lahey BB, Loeber R, et al. Developmental change in attention-deficit/hyperactivity disorder in boys: a four-year longitudinal study. J Abnorm Child Psychol 1995;23(6): 729–49.

[138] Spencer TJ, Biederman J, Mick E. Attention-deficit/hyperactivity disorder: diagnosis, lifespan, comorbidities, and neurobiology. J Pediatr Psychol 2007;32(6):631–42.

[139] Hill JC, Schoener EP. Age-dependent decline of attention-deficit/hyperactivity disorder. Am J Psychiatry 1996;153(9):1143–6.

[140] Biederman J, Mick E, Faraone SV. Age-dependent decline of symptoms of attention-deficit/ hyperactivity disorder: impact of remission definition and symptom type. Am J Psychiatry 2000;157(5):816–8.

[141] Barkley RA, Fischer M, Smallish L, et al. The persistence of attention-deficit/hyperactivity disorder into young adulthood as a function of reporting source and definition of disorder. J Abnorm Psychol 2002;111(2):279–89.

[142] Faraone SV, Biederman J, Mick E. The age-dependent decline of attention-deficit/hyperactivity disorder: a meta-analysis of follow-up studies. Psychol Med 2006;36(2):159–65.

[143] Spira EG, Fischel JE. The impact of preschool inattention, hyperactivity, and impulsivity on social and academic development: a review. J Child Psychol Psychiatry 2005;46(7): 755–73.

[144] Nolan EE, Gadow KD, Sprafkin J. Teacher reports of DSM-IV ADHD, ODD, and CD symptoms in schoolchildren. J Am Acad Child Adolesc Psychiatry 2001;40(2):241–9.

[145] Lahey BB, Pelham WE, Loney J, et al. Instability of the DSM-IV subtypes of ADHD from preschool through elementary school. Arch Gen Psychiatry 2005;62(8):896–902.

[146] Biederman J, Mick E, Faraone SV. Normalized functioning in youths with persistent attention-deficit/hyperactivity disorder. J Pediatr 1998;133(4):544–51.

[147] Mannuzza S, Klein RG, Bessler A, et al. Educational and occupational outcome of hyperactive boys grown up. J Am Acad Child Adolesc Psychiatry 1997;36(9):1222–7.

[148] Biederman J, Newcorn J, Sprich S. Comorbidity of attention-deficit/hyperactivity disorder with conduct, depressive, anxiety, and other disorders. Am J Psychiatry 1991;148(5): 564–77.

[149] Kadesjo C, Hagglof B, Kadesjo B, et al. Attention-deficit/hyperactivity disorder with and without oppositional–defiant disorder in 3- to 7-year-old children. Dev Med Child Neurol 2003;45(10):693–9.

[150] Mannuzza S, Klein RG, Bessler A, et al. Adult psychiatric status of hyperactive boys grown up. Am J Psychiatry 1998;155(4):493–8.

[151] Mannuzza S, Klein RG, Bonagura N, et al. Hyperactive boys almost grown up. V. Replication of psychiatric status. Arch Gen Psychiatry 1991;48(1):77–83.

[152] Biederman J, Wilens TE, Mick E, et al. Does attention-deficit/hyperactivity disorder impact the developmental course of drug and alcohol abuse and dependence? Biol Psychiatry 1998; 44(4):269–73.

[153] Milberger S, Biederman J, Faraone SV, et al. ADHD is associated with early initiation of cigarette smoking in children and adolescents. J Am Acad Child Adolesc Psychiatry 1997; 36(1):37–44.

[154] Wilens TE, Biederman J, Mick E. Does ADHD affect the course of substance abuse? Findings from a sample of adults with and without ADHD. Am J Addict 1998;7(2):156–63.

[155] Goldston DB, Walsh A, Mayfield Arnold E, et al. Reading problems, psychiatric disorders, and functional impairment from mid- to late adolescence. J Am Acad Child Adolesc Psychiatry 2007;46(1):25–32.

[156] Bonafina MA, Newcorn JH, McKay KE, et al. ADHD and reading disabilities: a cluster analytic approach for distinguishing subgroups. J Learn Disabil 2000;33(3):297–307.

[157] Dykman RA, Ackerman PT. Attention-deficit disorder and specific reading disability: separate but often overlapping disorders. J Learn Disabil 1991;24(2):96–103.

[158] Insel TR, Quirion R. Psychiatry as a clinical neuroscience discipline. JAMA 2005;294(17): 2221–4.

ELSEVIER
SAUNDERS

Child Adolesc Psychiatric Clin N Am
17 (2008) 309–323

CHILD AND
ADOLESCENT
PSYCHIATRIC CLINICS
OF NORTH AMERICA

Attention Deficit Hyperactivity Disorder and Substance Use Disorders

Claudia M. Szobot, MD[a,b,]*, Oscar Bukstein, MD[c]

[a]*Attention-Deficit/Hyperactivity Disorder Outpatient Clinic, Hospital de Clínicas de Porto Alegre (HCPA), Federal University of Rio Grande do Sul (UFRGS), Brazil*
[b]*Center for Drug and Alcohol Research HCPA, UFRGS, Centro de Pesquisa em Álcool e Drogas, Hospital de Clínicas de Porto Alegre. Rua Ramiro Barcelos, 2350, segundo andar, sala 2201A; Porto Alegre, Rio Grande do Sul, Brasil. CEP 90035-003*
[c]*Western Psychiatric Institute and Clinic, University of Pittsburgh School of Medicine, 200 Lothrop Street, Pittsburgh, PA 15213-2582, USA*

Attention deficit hyperactivity disorder (ADHD) is highly prevalent among adolescents who have substance use disorder (SUD). Several lines of evidence, although not conclusive, suggest that ADHD might have an independent effect on SUD liability. It is still to be determined, however, whether this association is mediated by conduct disorder. If ADHD would be an independent risk factor, this might have preventive implications. Because ADHD begins in early childhood, before the onset of SUD, these at-risk children can be identified and targeted for early and ongoing intervention to help prevent the onset of SUD. Regarding the treatment of adolescents who have ADHD plus SUD, few studies have evaluated pharmacologic interventions in this population. Up to now there is no clear algorithm for the pharmacologic treatment of adolescents who have ADHD plus SUD. If a stimulant medication is prescribed, there is an important concern regarding its potential for abuse/misuse/diversion in this specific population. Medications such as methylphenidate extended release and atomoxetine seem promising for this dually diagnosed population.

Conflict of interest: Dr. Szobot: Janssen-Cilag speaker's bureau. Dr.Bukstein: Shire Pharmaceuticals consultant, research support, and speaker's bureau; McNeil pediatrics speaker's bureau, consultant; Eli Lilly research support; Novartis speaker's bureau.

* Corresponding author. Programa de Déficit de Atenção/Hiperatividade (PRODAH), Hospital de Clínicas de Porto Alegre. Rua Ramiro Barcelos, 2350, segundo andar, sala 2201A, Porto Alegre, Brasil.

E-mail address: cmszobot@terra.com.br (C.M. Szobot).

In addition, more studies are needed to identify optimal psychosocial treatment approaches for adolescents who have ADHD and SUD.

Adolescent SUD is a major mental health concern [1,2] and one of the most prevalent disorders in adolescents [3]. It is well known that SUD has a multivariate etiology, with the influence of biologic and environmental variables [4,5]. Because a significant number of adults who have SUD have an onset of their SUD diagnosis before the age of 18 years [6], much attention has been given to the role of childhood psychopathology in the vulnerability to further SUD. Several studies have suggested ADHD as a risk factor for SUD because (1) ADHD is usually over-represented among adolescents who have SUD [7–9], and (2) ADHD onset is before age 7 years [10], this disorder usually is already present several years before drug experimentation.

Etiologic association

Theoretic and empiric reviews of the development of SUDs point to the early appearance of behavioral undercontrol characteristics, including the core symptoms of ADHD (inattention, impulsivity, and hyperactivity) in children before the onset of substance use [11–13]. In the Dunedin Health and Development Study, it was reported that behavioral undercontrol at age 3 years (impulsivity, impersistence, and difficulty sitting still) predicted alcohol dependence at age 21 years [14]. In the Montreal Longitudinal Study, novelty-seeking at ages 6 and 10 years (reported by teachers as restless, runs/jumps and doesn't keep still, squirmy and fidgety) predicted drug use and cigarette smoking in adolescence [15]. Also, in another study ADHD symptoms and poor response inhibition were related to adolescent problem drinking [16].

Recent prospective longitudinal studies of substance use and SUD in children who have ADHD support the hypothesis that children who have *Diagnostic and Statistical Manual of Mental Disorders (DSM)-III-R* or DSM-IV ADHD are at risk for adverse substance use outcomes. Two independent samples of adolescents followed from childhood (when they were diagnosed with ADHD) showed an increased risk for having used illicit drugs in the past 6 months, for heavy marijuana use and heavy cigarette use [17], heavy drinking [17,18], alcohol use disorder (AUD) symptoms [17], and AUD [18] in the mid to late teens.

Up to now, however, there is no agreement in the literature whether ADHD is an independent risk factor for SUD when results consider the presence of conduct disorder (CD), a well-known risk factor for SUD [19]. CD is highly prevalent among adolescents who have ADHD [20,21], and some evidence suggests that only those youths who have ADHD and who have comorbid CD would be at higher risk. Studies trying to disentangle the role of ADHD from the development of SUD have contradictory results. Table 1 summarizes the main studies on this topic.

Table 1
Studies on the association of attention deficit hyperactivity disorder and SUD

Author	Study design and sample	Main results
Sample: individuals who have SUD		
Carroll and Rounsaville, 1993 [22]	Prevalence; clinic; 298 adults; cocaine users	35% of the subjects had ADHD
Kuperman, et al, 2001 [23]	Prevalence; community-based; 54 adolescents who had AUD	Higher rate of ADHD than general population; ADHD preceded CD diagnosis, which preceded AUD
Szobot, et al, 2007 [9]	Case-control; community-based; 61 adolescents who had SUD and 183 normal control subjects	ADHD: significant OR (9.12) for SUD, even adjusting for the presence of CD
Sample: adults who have ADHD		
Biederman, et al, 1995 [24]	Longitudinal; compared; clinic; 120 ADHD and 120 control subjects	ADHD: Higher lifetime risk for psychoactive SUD (52%) than comparison subjects (27%)
Biederman, et al, 1998 [25]	Case-control; clinic; 239 ADHD and 268 control subjects	ADHD: a twofold increased risk for SUD
Murphy, et al, 2002 [26]	Case-control; 96 ADHD (clinic) and 64 control subjects (community)	ADHD: higher rates of SUD
Sample: adolescents who have ADHD		
Weiss, et al, 1985 [27]	Longitudinal (15 years); clinic; not blind; 63 ADHD and a control group	No higher rate of SUD among cases in comparison to control subjects
Biederman, et al, 1997 [21]	Longitudinal; clinic; 140 ADHD and 120 control subjects	Youths with and without ADHD had similar risk for SUD
Molina and Pelham, 2003 [17]	Longitudinal; clinic; 142 who had ADHD and 100 control subjects	Persistence of ADHD and CD were each associated with elevated substance use behaviors
Biederman, et al, 2006 [28]	Longitudinal (10 years); clinic; 140 ADHD and 120 control subjects	ADHD: more regular use of nicotine, alcohol, and illicit substances (HR = 2.7, 2.3, and 2.2, respectively)
August, et al, 2006 [29]	Longitudinal; community-based; 27 ADHD; 82 ADHD + CD or ODD and 91 control subjects	ADHD: more associated with SUD just in the presence of CD or ODD
Sample: adolescents who do not have ADHD or SUD		
Disney, et al, 1999 [30]	Prevalence; 626 17-year-old twins; community-based; both genders	ADHD: no effect over SUD when results were adjusted for the presence of CD

(continued on next page)

Table 1 (*continued*)

Author	Study design and sample	Main results
Tapert, et al, 2002 [31]	Longitudinal (8 years); community-based; 66 youths who did not have ADHD	Baseline attention/executive scores significantly predicted substance use and dependence symptoms 8 years later
Gau, et al, 2007 [32]	Longitudinal (3 years); 428 school children aged 12 years	ADHD independently associated with SUD (HR = 3.5)
Fergusson, et al, 2007 [33]	Longitudinal (25 years); community-based; birth cohort of 1265 New Zealand-born children	Early association between early attention problems and further SUD are mediated by conduct problems

Abbreviations: ADHD, attention deficit hyperactivity disorder; SUD, substance use disorder; AUD, alcohol use disorder; OR, odds ratio; HR, hazard ratio; CD, conduct disorder; ODD, oppositional defiant disorder.

Differences in methodology may account for the discordant results among the studies. Such differences include different definitions of drug problem, characteristics of the samples (eg, age, origin of the sample [clinical or community]), and history of ADHD treatment. If ADHD pharmacotherapy is protective for the development of substance use and SUD in adolescents as suggested by Biederman and colleagues [34] and Wilens and colleagues [35], an effect of ADHD on higher SUD risk may be reduced, and the effect of CD would be more evident in samples including treated subjects for ADHD.

Considering a multivariate etiologic model of adolescent ADHD, it seems reasonable to consider that untreated ADHD could be an independent risk factor for further SUD. Different lines of evidence support this possibility.

Developmental perspective

From a developmental perspective for adolescent psychopathology, ADHD has an earlier age of onset than either CD or SUD. Some of the ADHD-associated impairments (such as peer rejection and academic problems) through childhood and adolescence are consistently mentioned in the literature as enhancing the adolescent SUD liability [36]. Since CD onset usually occurs some years after ADHD onset, an untreated ADHD child may manifest several impairments, clearly associated with higher risk SUD, before a diagnosis of CD or antisocial behavior.

Neurobiologic perspective

From a neurobiologic perspective, it is also possible to consider ADHD as an early antecedent of SUD. Children who have ADHD have dysfunctions in the dopaminergic circuits, mostly in basal ganglia and frontal cortex [37], with defects in executive function [38] and in the reward system (RS) [39]. The dopamine system has long been implicated also in alcohol and illicit drug addiction [40–43]. For example, dopaminergic system genes have been involved in ADHD [44,45] and drug problems [46–49].

Dopamine-regulated areas such as the basal ganglia and frontal areas are affected in patients who have ADHD and SUD [50]. Executive [51] and RS functions [50] have a strong influence on SUD liability. Children who have ADHD thus have cognitive dysfunctions that may impair them in high-risk drug use situations, like their tendency in overestimating their competence [52,53] and in sustaining a behavior despite negative consequences [54]. An adolescent who has ADHD might have more difficulties in accurately evaluating the negative consequences of drug use or a high risk situation for drug use, which is an important mechanism to avoid drug use. If the adolescent realizes that drug use is resulting in negative consequences, such as family problems, they might have more difficulty in changing to a healthier behavior because of their impaired cognitive flexibility. Furthermore, ADHD and SUD may have similar dysfunctions in the brain RS. The RS is associated with motivation, salience of a stimulus [55], and delay capacity [39]. As a result, a youth who has ADHD may choose a more immediate but ultimately worse reward rather than delayed gratification for future benefit. Impulsive behavior and choices are associated with drug use. Subjects who have SUD may decide on choices with high immediate gains despite higher future losses [56].

Self-medication

Some ADHD symptoms might be attenuated with drug use. After drug experimentation, some adolescents therefore may feel or behave better, which may further reinforce drug use. For example, the acute use of nicotine, a substance with stimulant properties, is associated with an improvement in some cognitive functions [57]. As a consequence, individuals who have ADHD, after nicotine experimentation might feel a cognitive improvement, leading to repeated use. Not surprisingly, individuals who have ADHD are at higher risk for nicotine regular use [58,59]. In several prospective longitudinal studies, childhood ADHD has predicted an increased risk for cigarette smoking by adolescence and by young adulthood. These studies include children ascertained in clinic samples [17,60] and in a community sample in which most children were diagnosed as hyperactive by community practitioners in addition to research criteria [61].

More studies are needed to better elucidate the possibility of an independent effect of ADHD on the etiology of SUD. These studies should preferably adjust the results for the effect of ADHD treatment and for the presence of CD. Also, it is important to have enough sample size to estimate the effect of attention and hyperactivity/impulsivity dimensions of ADHD on further SUD. Although the debate is still open, it is reasonable to pay attention to ADHD impairments that might make a link with SUD, such as poor academic performance or impulsive choices. Clinicians also should be aware of ADHD symptoms that can be initially attenuated with first drug contacts (eg, impulsivity and cannabis; inattention and nicotine).

Pharmacologic treatment

As described, there is a significant association between ADHD and SUD in adolescents, regardless of the existence or not of direct cause–effect relation or whether this relationship is mediated by the presence of CD. The comorbidity is clinically relevant, because ADHD is associated with a worse SUD prognosis, for different categories of substances. There is evidence for an association between childhood ADHD and smoking cessation treatment failure [62], for earlier and more frequent alcohol relapses [63], and for a lower likelihood of cannabis treatment completion in adolescents [64]. Despite the clinical relevance of ADHD treatment in adolescents who have current SUD, few treatment studies have been conducted in this comorbid population. Because of the absence of psychosocial treatment studies, the authors present a summary of the literature on pharmacologic studies.

Stimulants

Several evidence-based guidelines suggest that stimulants (eg, methylphenidate [MPH]) should be the first option for treatment of ADHD (see, for instance, reference [65]), but ADHD treatment studies typically exclude individuals who have drug use/misuse or SUD. Because ADHD [66], MPH [67], and most abused drugs [50,68–70] are associated with dysfunctions and actions on the dopaminergic system, MPH clinical and neurobiologic effects might not necessarily be generalized to this dually-diagnosed population. Cocaine, for example, increases dopamine (DA) by blocking striatal dopamine transporter (DAT) [71], the same target of MPH. Moreover, there is a body of evidence describing that cannabis, the most abused illicit drug worldwide [72], affects dopamine regulation [68,70,73]. MPH clinical effects thus might not be the same in the context of acute or chronic drug exposure, highlighting the need of treatment protocols derived from studies based on ADHD/SUD samples and not just on ADHD or ADHD plus other comorbidities.

The lack of studies with stimulants in adolescents who have ADHD/SUD might reflect a concern regarding its abuse potential, already described in human studies [74,75]. There is evidence suggesting, however, that childhood treatment with MPH is associated with a protection for SUD development. A longitudinal study of children who had ADHD treated with stimulants and followed for approximately 13 years found no evidence that stimulant treatment leaded to an increased risk for substance experimentation, use, abuse, or dependence by adulthood [76]. In a meta-analytic review of the literature, the pooled estimate of the odds ratio indicated a 1.9-fold reduction in risk for SUD in youths who received pharmacotherapy for ADHD [35]. More recent reports from a large prospective study of ADHD youths, however, found that although a history of treatment with a psychostimulant had no effect on substance use in adolescents who had ADHD, a history of psychostimulant treatment seemed to be associated with increased marijuana use, cigarette use, and binge drinking in young adults [77].

The authors were not able to find many treatment studies with stimulants, independent of the formulation, for adolescents who have ADHD/SUD. In a randomized, double-blind, placebo-controlled trial of the stimulant pemoline (discontinued in the United States in October 2005 because of liver toxicity) in adolescents who had comorbid ADHD and SUD, the stimulant medication was shown to improve ADHD symptoms but to have little, if any, effect on substance use [78]. Recently the effectiveness of a long-acting formulation of methylphenidate (MPH-SODAS) on ADHD symptoms was evaluated in an outpatient sample of adolescents who had ADHD and illicit SUD in a crossover, placebo-controlled trial. In this study, subjects (mostly cannabis users) had a significantly higher reduction in the Swanson, Nolan and Pelham Scale, version IV (SNAP-IV) and the Clinical Global Impression Scale (CGI) scores ($P<.001$ for all analyses) during MPH-SODAS treatment when compared with placebo. There was no significant effect over drug use, and MPH-SODAS was well tolerated, but it was associated with more severe appetite reduction than placebo ($P<.001$) [79].

The few available randomized clinical trials (RCTs) were conducted only on adults, and some did not find a superior effect of MPH over placebo [80–82]. Schubiner and colleagues [83] reported significant reductions in ADHD symptoms ($P = .0039$) and a decline in cocaine craving with MPH use when compared with placebo, although there was no difference in cocaine use. Approximately 47% of the sample dropped out from the study, however. These findings may not necessarily be translated to adolescents, because there are reports of different MPH [84] and drug responses between adults and adolescents [85–87].

Bupropion

Although bupropion is not a first-line ADHD medication [65], it is the most studied medication in adolescents who have ADHD/SUD, probably because it is considered safer from misuse and abuse. Bupropion seems to have a low abuse potential on physiologic measures compared with dextroamphetamine [88]. The approval by the Food and Drug Administration (FDA) for the use of bupropion for smoking cessation and its efficacy in controlled clinical trials [89] suggests the potential value of this agent for addictive disorders. Only open trials with this medication were conducted in adolescents who had ADHD plus SUD, however, up to now. Riggs and colleagues [90] evaluated bupropion effects on 13 adolescents who had ADHD/SUD/CD in a residential program. In this 5-week open trial, there was a significant reduction in scores of ADHD outcome measures. Solhkhah and colleagues [91] evaluated effects of bupropion SR over ADHD symptoms in 14 adolescents who had ADHD/SUD associated with mood disorder in a 6-month open trial. The investigators reported a significant reduction in drug use and ADHD symptoms. The authors of this article were not able to find controlled studies with bupropion in adolescents who have ADHD/SUD.

Other non-stimulants

Because of the absence of evidence regarding abuse potential, atomoxetine was not listed as a scheduled drug by the Drug Enforcement Agency (DEA). Further evidence of atomoxetine's lack of abuse potential is provided by a finding of lack of increased extra cellular dopamine in the nucleus accumbens of rats [92]. The nucleus accumbens is involved in the reward aspects of drug use, which seems to be mediated through dopamine. Heil and colleagues [93] reported that atomoxetine did not produce subjective effects similar to methylphenidate, thus suggesting its absence of abuse liability. The authors, however, were not able to find atomoxetine studies on adolescents who have ADHD plus SUD.

Modafinil, marketed for the treatment of daytime sleepiness in narcolepsy, has effects on glutamate and GABA neurotransmitter systems that may oppose some effects of chronic cocaine administration and may have an alerting effect that may ameliorate some of the vegetative symptoms of cocaine withdrawal and may blunt cocaine euphoria [94]. Moreover, dose-related effects on prepotent inhibition in normal volunteers and in patients who have ADHD suggests a positive effect of modafinil in reducing impulsive responding [95,96]. A double-blind, placebo-controlled trial in 62 cocaine-dependent men and women reported increased cocaine abstinence in the modafinil group [97]. Trials in children and adolescents who have ADHD show improvement in ADHD symptoms for modafinil over placebo while demonstrating its safety and tolerability [98,99].

Stimulant abuse/diversion

When considering an algorithm for pharmacologic treatment of ADHD, stimulant abuse/diversion data should be considered. It is well known that adolescents who have SUD can divert or misuse stimulants [100,101], creating an intriguing scenario for ADHD pharmacologic treatment in youths who already have drug problems. The misuse of stimulants as "study drugs" [102] is not uncommon on college campuses. A recent Web-based survey found a 6% past-year prevalence and a lifetime prevalence of 8% of stimulant misuse in 4580 college students (75% used amphetamines, 25% methylphenidate) [103]. A mail-in survey of 11,000 college students at 119 institutions reported a 4% past-year prevalence for nonmedical use of stimulants (7% lifetime) [104]. Most undergraduates (60%) who reported MPH misuse in a cohort at one college (prevalence: 5.4% of 9000 surveyed) reported that stimulants "help me concentrate," and 40% said stimulant use "helps increase my awareness"; another 40% reported that use of immediate-release stimulants "gives me a high" [105].

Recently Wilens and colleagues [106] evaluated the characteristics of adolescents and young adults who have ADHD who divert or misuse their prescribed medications. Regarding immediate-release methylphenidate (the only formulation of MPH reported in the sample), 11% of the subjects (all of whom had an additional diagnosis of CD, SUD, or both) sold the medication to others, and 22% (of whom 83% also had CD, SUD, or both) misused the medication. The presence of comorbid CD and SUD was thus a significant risk factor for misuse and diversion.

The route of administration and the rates of onset and offset in the brain play critical roles in determining the risk for chemical dependency [71]. A recent brain imaging study supports that the abuse potential of sustained-release formulations may be less than that for immediate-release formulations [67]. These findings suggest that the newer, longer-acting stimulants, such as extended-release methylphenidate, dexmethylphenidate extended release, lisdexamphetamine, or the extended-release formulation of mixed amphetamine salts, may have a lower abuse/misuse/diversion potential than immediate-release preparations of psychostimulants. In addition, once-a-day medications may be easier to monitor in compliance and possible diversion. Up to now, however, there are no empiric data derived from adolescents to support this possibility.

Summary

Although we do not have enough RCTs describing treatment effects over ADHD symptoms, drug use, and medication abuse/diversion in adolescents who have ADHD plus SUD, clinicians are challenged with intriguing issues, such as: (1) Should they prescribe bupropion, avoiding concerns about abuse or diversion but offering a medication with smaller effect size for ADHD than stimulants? This is intriguing, because, as already reported, there is evidence that untreated ADHD is associated with a worse SUD prognosis. (2) Should they prescribe stimulants, risking abuse or diversion?

Up to now there are not enough data in the adolescent literature to support a treatment algorithm for adolescents who have ADHD plus SUD. Given concerns about abuse/misuse/diversion, the mixed literature on the effectiveness of treating ADHD in patients who have SUD does not support the use of specific drugs, the exact time for initiating treatment for ADHD, and the length of treatment. In adolescents, open-label trials with bupropion and clinical experience are providing some guidance. Some investigators have proposed that non-stimulant agents (atomoxetine) and antidepressants (bupropion) might be alternatives to stimulants in adolescents who have ADHD and active SUD symptoms and behaviors. For those who have stabilized SUD or merely a past history of SUD or recreational/experimental substance use (assuming non-amphetamine/methylphenidate SUD), the use of extended-release or longer acting stimulants with lower potential for abuse liability and diversion is recommended for treatment of ADHD. There are no evidence-based data to support this recommendation, however.

In the absence of clear evidence of ongoing diversion (misuse and reselling) or high-risk situations (eg, family member who has an active SUD or antisocial personality disorder in the patient or family members), the threat of or potential for diversion should not be the sole reason for withholding or not using stimulant medications. Rather, the clinician should always evaluate risk factors for diversion and set up a clear plan of control and administration of the stimulant (or other) medication. Clinicians should monitor prescriptions carefully with high suspicion directed toward early requests for refills or lost prescriptions. The treating physician must require frequent follow-up for all patients who have ADHD–SUD; questionnaires, objective toxicology screens, and contingency plans are suggested. Finally, despite variable improvements in ADHD symptoms, the existing studies rarely produced significant improvements in substance use. Specific treatment for an active SUD is therefore critical [1].

References

[1] Bukstein OG, Bernet W, Arnold V, et al. Practice parameter for the assessment and treatment of children and adolescents with substance use disorders. J Am Acad Child Adolesc Psychiatry 2005;44:609–21.
[2] Galduroz JC, Noto AR, Nappo SA, et al. Household survey on drug abuse in Brazil: study involving the 107 major cities of the country—2001. Addict Behav 2005;30:545–56.
[3] Costello EJ, Mustillo S, Erkanli A, et al. Prevalence and development of psychiatric disorders in childhood and adolescence. Arch Gen Psychiatry 2003;60(8):837–44.
[4] Kendler KS, Jacobson KC, Prescott CA, et al. Specificity of genetic and environmental risk factors for use and abuse/dependence of cannabis, cocaine, hallucinogens, sedatives, stimulants, and opiates in male twins. Am J Psychiatry 2003;160(4):687–95.
[5] Callas PW, Flynn BS, Worden JK. Potentially modifiable psychosocial factors associated with alcohol use during early adolescence. Addict Behav 2004;29(8):1503–15.
[6] Kim-Cohen J, Caspi A, Moffitt TE, et al. Prior juvenile diagnoses in adults with mental disorder: developmental follow-back of a prospective-longitudinal cohort. Arch Gen Psychiatry 2003;60:709–17.
[7] Horner BR, Scheibe KE. Prevalence and implications of attention-deficit hyperactivity disorder among adolescents in treatment for substance abuse. J Am Acad Child Adolesc Psychiatry 1997;36(1):30–6.
[8] DeMilio L. Psychiatric syndromes in adolescent substance abusers. Am J Psychiatry 1989; 146(9):1212–4.

[9] Szobot CM, Rohde LA, Bukstein O, et al. Is attention-deficit/hyperactivity disorder associated with illicit substance use disorders in male adolescents? A community-based case-control study. Addiction 2007;102(7):1122–30.

[10] American Psychiatric Association. Diagnostic and statistical manual of mental disorders. 4th edition. Washington, DC: American Psychiatric Association; 1994.

[11] Sher KJ. Children of alcoholics: a critical appraisal of theory and research. Chicago: University of Chicago Press; 1991.

[12] Zucker RA, Gomberg ES. Etiology of alcoholism reconsidered. The case for a biopsychosocial process. Am Psychol 1986;41(7):783–93.

[13] Zucker RA. Alcohol use and the alcohol use disorders: a developmental biopsychosocial systems formulation covering the life course. In: Cicchetti D, Cohen DJ, editors. Developmental psychopathology. Vol. 3. Risk, disorder, and adaptation. 2nd edition. Hoboken (NJ): Wiley & Sons; 2006. p. 620–56.

[14] Caspi A, Moffitt TE, Newman DL, et al. Behavioral observations at age 3 years predict adult psychiatric disorders. Longitudinal evidence from a birth cohort. Arch Gen Psychiatry 1996;53:1033–9.

[15] Masse LC, Tremblay RE. Behavior of boys in kindergarten and the onset of substance use during adolescence. Arch Gen Psychiatry 1997;54:62–8.

[16] Nigg JT, Wong MM, Martel MM, et al. Poor response inhibition as a predictor of problem drinking and illicit drug use in adolescents at risk for alcoholism and other substance use disorders. J Am Acad Child Adolesc Psychiatry 2006;45(4):468–75.

[17] Molina B, Pelham WE. Childhood predictors of adolescent substance use in a longitudinal study of children with ADHD. J Abnorm Psychol 2003;112(3):497–507.

[18] Molina BSG, Pelham WE, Gnagy EM, et al. ADHD risk for heavy drinking and alcohol use disorder is age-specific. Alcohol Clin Exp Res 2007;31(4):643–54.

[19] Myers MG, Stewart DG, Brown SA. Progression from conduct disorder to antisocial personality disorder following treatment for adolescent substance abuse. Am J Psychiatry 1998;155(4):479–85.

[20] Clark DB, Cornelius JR, Kirisci L, et al. Childhood risk categories for adolescent substance involvement: a general liability typology. Drug Alcohol Depend 2005;77:13–21.

[21] Biederman J, Wilens T, Mick E, et al. Is ADHD a risk factor for psychoactive substance use disorders? Findings from a four-year prospective follow-up study. J Am Acad Child Adolesc Psychiatry 1997;36:21–9.

[22] Carroll KM, Rounsaville BJ. History and significance of childhood attention deficit disorder in treatment-seeking cocaine abusers. Compr Psychiatry 1993;34(2):75–82.

[23] Kuperman S, Schlosser SS, Kramer JR, et al. Developmental sequence from disruptive behavior diagnosis to adolescent alcohol dependence. Am J Psychiatry 2001;158(12): 2022–6.

[24] Biederman J, Wilens T, Mick E, et al. Psychoactive substance use disorders in adults with attention deficit hyperactivity disorder (ADHD): effects of ADHD and psychiatric comorbidity. Am J Psychiatry 1995;152(11):1652–8.

[25] Biederman J, Wilens TE, Mick E, et al. Does attention-deficit hyperactivity disorder impact the developmental course of drug and alcohol abuse and dependence? Biol Psychiatry 1998; 44(4):269–73.

[26] Murphy KR, Barkley RA, Bush T. Young adults with attention deficit hyperactivity disorder: subtype differences in comorbidity, educational, and clinical history. J Nerv Ment Dis 2002;190(3):147–57.

[27] Weiss G, Hechtman L, Milroy T, et al. Psychiatric status of hyperactives as adults: a controlled prospective 15-year follow-up of 63 hyperactive children. J Am Acad Child Psychiatry 1985;24(2):211–20.

[28] Biederman J, Monuteaux MC, Mick E, et al. Young adult outcome of attention deficit hyperactivity disorder: a controlled 10-year follow-up study. Psychol Med 2006;36(2):167–79.

[29] August GJ, Winters KC, Realmuto GM, et al. Prospective study of adolescent drug use among community samples of ADHD and non-ADHD participants. J Am Acad Child Adolesc Psychiatry 2006;45(7):824–32.

[30] Disney ER, Elkins IJ, McGue M, et al. Effects of ADHD, conduct disorder, and gender on substance use and abuse in adolescence. Am J Psychiatry 1999;156:1515–21.

[31] Tapert SF, Baratta MV, Abrantes AM, et al. Attention dysfunction predicts substance involvement in community youths. J Am Acad Child Adolesc Psychiatry 2002;41(6):680–6.

[32] Gau SS, Chong MY, Yang P, et al. Psychiatric and psychosocial predictors of substance use disorders among adolescents: longitudinal study. Br J Psychiatry 2007;190:42–8.

[33] Fergusson DM, Horwood LJ, Ridder EM. Conduct and attentional problems in childhood and adolescence and later substance use, abuse and dependence: results of a 25-year longitudinal study. Drug Alcohol Depend 2007;88(Suppl 1):S14–26.

[34] Biederman J, Wilens T, Mick E, et al. Pharmacotherapy of attention-deficit/hyperactivity disorder reduces risk for substance use disorder. Pediatrics 1999;104(2):E20.

[35] Wilens TE, Faraone SV, Biederman J, et al. Does stimulant therapy of attention-deficit/hyperactivity disorder beget later substance abuse? A meta-analytic review of the literature. Pediatrics 2003;111:179–85.

[36] Tarter RE. Etiology of adolescent substance abuse: a developmental perspective. Am J Addict 2002;11:171–91.

[37] Seidman LJ, Valera EM, Makris N. Structural brain imaging of attention-deficit/hyperactivity disorder. Biol Psychiatry 2005;57:1263–72.

[38] Fischer M, Barkley RA, Smallish L, et al. Executive functioning in hyperactive children as young adults: attention, inhibition, response perseveration, and the impact of comorbidity. Dev Neuropsychol 2005;27:107–33.

[39] Sonuga-Barke EJ. Psychological heterogeneity in AD/HD—a dual pathway model of behaviour and cognition. Behav Brain Res 2002;10:29–36.

[40] Koob GF, Bloom FE. Cellular and molecular mechanisms of drug dependence. Science 1988;242:715–23.

[41] Volkow ND, Wang GJ, Fowler JS, et al. Imaging the effects of methylphenidate on brain dopamine: new model on its therapeutic actions for attention-deficit/hyperactivity disorder. Biol Psychiatry 2005;57(11):1410–5.

[42] Volkow ND, Wang GJ, Begleiter H, et al. High levels of dopamine D2 receptors in unaffected members of alcoholic families: possible protective factors. Arch Gen Psychiatry 2006;63(9):999–1008.

[43] Wise RA, Bozarth MA. A psychomotor stimulant theory of addiction. Psychol Rev 1987; 94:469–92.

[44] Cook EH, Stein MA, Ellison T, et al. Attention-deficit hyperactivity disorder and whole-blood serotonin levels—effects of comorbidity. Psychiatry Res 1995;57(1):13–20.

[45] LaHoste GJ, Swanson JM, Wigal SB, et al. Dopamine D4 receptor gene polymorphism is associated with attention deficit hyperactivity disorder. Mol Psychiatry 1996;1:121–4.

[46] Goldman D. Genetic transmission. In: Galanter M, editor. Alcoholism. vol. 11. New York: Plenum; 1993. p. 232–44.

[47] Robinson TE, Berridge KC. The neural basis of drug craving: an incentive-sensitization theory of addiction. Brain Res Brain Res Rev 1993;18:247–91.

[48] Pato CN, Macciardi F, Pato MT, et al. Review of the putative association of dopamine D2 receptor and alcoholism: a meta-analysis. Am J Med Genet 1993;48:78–82.

[49] Persico AM, Uhl GR. Polymorphisms of the D2 dopamine receptor gene in polysubstance abusers. In: Blum K, Noble EP, editors. Handbook of psychiatric genetics. Boca Raton (FL): CRC Press, Inc.; 1997. p. 353–66.

[50] Volkow ND, Fowler JS, Wang GJ. The addicted human brain viewed in the light of imaging studies: brain circuits and treatment strategies. Neuropharmacology 2004;47:3–13.

[51] Tarter RE, Kirisci L, Mezzich A, et al. Neurobehavioral disinhibition in childhood predicts early age at onset of substance use disorder. Am J Psychiatry 2003;160:1078–85.

[52] Gerdes AC, Hoza B, Pelham WE. Attention-deficit/hyperactivity disordered boys' relationships with their mothers and fathers: child, mother, and father perceptions. Dev Psychopathol 2003;15:363–82.

[53] Hoza B, Gerdes AC, Hinshaw SP, et al. Self-perceptions of competence in children with ADHD and comparison children. J Consult Clin Psychol 2004;72(3):382–91.

[54] Nigg JT, Casey BJ. An integrative theory of attention-deficit/hyperactivity disorder based on the cognitive and affective neurosciences. Dev Psychopathol 2005;17:785–806.

[55] Kalivas PW, Volkow ND. The neural basis of addiction: a pathology of motivation and choice. Am J Psychiatry 2005;162:1403–13.

[56] Bechara A, Martin EM. Impaired decision-making related to working memory deficits in individuals with substance addictions. Neuropsychology 2004;18:152–62.

[57] Weiss S, Nosten-Bertrand M, McIntosh JM, et al. Nicotine improves cognitive deficits of dopamine transporter knockout mice without long-term tolerance. Neuropsychopharmacology 2007; 32(12):2465–78.

[58] Kollins SH, McClernon FJ, Fuemmeler BF. Association between smoking and attention-deficit/hyperactivity disorder symptoms in a population-based sample of young adults. Arch Gen Psychiatry 2005;62(10):1142–7.

[59] Sartor CE, Lynskey MT, Heath AC, et al. The role of childhood risk factors in initiation of alcohol use and progression to alcohol dependence. Addiction 2007;102(2):216–25.

[60] Burke JD, Loeber R, Lahey BB. Which aspects of ADHD are associated with tobacco use in early adolescence? J Child Psychol Psychiatry 2001;42:493–502.

[61] Lambert NM, Hartsough CS. Prospective study of tobacco smoking and substance dependencies among samples of ADHD and non-ADHD participants. J Learn Disabil 1998; 31(6):533–44.

[62] Humfleet GL, Prochaska JJ, Mengis M, et al. Preliminary evidence of the association between the history of childhood attention-deficit/hyperactivity disorder and smoking treatment failure. Nicotine Tob Res 2005;7(3):453–60.

[63] Ercan ES, Coskunol H, Varan A, et al. Childhood attention deficit/hyperactivity disorder and alcohol dependence: a 1-year follow-up. Alcohol Alcohol 2003;38(4):352–6.

[64] White AM, Jordan JD, Schroeder KM, et al. Predictors of relapse during treatment and treatment completion among marijuana-dependent adolescents in an intensive outpatient substance abuse program. Subst Abus 2004;25(1):53–9.

[65] Pliszka SR, Crismon ML, Hughes CW, et al, Texas Consensus Conference Panel on Pharmacotherapy of Childhood Attention Deficit Hyperactivity Disorder. The Texas Children's Medication Algorithm Project: revision of the algorithm for pharmacotherapy of attention-deficit/hyperactivity disorder. J Am Acad Child Adolesc Psychiatry 2006;45(6):642–57.

[66] Spencer TJ, Biederman J, Mick E. Attention-deficit/hyperactivity disorder: diagnosis, lifespan, comorbidities, and neurobiology. Ambul Pediatr 2007;7(1 Suppl):73–81.

[67] Spencer TJ, Biederman J, Ciccone PE, et al. PET study examining pharmacokinetics, detection and likeability, and dopamine transporter receptor occupancy of short—and long-acting oral methylphenidate. Am J Psychiatry 2006;163(3):387–95.

[68] Rodriguez de Fonseca F, Del Arco I, Bermudez-Silva FJ, et al. The endocannabinoid system: physiology and pharmacology. Alcohol Alcohol 2005;40(1):2–14.

[69] Koob GF. The neurobiology of addiction: a neuroadaptational view relevant for diagnosis. Addiction 2006;101(Suppl 1):23–30.

[70] Tzavara ET, Li DL, Moutsimilli L, et al. Endocannabinoids activate transient receptor potential vanilloid 1 receptors to reduce hyperdopaminergia-related hyperactivity: therapeutic implications. Biol Psychiatry 2006;59(6):508–15.

[71] Volkow ND, Ding YS, Fowler JS, et al. Is methylphenidate like cocaine? Studies on their pharmacokinetics and distribution in the human brain. Arch Gen Psychiatry 1995;52(6): 456–63.

[72] World Health Organization (WHO). Available at: http://www.who.int/substance_abuse/facts/cannabis/en/index.html. Accessed January 08, 2006.

[73] Price DA, Owens WA, Gould GG, et al. CB(1)-independent inhibition of dopamine transporter activity by cannabinoids in mouse dorsal striatum. J Neurochem 2007;101(2): 389–96.

[74] Rush CR, Essman WD, Simpson CA, et al. Reinforcing and subject-rated effects of methylphenidate and d-amphetamine in non-drug-abusing humans. J Clin Psychopharmacol 2001;21(3):273–86.

[75] Stoops WW, Lile JA, Fillmore MT, et al. Reinforcing effects of methylphenidate: influence of dose and behavioral demands following drug administration. Psychopharmacology (Berl) 2005;177(3):349–55.

[76] Barkley RA, Fischer M, Smallish L, et al. Does the treatment of attention-deficit/hyperactivity disorder with stimulants contribute to drug use/abuse? A 13-year prospective study. Pediatrics 2003;111(1):97–109.

[77] Molina BSG, Marshal MP, Pelham WE, et al. Coping skills and parent support mediate the association between childhood ADHD and adolescent cigarette use. J Pediatr Psychol 2005; 30(4):345–57.

[78] Riggs PD, Hall SK, Mikulich-Gilbertson SK, et al. A randomized controlled trial of pemoline for attention-deficit/hyperactivity disorder in substance-abusing adolescents. J Am Acad Child Adolesc Psychiatry 2004;43(4):420–9.

[79] Szobot CM, Rohde LA, Katz B, et al. A randomized crossover clinical study showing that methylphenidate-SODAS improves attention-deficit/hyperactivity disorder symptoms in adolescents with substance use. Brazilian Journal of Medical and Biological Research, in press.

[80] Carpentier PJ, de Jong CA, Dijkstra BA, et al. A controlled trial of methylphenidate in adults with attention deficit/hyperactivity disorder and substance use disorders. Addiction 2005;100(12):1868–74.

[81] Levin FR, Evans SM, Brooks DJ, et al. Treatment of cocaine dependent treatment seekers with adult ADHD: double-blind comparison of methylphenidate and placebo. Drug Alcohol Depend 2007;87(1):20–9.

[82] Levin FR, Evans SM, Brooks DJ, et al. Treatment of methadone-maintained patients with adult ADHD: double-blind comparison of methylphenidate, bupropion and placebo. Drug Alcohol Depend 2006;81(2):137–48.

[83] Schubiner H, Saules KK, Arfken CL, et al. Double-blind placebo-controlled trial of methylphenidate in the treatment of adult ADHD patients with comorbid cocaine dependence. Exp Clin Psychopharmacol 2002;10(3):286–94.

[84] Kuperman S, Perry PJ, Gaffney GR, et al. Bupropion SR vs. methylphenidate vs. placebo for attention deficit hyperactivity disorder in adults. Ann Clin Psychiatry 2001;13(3): 129–34.

[85] Chambers RA, Taylor JR, Potenza MN. Developmental neurocircuitry of motivation in adolescence: a critical period of addiction vulnerability. Am J Psychiatry 2003;160(6): 1041–52.

[86] Stansfield KH, Kirstein CL. Neurochemical effects of cocaine in adolescence compared to adulthood. Brain Res Dev Brain Res 2005;159(2):119–25.

[87] Badanich KA, Adler KJ, Kirstein CL. Adolescents differ from adults in cocaine conditioned place preference and cocaine-induced dopamine in the nucleus accumbens septi. Eur J Pharmacol 2006;550(1–3):95–106.

[88] Griffith JD, Carranza J, Griffith C, et al. Bupropion: clinical essay for amphetamine-like potential. J Clin Psychiatry 1983;44:206–8.

[89] Goldstein MG. Bupropion sustained release and smoking cessation. J Clin Psychiatry 1998; 59:66–72.

[90] Riggs PD, Leon SL, Mikulich SK, et al. An open trial of bupropion for ADHD in adolescents with substance use disorders and conduct disorder. J Am Acad Child Adolesc Psychiatry 1998;37(12):1271–8.

[91] Solhkhah R, Wilens TE, Daly J, et al. Bupropion SR for the treatment of substance-abusing outpatient adolescents with attention-deficit/hyperactivity disorder and mood disorders. J Child Adolesc Psychopharmacol 2005;15(5):777–86.

[92] Bymaster FP, Katner JS, Nelson DL, et al. Atomoxetine increases extracellular levels of norepinephrine and dopamine in prefrontal cortex of rat: a potential mechanism for efficacy inattention deficit/hyperactivity disorder. Neuropsychopharmacology 2002;27: 699–711.

[93] Heil SH, Holmes HW, Bickel WK, et al. Comparison of the subjective, physiological, and psychomotor effects of atomoxetine and methylphenidate in light drug users. Drug Alcohol Depend 2002;67(2):149–56.

[94] Dackis CA, Lynch KG, Yu E, et al. Modafinil and cocaine: a double-blind, placebo-controlled drug interaction study. Drug Alcohol Depend 2003;70(1):29–37.

[95] Turner DC, Robbins TW, Clark L, et al. Cognitive enhancing effects of modafinil in healthy volunteers. Psychopharmacology 2003;165:260–9.

[96] Turner DC, Clark L, Dowson J, et al. Modafinil improves cognition and response inhibition in adult attention deficit/hyperactivity disorder. Biol Psychiatry 2004;55:1031–40.

[97] Dackis CA, Kampman KM, Lynch KG, et al. A double-blind, placebo-controlled trial of modafinil for cocaine dependence. Neuropsychopharmacology 2005;30:205–11.

[98] Rugino TA, Copley TC. Effects of modafinil in children with attention-deficit/hyperactivity disorder: an open-label study. J Am Acad Child Adolesc Psychiatry 2001;40(2):230–5.

[99] Biederman J, Swanson JM, Wigal SB, et al. Comparison of once-daily and divided doses of modafinil in children with attention-deficit/hyperactivity disorder: a randomized, double-blind, and placebo-controlled study. J Clin Psychiatry 2006;67(5):727–35.

[100] Gordon SM, Tulak F, Troncale J. Prevalence and characteristics of adolescents patients with co-occurring ADHD and substance dependence. J Addict Dis 2004;23(4):31–40.

[101] Williams RJ, Goodale LA, Shay-Fiddler MA, et al. Methylphenidate and dextroamphetamine abuse in substance-abusing adolescents. Am J Addict 2004;13(4):381–9.

[102] Sussman S, Pentz MA, Spruijt-Metz D, et al. Misuse of "study drugs:" prevalence, consequences, and implications for policy. Subst Abuse Treat Prev Policy 2006;9(1):15.

[103] Teter CJ, McCabe SE, LaGrange K, et al. Illicit use of specific prescription stimulants among college students: prevalence, motives, and routes of administration. Pharmacotherapy 2006;26(10):1501–10.

[104] McCabe SE, Knight JR, Teter CJ, et al. Non-medical use of prescription stimulants among US college students: prevalence and correlates from a national survey. Addiction 2005;100: 96–106.

[105] Teter CJ, McCabe SE, Cranford JA, et al. Prevalence and motives for illicit use of prescription stimulants in an undergraduate student sample. J Am Coll Health 2005;53:253–62.

[106] Wilens TE, Gignac M, Swezey A, et al. Characteristics of adolescents and young adults with ADHD who divert or misuse their prescribed medications. J Am Acad Child Adolesc Psychiatry 2006;45(4):408–14.

ELSEVIER
SAUNDERS

Child Adolesc Psychiatric Clin N Am
17 (2008) 325–346

CHILD AND
ADOLESCENT
PSYCHIATRIC CLINICS
OF NORTH AMERICA

Frontiers Between Attention Deficit Hyperactivity Disorder and Bipolar Disorder

Cathryn A. Galanter, MD[a],*, Ellen Leibenluft, MD[b]

[a]Division of Child and Adolescent Psychiatry, Columbia University/New York State
Psychiatric Institute, 1051 Riverside Drive, #78, New York, NY 10032, USA
[b]Section on Bipolar Spectrum Disorders, Emotion and Development Branch,
Mood and Anxiety Disorders Program, National Institute of Mental Health,
Building 15K, Room MSC-2670, Bethesda, MD 20892–2670, USA

The co-occurrence of attention deficit hyperactivity disorder (ADHD) and bipolar disorder (BD) has received much recent attention in the literature. First, there is symptom overlap between the two illnesses (Table 1) [1], including disordered attention, activity, and speech. Second, children who have BD are often irritable during and between episodes of mania and depression [2]. Irritability can be associated with ADHD and other childhood psychopathologies that are often comorbid with ADHD, however, including oppositional defiant disorder (ODD), major depressive disorder (MDD), and generalized anxiety disorder [1]. Questions have arisen as to how to differentiate irritable children who have ADHD from children who have BD.

ADHD is a non-episodic illness, whereas BD is an episodic illness. A closely related scientific question concerns whether severe and chronic (ie, persistent, non-episodic) irritability is a developmental presentation of mania [3,4]. Clinicians and researchers are usually able to recognize children who have episodic BD with euphoric mood, and they are usually able to recognize children who have ADHD and no mood disturbance. Diagnosing children who have ADHD and severe irritability can be difficult, however.

We review the literature examining associations between ADHD and BD in children and data concerning severe irritability in youth who have

This work was supported by grant No. 1 K23 MH071337-3 from the National Institutes of Mental Health. Dr. Galanter has received funding from the American Psychiatric Institute for Research and Education Young Minds in Psychiatry Award, which is funded by AstraZeneca. Dr. Leibenluft has no financial relationships to disclose.

* Corresponding author.
E-mail address: cg168@columbia.edu (C.A. Galanter).

1056-4993/08/$ - see front matter © 2008 Elsevier Inc. All rights reserved.
doi:10.1016/j.chc.2007.11.001

Table 1
Attention deficit hyperactivity disorder and bipolar disorder criteria from the DSM-IV-TR with
overlapping symptoms highlighted

ADHD	Bipolar disorder
Inattention (≥ 6 symptoms for ≥ 6 mo)	A Criteria (lasting ≥ 1 wk; less
Fails to give attention to detail or	if hospitalization is required)
makes careless mistakes	Distinct period of abnormally and
Difficulty with sustained attention	persistently elevated, expansive, or
Often does not seem to listen when	[a]irritable mood
spoken to	B Criteria (≥ 3 are present during period
Often does not follow through on	of mood disturbance; ≥ 4 if mood
instructions or fails to finish activities	disturbance is irritability)
Often has difficulty organizing tasks	[a]Increased self-esteem or grandiosity
Often avoids, dislikes tasks that require	Decreased need for sleep
sustained attention	***More talkative or pressured speech***
Often loses things	Flight of ideas or racing thoughts
Is often easily distractible by	***Distractibility***
extraneous stimuli	***Increased goal-directed activity,***
Is often forgetful	***psychomotor* agitation**
Fails to give attention to detail	[a]Excessive involvement in risky,
or makes careless mistakes	pleasurable activities
Difficulty with sustained attention	
Hyperactivity/impulsivity (≥ 6 symptoms	
for ≥ 6 mo)	
Often fidgets	
Often leaves seat when staying in seat	
is expected	
Often runs about or climbs in	
inappropriate situations	
Often has difficulty playing quietly	
Is often "on the go" or "driven by	
a motor"	
Often talks excessively	
Often blurts out answers	
Often has difficulty awaiting turn	
Often interrupts, intrudes	
Selected diagnostic and associated features	
[a]Engaging in risky activities secondary	Episodic antisocial behavior
to impulsivity	Rapid mood shifts
[a]Low frustration tolerance	
[a]Bossiness	
Temper outbursts	
Mood lability	

Bold face italicized text indicates overlapping symptoms.
[a] Bipolar symptoms that overlap with associated features of ADHD.
Modified from American Psychiatric Association. Diagnostic and statistical manual of mental
disorders. 4th edition. Text revision. Washington, DC: American Psychiatric Association; 2000.

ADHD. We focus on (1) population-based studies that examined ADHD and BD or ADHD and co-occurring irritability, (2) the co-occurrence and prospective relationships of ADHD and BD in clinical samples, (3) phenomenology and assessment of BD and ADHD, including recommendations for differentiating DSM-IV-TR BD from ADHD, (4) treatment of comorbid ADHD and BD, (5) family and genetic studies of ADHD and BD, and (6) pathophysiologic comparisons between children who have ADHD and irritability and BD.

Attention deficit hyperactivity disorder and bipolar disorder in population-based samples

Cross-sectional studies

Six studies reported population-based rates of ADHD and BD in youth, three of which showed elevated rates of BD in participants who have ADHD (Table 2). The negative studies included the Great Smoky Mountains Study [6], which found low rates of mania (0 cases of mania; 0.1% had hypomania) and ADHD (1.9%). Second, in a nonreferred sample of twins enriched for ADHD and a random control twin sample, 0.2% of youth from the control twin sample had possible BD and 0.84% of those diagnosed with ADHD had possible BD [7]. Among youth who had BD or subthreshold BD, 33% had ADHD. This finding suggests that youth who have ADHD are not at elevated risk for BD, but youth who have BD are at elevated risk for ADHD. Third, in a Finnish birth cohort of 457 16- to 18-year-old patients, also enriched for ADHD, only 2 adolescents had BD, neither of whom also had ADHD [9]. These studies have low rates of BD, and the lack of correlation with BD and ADHD should be interpreted cautiously.

Three studies indicated that people who have ADHD are more likely than people without to have comorbid BD and that people who have BD are more likely than people without to have comorbid ADHD. In a sample of 1709 high school seniors, 1% had a lifetime diagnosis of BD (primarily BD II and cyclothymia) and 3% had a lifetime diagnosis of ADHD [5]. Of those who had ADHD, 3.8% had BD. Of those who had BD, 11.1% had ADHD. The Children in the Community study, a prospective epidemiologic sample of 776 youth, had similar findings [11]. Specifically, 12% of early adolescents had ADHD and 6.2% had BD; however, 18.3% of the youth who had ADHD had BD, and 35.4% of the youth who had BD had ADHD. Finally, in an adult sample ($N = 3199$), participants who had ADHD had elevated rates of BD, and participants who had BD had elevated rates of ADHD [8]. Specifically, 19.4% of adults who had ADHD had BD and 21% of adults who had BD had ADHD.

Taken together, the data suggest preliminarily that children, adolescents, and adults who have ADHD, compared with individuals who do not have

Table 2
Epidemiologic studies citing rates of comorbidity between attention deficit hyperactivity disorder and bipolar disorder or mood disorders

Reference	Sample (n)	Sample Age (y)	Assessment	Informant(s)	Rate of ADHD (%)	Rate of BD (%)	Comorbidity and predictive findings
Cross-sectional studies							
Lewinsohn, et al, 1995 [5]	1709	14–18	K-SADS	youth	3.1	1 (2 BD-I, 11 BD-II, 5 cyclothymia)	3.8% of persons with ADHD had BD 11.1% of persons with BD had ADHD
Costello, et al, 1996 [6]	1015	9–13	CAPA	parent, youth	1.9	0 (mania) 0.1 (hypomania)	17.8% of persons with behavioral disorders had emotional disorders; 55.2% of persons with depressive disorders had behavioral disorders
Reich, et al, 2005 [7]	1610 (MZ and DZ twins; enriched for ADHD)	7–18	MAGIC	parent	22.3	0.2 (1 BD-I, 1 BD-II, 1 hypomania)	0.84% of persons with ADHD had BD 33% of persons with BD had ADHD
Kessler, et al, 2006 [8]	3199	18–44	DIS	adult	4.4	2.6	19.4% of persons with ADHD had BD 21% of persons with BD had ADHD

Study	N	Age	Instrument	Informants			Findings
Hurtig, et al, 2007 [9]	457 (from a birth cohort of 6622; enriched for ADHD)	16–18	K-SADS-PL	parent, youth	23	0.4	Neither of the two individuals with BD had ADHD
Prospective studies Kim-Cohen, et al, 2003 [10]	925 at age 11	11–15, 26 at follow-up	DISC (ages 11–15) DIS (ages 18–26)	parent, youth (ages 11–15) adult (ages 18–26)	approximately 6 (aged 11–15)	Not assessed in childhood 2.2 at age 26	approximately 4% of adults with mania had childhood ADHD Childhood ADHD did not predict BD at age 26
Galanter, et al, 2003 [11]	776 at mean age 13.7	Mean ages: T1: 13.7 ± 2.8 T2: 16.2 ± 2.8 T3: 22.1 ± 2.7 T4: 33.1 ± 2.9	DISC (T1, T2) SCID-IV-NP and ADHD symptom checklist (T3, T4)	Parent, youth (T1, T2) adult (T3, T4)	12.0 (T1) 7.6 (T2) 1.1 (T3) 2.4 (T4)	6.2 (T1) 5.8 (T2) 4.6 (T3) 1.5 (T4)	Individuals with ADHD compared with those without ADHD had greater rates off BD at all four assessments; ADHD at T1 predicted BD at mean age T2, and T3, but only at T2 when controlling for baseline ADHD

Abbreviations: CAPA, Children and Adolescent Psychiatric Assessment; DIS, Diagnostic Interview Schedule; DISC, Diagnostic Interview Schedule for Children; DZ, dizygotic; K-SADS(-PL), Schedule for the Affective Disorders and Schizophrenia for School-Age Children (Present and Lifetime Version); MAGIC, Missouri Assessment of Genetics Interview of Children; MZ, monozygotic; SCID-IV-NP, Structured Clinical Interview for DSM-IV Axis I Disorders, Non-Patient Version; T1, time of first diagnostic assessment; T2, time of second diagnostic assessment; T3, time of third diagnostic assessment; T4, time of fourth diagnostic assessment.

ADHD, may have elevated rates of BD. Individuals of all ages who have BD also seem to have high rates of ADHD.

Longitudinal studies

Two prospective epidemiologic studies examined whether ADHD in youth predicts BD in adolescence or adulthood. In the Dunedin Multidisciplinary Health and Development Study, ADHD at age 11 to 15 did not predict BD at age 26 years, but depression and conduct/ODD did [10]. In the Children in the Community sample, when the data were controlled for baseline BD, ADHD at mean age 13.7 (SD = 2.8) predicted BD at mean age 16.3 (SD = 2.8) but not at mean age 22.1 (SD = 2.7) or 33.1 (SD = 2.9) [11]. These data do not indicate that having ADHD in youth is a risk factor for adult BD.

Because investigators have suggested that children and adolescents who have ADHD and non-episodic severe irritability are exhibiting a developmental phenotype of BD, it is also important to study the diagnostic outcome of such youth. Leibenluft and colleagues [12] examined data from the Children in the Community sample and found that episodic irritability at mean age 13.7 (SD = 2.8) was associated with mania and anxiety disorders at mean age 16.3 (SD = 2.8), whereas chronic irritability at mean age 13.7 (SD = 2.8) was associated with ADHD at mean age 16.3 (SD = 2.8) and MDD at mean age 22.1 (SD = 2.7). These investigators also analyzed data from the Great Smoky Mountains Study to determine the diagnostic correlates of childhood severe mood dysregulation (SMD), a construct that includes irritable mood, emotional reactivity, and hyperarousal [13]. Lifetime prevalence of SMD was 3.3%, and 26.9% of youth who had SMD had ADHD. Youth who had SMD at wave one (mean age 10.6, SD = 1.4) were more likely than youth who never met criteria for SMD to meet criteria for depressive disorder at the last wave (mean age 18.3, SD = 2.1) (OR = 7.21, CI, 1.34–38.85). The low association between wave one SMD and last wave BD may be partly caused by the study's overall low rates of BD, and some participants with depressive disorder eventually may develop BD. These studies indicated that youth with severe irritability may not have BD as adults but are at elevated risk for depressive disorders. They are post hoc analyses, however, and prospective studies are needed.

Clinical samples

In assessing ADHD in clinical samples of youth who have BD or rates of BD in youth who have ADHD, it is important to note that assessment techniques of BD vary across research groups, leading to variations in the characteristics of the diagnosed sample. One approach is to use DSM-IV-TR (adult) criteria and adhere to mood and episode requirements (the "A" criterion; see

Table 1) [14,15]. Other investigators waive the "A" episodicity criterion for mania if a child presents with particularly severe irritability [16,17]. A third approach requires elevated mood or grandiosity for the diagnosis of mania and redefines an episode as a mood state that is at least 2 weeks long or has the onset to offset of a period of cycling and a cycle as mood switches during an episode [18]. These and other variations in assessment are likely to affect the characteristics of the recruited patients and the rates of BD.

Bipolar disorder in patients who have attention deficit hyperactivity disorder

Cross-sectional studies
   Several clinical studies have found rates of BD ranging from 11% to 23% in youth who have ADHD [16,17,19]. Of note, most of these studies were at one site—a tertiary care medical center that specializes in studies of ADHD and BD; studies in different settings are needed.

Longitudinal studies
   Longitudinal studies that examine the development of BD in clinical samples of youth who have ADHD have yielded conflicting results. Several studies that examined the adult outcome of children who have ADHD have not found increased rates of BD [20–22]. In contrast, Biederman and colleagues [16] found that compared with controls, youth who had ADHD had higher baseline rates of BD (11% versus 0%) and higher conversion rates to BD by year 4 (13/128 versus 2/109). Similarly, Tillman and Geller [23] found that 28.5% of 81 children who had ADHD, who were first assessed at mean age 9.7 (SD = 2.0), developed BD over 6-year follow-up. These variations from the earlier negative studies may result from differences in the techniques used to diagnose BD. Several investigators have examined children who have ADHD prospectively and found that the presence of some manic symptoms is not associated with increased risk for later BD (Galanter and colleagues, unpublished data) [24–26].

Attention deficit hyperactivity disorder in patients who have bipolar disorder

   Clinical studies generally demonstrate high rates of ADHD in patients who have BD. Rates vary widely across samples, from 4% to 98% [14,27,28]. Setting, participant age, age of onset of BD, referral source, and ascertainment bias affect these rates. Bipolar type also may affect rates of comorbidity. For example, in a large study that examined the course and phenomenology of children and adolescents who have BD, youth who had BD II were less likely to have ADHD than youth who had BD I or BD not otherwise specified (BD-NOS) (31.6% versus 61.2% and 59.8%) [14]. Some of these studies did not specifically assess ADHD symptoms during euthymic periods, which might artificially inflate the rates of ADHD.

Few studies described the ages of onset of ADHD and BD. Two studies demonstrated that ADHD preceded prepubertal BD by approximately 2 years [17,29]. In one study, mean age of onset was 4.8 years (SD = 1.5) for ADHD and 6.8 years (SD = 3.4) for the first manic episode [29], whereas in another study, mean age of onset was 2.5 years (SD = 1.9) for ADHD and 4.4 years (SD = 3.1) for mania [17]. These studies are remarkable for the early age of onset of BD, and several studies indicated that earlier onset of BD is associated with higher rates of ADHD. In patients who have BD, Faraone and colleagues [30] found that rates of ADHD were 93% in children, 88% in adolescents who had childhood-onset mania, and 59% in adolescents who had adolescent-onset BD. In 1000 adults who had BD, Perlis and colleagues [31] found that ADHD was more common in the prepubertal-onset group (< 13 years old; 53/272, 20.4%) than in the adolescent-onset (13–18 years old; 27/370, 7.6%) or adult-onset (> 18 years old; 19/341, 5.7%) groups [31].

Finally, data indicate that comorbid ADHD in patients who have BD is associated with greater psychosocial impairment [32], fewer periods of wellness, more frequent episodes of depression, and higher rates of comorbidity with other psychiatric disorders, including anxiety and substance use disorders [33].

Summary

Data are mixed as to whether having ADHD increases one's risk for developing BD, but overall, community and clinical data show an increased risk of BD in people who have ADHD. Having ADHD with some manic symptoms seems not to increase one's risk for future BD, although some studies may be too small to detect increased risk of moderate or small magnitude. It is clear that youth who have BD are more likely to have ADHD than youth who do not have BD, although the precise degree of risk is unclear. For participants who have BD, rates of comorbid ADHD seem to be greater with younger age of onset, and comorbid ADHD is associated with greater morbidity.

Assessment

In this section, we review the literature relevant to the assessment and differentiation of ADHD and BD and focus on the identification of episodes, symptoms that differentiate ADHD from BD, the differential diagnosis of irritability in a child who has ADHD, and the use of screening tools. Although we focus on the diagnosis of BD I and II, clinicians often give children the diagnosis of BD-NOS. The DSM-IV-TR does not operationalize BD-NOS but notes that the category includes disorders with bipolar features that do not meet criteria for any specific BD [1]. For clinicians who wish to diagnose a child with BD-NOS, it is important to specify which criteria for BD the child meets and why the child does not meet full criteria for BD I or II. In practice, there are two common usages for the BD-NOS diagnosis on youth. First, it is assigned often when children have distinct episodes that meet criteria for hypomania or mania but the episodes are too short to meet DSM-IV criteria. In the Course of Bipolar Youth study, specific criteria were defined to capture this group, and data indicated that approximately one third of these youth meet full criteria for BD within 2 years [14]. The second major use of BD-NOS is for youth who do not have distinct episodes of mania but instead have non-episodic, impairing irritability. In the case of these youth, data indicate that they may have a particularly high risk for major depression in early adulthood rather than BD [12,13]. Clinicians who assign the diagnosis of BD-NOS should be aware that the term is used frequently for several populations of patients who may have different outcomes, and they should document clearly the reasoning behind their assignment of this diagnosis.

Episodes

By definition, BD is episodic. That is, to fulfill DSM-IV-TR criteria for bipolar I disorder, a child must have a distinct period (ie, an episode) of elevated, expansive, or irritable mood that lasts at least 7 days and three of the "B" symptoms of mania (four if the mood is irritable), with the "B" criteria occurring at the same time as the change in mood [1]. (See Table 1 for a description of diagnostic criteria of BD and ADHD.) For BD II, the episode must last for at least 4 days and be noticeable to others rather than be severely impairing, as in mania. Consistent with the practice parameters of the American Academy of Child and Adolescent Psychiatry, we recommend that clinicians adhere to DSM-IV-TR criteria when diagnosing mania in youth. That is, only diagnose BD when episodes are present and, in the absence of elevated or expansive mood, only diagnose BD if the irritability is episodic and worsens in concert with the onset of the associated "B" symptoms [34].

One effective way to ascertain whether episodes have occurred is for the clinician to meet with the child and guardian together and ask them to identify a period of time when the child had a distinct period of abnormally and persistently elevated, expansive, or irritable mood that lasted the requisite duration. During the episode, the child's behavior should differ from baseline to an extent that is noticeable to others (hypomania) or is impairing (mania). It is often helpful to inquire about the most recent episode and the most severe and to anchor episodes to events that the child is likely to remember (eg, start of school, Halloween).

Once a period of mood change has been identified, the clinician can determine whether the child has the other symptoms of BD ("B" criteria) at the same time. For example, the clinician might say, "During the period when your son was extremely irritable, did he sleep less but still wake up feeling rested?" If clinician and family cannot discern a period when the child's mood was different from his or her baseline (ie, if the child's mood is chronically irritable without discernable periods of several days or weeks when the irritability worsened), it is unlikely that the child has BD. Instead, the child's irritability is probably caused by another condition, such as ODD, which is a chronic non-episodic condition.

Differentiating attention deficit hyperactivity disorder and bipolar disorder symptoms

Several investigators have tried to discern which symptoms are the most helpful in distinguishing ADHD from BD. Geller and colleagues [35], who required elation or grandiosity for the diagnosis of BD, found that five symptoms (elation, grandiosity, flight of ideas/racing thoughts, decreased need for sleep, and hypersexuality) best discriminated children who had BD from children who had ADHD or from a community control group. For example, 83 of 93 (89.3%) children who had BD had elated mood compared with 11 of 81 (13.6%) children who had ADHD and 0 ($N = 94$) controls. Irritability, hyperactivity, accelerated speech, and distractibility were frequent in both patient groups [35].

Children who have comorbid ADHD and BD may report that their ADHD-like symptoms are worse during a manic episode. A child who has ADHD and always has been active may be even more so during a manic phase. For example, when a patient who has comorbid ADHD and BD presents to a clinician's office in a euthymic phase, he or she may shift around in his or her seat or start playing with things in the office that do not belong to him or her, whereas in a manic phase the patient may be unable to stay in his or her chair and do push-ups. Children who have ADHD are often distractible and sometimes may be hard to follow as they jump from one topic to another, but children who have BD have even more severely discordant thoughts. For example, they may describe racing thoughts in terms such as "my brain feels like it is on fast forward." Children who have ADHD often have difficulty getting ready for bed and falling asleep [36]. In contrast, children who have BD may have decreased need for sleep, staying up late playing and being well rested after little sleep.

The differential diagnosis of attention deficit hyperactivity disorder and irritability

ODD, conduct disorder (CD), MDD, and anxiety disorders are frequently comorbid with ADHD and are associated with irritability. In a child who has ADHD, anxiety disorders and MDD can be difficult to differentiate from BD because of overlapping symptoms (eg, irritability, psychomotor agitation, and sleep disturbances). To differentiate BD from other mood and anxiety disorders, it is important to elicit the predominant mood and specific examples of precipitants for irritability or outbursts. For example, children who have severe irritability in response to separations or other anxiety-provoking situations may have an anxiety disorder. To differentiate

MDD from BD, in addition to eliciting mood symptoms, it is helpful to examine other criteria for each illness, such as decreased need for sleep (mania) versus difficulty sleeping and feeling tired (MDD) or inflated (mania) versus decreased (MDD) self-esteem. Mood lability ("mood swings") manifested by changes from euthymia to depression in the absence of other manic symptoms is more likely to be evidence of depression than BD.

ODD and CD also can be difficult to discern from BD because of shared symptoms, such as irritability, defiance (a symptom of ODD that may be difficult to discern from grandiosity of BD), and reckless behavior. Differentiating between episodic and non-episodic irritability and between episodic and non-episodic grandiosity/oppositionality can be especially helpful in distinguishing BD from ODD and CD. Children who have symptoms of ADHD and of a pervasive developmental disorder can become irritable because of rigidity and difficulties with transitions. Children who have ADHD and a learning disorder may be more irritable or disruptive because they have the wrong classroom placement.

In sum, children who have ADHD and irritability may have one of several comorbid diagnoses. Distinguishing between chronic and episodic symptoms, assessing carefully the associated BD criteria, eliciting details around precipitants for irritability, and ruling in or out commonly associated comorbid conditions through interviews and with screening tools are helpful techniques in clarifying a child's diagnosis.

Screening tools

Several rating scales, including the Young Mania Rating Scale [37], the Child Mania Rating Scale [38], the General Behavior Inventory [39], the Mood Disorders Questionnaire [40,41], and the Child Behavior Checklist (CBCL) [42], can be effective screening tools for BD and may assist clinicians in differentiating BD from ADHD and other behavioral disorders. Youngstrom and colleagues [43] compared several rating tools and determined that the parent–General Behavior Inventory and the parent–Mood Disorders Questionnaire were the most efficient in predicting BD in a community mental health center setting. Several studies also showed that screening instruments completed by caregivers are more effective than instruments completed by teachers or children and that combining screening instrument data from multiple informants does not provide additional information [44]. The CBCL is not specific for identifying BD in community samples [42], and the CBCL-juvenile BD (CBCL-JBD) profile (elevated scores on the attention, aggression, and anxious/depressed subscales) often identifies youth with other disorders [45]. In addition to a thorough clinical assessment that includes parent and child interviews, clinicians should use a parent-report rating scale, such as the Mood Disorders Questionnaire, General Behavior Inventory, or Child Mania Rating Scale, to support decision making, especially in patients with complicated presentations.

Treatment

*Treating attention deficit hyperactivity disorder in children
and adolescents who have bipolar disorder*

Two studies addressed treating ADHD in youth who have BD. In one
study ($N = 40$), mixed amphetamine salts, added to divalproex sodium,
were more effective than placebo in treating the symptoms of ADHD,
and no significant worsening of manic symptoms emerged [46]. The second
study was a chart review ($N = 38$) that concluded that mood stabilization
was a prerequisite for ADHD treatment [47].

*Treating attention deficit hyperactivity disorder with irritability
and subthreshold bipolar disorder*

Post hoc analyses indicate that children who have ADHD and some manic
symptoms (but who do not meet full criteria for BD) can be treated effectively
with stimulants. In the Multimodal Treatment Study of Children with ADHD
($N = 289$), children who had some manic symptoms (who did not meet full criteria for BD) responded well to treatment with stimulants [24,48]. Similarly,
Carlson and colleagues [25] demonstrated that of 75 6- to 12-year-old boys
treated for hyperkinetic reaction of childhood, the 23% who had symptoms
that suggested childhood mania (eg, irritability) did not differ in their response
to methylphenidate and were no more likely than youth without manic symptoms to develop BD at ages 21 to 23. Stimulants generally decrease irritability
and aggression in children who have ADHD [49]. Of note, children who have
ADHD may exhibit affective symptoms as their stimulant wears off, and this
"rebound" may be misdiagnosed as BD [50].

*Treating bipolar disorder with comorbid attention deficit hyperactivity
disorder*

Two studies demonstrated that adolescents who have BD and comorbid
ADHD are less likely than youth without comorbid ADHD to respond well
to antimanic medication. In one chart review of adolescents hospitalized for
mania, a history of ADHD was associated with a diminished response to
divalproex sodium or lithium [51]. In a naturalistic treatment study of 40
adolescents who had BD, ADHD, and CD, baseline severity correlated
with nonresponse [52]. In another treatment study of 48 adolescents who
had BD, however, a history of ADHD was not associated with a poor lithium response [53].

Stimulants precipitating mania or bipolar disorder

Case studies describe stimulants precipitating manic symptoms in children [54]. In reviewing several pharmaceutical company–sponsored trials,
the US Food and Drug Administration found that stimulant-associated

psychotic-like and manic-like symptoms occurred rarely—in approximately 0.25% of children treated with stimulants [55]. In 55 of 60 reported cases of psychotic-like or manic-like symptoms in response to stimulants, the symptoms resolved when the stimulant was discontinued [55]. In the five cases that did not, the patients were rediagnosed with schizophrenia or BD. In some cases, children may tolerate a carefully monitored rechallenge of stimulant at a lower dose [55].

Investigators have hypothesized that stimulants may hasten the onset of mania. Reichart and Nolen [56] estimated that the rate of BD in the Netherlands was much lower than that in the United States and proposed that medication exposure may hasten the onset of BD, especially in youth with a family history of BD [56]. In a retrospective analysis of 80 hospitalized manic adolescents, stimulant exposure was associated with more severe hospital course, younger age, ADHD, and ODD [57]. In another study from the same institution, prior stimulant treatment was associated with earlier onset of BD; however, ADHD was not associated with age of onset of BD [58]. These studies were retrospective and uncontrolled (ie, more severe ADHD may be associated independently with stimulant treatment and earlier BD onset). In contrast, in one prospective study of 81 children who had ADHD, 28.5% switched to BD, and less stimulant use was associated with developing BD [23]. Future studies should examine treated and untreated children who have ADHD and investigate irritability, comorbidity, and onset of new psychopathology.

Family and genetic studies

Top-down studies

A number of "top-down" studies have examined offspring of bipolar parents for ADHD. Several have not found increased risk for ADHD [59] or ADHD symptoms [60], whereas others have. For example, Carlson and Weintraub [61] found that children of parents who had BD and children of psychiatric controls had greater rates of attention and behavior problems than the children of normal controls [61]. Childhood attention problems were related to young adult mood disorder only in the BD offspring group. Another group found that children of parents who had BD had higher rates of ADHD than children of parents who had panic disorder or MDD [62]. In a study of 60 children of parents who had BD, Chang and colleagues [63] also found high rates of ADHD (28%).

Bottom-up studies

Several investigators examined rates of BD and ADHD in first-degree relatives of youth who have these illnesses ("bottom-up" studies). Faraone and colleagues [30] found that first-degree relatives of youth who have BD and ADHD were more likely to have comorbid ADHD and BD than were the relatives of probands with ADHD alone or controls, which suggests cofamiliality of BD and ADHD. Other research from this group indicated that antisocial and bipolar ADHD subtypes may be different manifestations of the same condition [64].

Several investigators examined the first-degree relatives of youth who have BD for psychopathology [65,66]. Geller and colleagues [65] found that probands with BD have first-degree relatives with greater morbidity risk of BD than relatives of ADHD or healthy controls and that the risk of BD was similar in the relatives of probands with ADHD and the relatives of healthy controls. In a pilot study, Wozniak and colleagues [66] found that first-degree relatives of children who have BD (most with comorbid ADHD) had higher rates of ADHD than the normal control group and higher rates of BD than the nonbipolar ADHD group and that ADHD cosegregated in these relatives. In another study, investigators found that the most common diagnosis in the first-degree relatives of youth who have BD was MDD, but there were also high rates of BD, anxiety, ADHD, CD, substance use, and suicidal ideation, especially in the relatives of youth who have childhood-onset BD [67]. These studies indicated that rates of ADHD are elevated in family members of children who have BD (many of whom had comorbid ADHD). They did not demonstrate elevated rates of BD in children who have ADHD, although this negative finding may be because the studies were not powered to detect this elevation.

Twin studies

In a large sample of Dutch twin pairs examined prospectively [67], investigators found that the CBCL-JBD phenotype identified by high scores on attention, anxious-depressed, and aggression subscales, was present in approximately 1% of the population overall and in 20% of individuals with high scores on the CBCL attention problems scale. They also found that ADHD was more genetically influenced, whereas the CBCL-JBD phenotype had a stronger environmental contribution.

Molecular studies

One study found no common genes between ADHD and BD when scanning an estrogen receptor and thyroid hormone receptor gene [68]. Several studies proposed that dopamine transporter genes are implicated in ADHD [69,70] and BD [71-73]. Several studies have shown that the brain-derived neurotrophic factor (BDNF) gene is involved in the pathogenesis of ADHD [74] and BD [75]. However, there are also studies which show a lack of association between the Val66Met polymorphism of BDNF, including a meta-analysis [76], so the data are not currently conclusive. One study also identified ADHD subjects with the A559V variant of the dopamine transporter gene [77], which was previously identified in a subject who had BD [78].

Pathophysiology

Pathophysiologic studies are needed to compare patients who have ADHD or BD (with and without comorbid ADHD) and controls. One important question concerns whether ADHD that occurs in the setting of BD is similar pathophysiologically to ADHD that occurs alone or, alternatively, represents a phenocopy. It is important to determine whether neuropsychological tests and imaging can assist in making clinical diagnoses and whether pathophysiology might ultimately help guide our interventions.

The literature is mixed as to whether youth who have ADHD, BD with ADHD, and BD without ADHD can be differentiated neuropsychologically. One study found that patients who had ADHD with and without BD showed more deficits than patients who had BD alone or controls on processing speed, automatized naming speed, memory, and executive functioning [79]. A second study of neurologic examination abnormalities found that children who had ADHD alone were impaired on repetitive task reaction time, whereas children who had BD—with and without comorbid ADHD—were impaired on sequential task reaction time [80]. Two studies examined executive function in youth with BD with and without ADHD and in healthy controls [81,82]. These studies demonstrated that youth with BD, with and without comorbid ADHD, had impaired executive function and that those youth with both disorders had poorer function. Other studies did not find differences between the BD groups with and without ADHD when examining factors such as biologic risk factors [83], prepulse inhibition [84], limbic hyperactivation while processing neutral faces [85], and cognitive flexibility [86].

With regard to neuroimaging, one study of 368 youth hospitalized with various DISC-defined diagnoses found that individuals who had BD ($N = 56$) or ADHD/CD ($N = 94$) had significantly more white matter hyperintensities than controls, but the two groups did not differ significantly from each other [87]. Moore and colleagues [88] examined brain chemistry in children and adolescents who had ADHD with and without comorbid BD. They found that children who had ADHD alone had significantly higher ratios of glutamate plus glutamine to myo-inositol than did children who had ADHD and BD, which suggested a means for differentiating the two illnesses. Two studies that compared youth with BD with and without comorbid ADHD found possible differences in neural activation during attentional or motor inhibitory tasks [89,90], although a different study found no differences between ADHD and BD groups [85].

Overall, these studies indicate that some neuropsychological, neurologic, and neuroimaging measures may differentiate BD from ADHD. Many of the "negative studies" were post hoc analyses in BD samples either controlling for ADHD or comparing participants with and without ADHD, and they may not have been adequately powered to detect differences. Further research is needed before using these pathophysiologic measures to guide diagnosis.

Summary

Often when a child has ADHD and mood dysregulation, it can be difficult to make an accurate diagnosis and decide on an evidence-based treatment plan. Research in epidemiology, assessment, treatment, family studies, genetics, and pathophysiology can help guide our diagnostic and treatment decisions. We draw from this research to make clinical recommendations while highlighting important directions for future research.

Clinical recommendations

1. Keep base rates in mind when considering a diagnosis. ADHD is a common childhood disorder. BD is much less common, although it may occur more frequently than we once thought. Statistically speaking, a child is much less likely to have BD than ADHD. These likelihoods differ according to setting. For example, a child in a pediatric office who has ADHD is much less likely to have BD than one in a tertiary care clinic that specializes in BD or in an inpatient psychiatric unit. Similarly, if a child has ADHD and irritability, consider not only BD but also ODD, CD, generalized anxiety disorder, and MDD, which are much more common than BD.

2. Conduct a thorough diagnostic interview with both child and guardian when assessing for possible BD in children who have ADHD or possible ADHD in children who have BD. To diagnose BD, look for an episode of extremely elevated or expansive mood. If none exists, look for an episode of irritability that is more severe than the child's baseline. Then determine if the child had the associated "B" symptoms of mania at the same time as the mood symptoms. Those B symptoms that are not shared by ADHD (grandiosity, flight of ideas/racing thoughts, decreased need for sleep, and hypersexuality) are especially helpful in discriminating between the two disorders. When looking for ADHD in a child who has BD, look for decreased attention and increased activity which are non-episodic and occur at times other than during a mood episode.

3. Use rating scales to support clinical decision making. If you suspect BD, parent-report rating scales with symptoms specific to BD are the best predictors.

4. The data are limited as to how to best treat a child or adolescent with both BD and ADHD. A good diagnostic assessment is essential, because the treatment of ADHD and BD may be different than the treatment of ADHD and irritability secondary to another condition. Children who have ADHD and irritability who do not meet criteria for BD may benefit

from medications that we are wary of prescribing to patients who have BD. For example, children who have ADHD and irritability may respond to stimulants with decreased irritability [91]. Children who have ADHD and anxiety or irritable depression may benefit with treatment for their anxiety or depression, such as a selective serotonin reuptake inhibitor or psychotherapy. If a child has ADHD and BD, the limited data indicate that first you should stabilize the BD and, if residual ADHD symptoms remain, then treat the ADHD. Take into account the risk of adverse effects or destabilization from medication and discuss this with families, but do not overweigh the possibility of risk when making a recommendation.

Directions for future research

1. Although there is some indication of elevated rates of BD in ADHD samples and strong data to support elevated rates of ADHD in BD samples, further research is needed to investigate the rates of comorbidity in younger population-based samples. Few data are available for school-aged children or toddlers and in clinical samples in varied settings. Similarly, more data are needed on the longitudinal relationship between ADHD and BD in youth, specifically examining onset and offset of the two illnesses, symptoms or risk factors that predispose a child with ADHD to developing BD, and the question of whether ADHD with severe irritability is continuous with ADHD or BD.

2. The assessment of ADHD and BD and the use of diagnostic instruments may vary from site to site in research settings. The field would benefit from greater standardization of instruments, symptom description, and symptom interpretation, which would lead to improved capacity to compare results across settings.

3. Similarly, clinicians would benefit from screening tools and diagnostic instruments that are designed to differentiate between BD and ADHD in clinical settings.

4. Further treatment trials of BD with comorbid ADHD are needed. In particular, are some medications particularly effective in treating both disorders? Are some ADHD treatments more or less likely to destabilize children with BD? If a child has ADHD but is at risk for BD because of family history or symptom profile, should the prescribing clinician avoid stimulants or only prescribe stimulants after a child has been stabilized on other medications? If a child has an adverse "manic-like" reaction to an ADHD medication, does this have diagnostic implications?

5. Further family studies and genetic studies are needed. Specific questions include quantifying the risk of developing BD in a child who has ADHD and a first-degree relative who has BD. High-risk studies may permit us to see the antecedents of BD in a child who has ADHD and may lead to opportunities for intervention. Studies also should investigate the possibility of shared risk-related genes.

6. Further pathophysiologic and neuroimaging studies are needed to compare youth who have BD (with and without comorbid ADHD), youth who have ADHD alone (with and without irritability), and controls. Studying the underlying mechanisms of behavior and contrasting these different groups may allow us to determine whether ADHD in children who have BD is a phenotypic copy of ADHD in non-BD patients, create better treatment interventions, and ultimately develop laboratory tests to assist in differentiating between the two disorders in clinical practice.

Acknowledgments

The authors wish to thank Peter Oberg for his assistance in the preparation of the manuscript.

References

[1] American Psychiatric Association. Diagnostic and statistical manual of mental disorders. 4th edition. Text revision. Washington, DC: American Psychiatric Association; 2000.

[2] Leibenluft E, Blair RJ, Charney DS, et al. Irritability in pediatric mania and other childhood psychopathology. Ann N Y Acad Sci 2003;1008:201–18.

[3] Leibenluft E, Charney DS, Towbin KE, et al. Defining clinical phenotypes of juvenile mania. Am J Psychiatry 2003;160(3):430–7.

[4] Biederman J, Klein RG, Pine DS, et al. Resolved: mania is mistaken for ADHD in prepubertal children. J Am Acad Child Adolesc Psychiatry 1998;37(10):1091–6 [discussion: 1096–9].

[5] Lewinsohn PM, Klein DN, Seeley JR. Bipolar disorders in a community sample of older adolescents: prevalence, phenomenology, comorbidity, and course. J Am Acad Child Adolesc Psychiatry 1995;34(4):454–63.

[6] Costello EJ, Angold A, Burns BJ, et al. The Great Smoky Mountains Study of Youth: goals, design, methods, and the prevalence of DSM-III-R disorders. Arch Gen Psychiatry 1996; 53(12):1129–36.

[7] Reich W, Neuman RJ, Volk HE, et al. Comorbidity between ADHD and symptoms of bipolar disorder in a community sample of children and adolescents. Twin Res Hum Genet 2005;8(5):459–66.

[8] Kessler RC, Adler L, Barkley R, et al. The prevalence and correlates of adult ADHD in the United States: results from the National Comorbidity Survey Replication. Am J Psychiatry 2006;163(4):716–23.

[9] Hurtig T, Ebeling H, Taanila A, et al. ADHD and comorbid disorders in relation to family environment and symptoms severity. Eur Child Adolesc Psychiatry 2007;16:362–9.

[10] Kim-Cohen J, Caspi A, Moffitt TE, et al. Prior juvenile diagnoses in adults with mental disorder: developmental follow-back of a prospective-longitudinal cohort. Arch Gen Psychiatry 2003;60(7):709–17.

[11] Galanter CG, Cohen P, Jensen PS, et al. ADHD does not predict adult bipolar disorder using longitudinal epidemiological data. Presented at the Annual Meeting of the American Academy of Child and Adolescent Psychiatry. New York, October, 2003.

[12] Leibenluft E, Cohen P, Gorrindo T, et al. Chronic versus episodic irritability in youth: a community-based, longitudinal study of clinical and diagnostic associations. J Child Adolesc Psychopharmacol 2006;16(4):456–66.

[13] Brotman MA, Schmajuk M, Rich BA, et al. Prevalence, clinical correlates, and longitudinal course of severe mood dysregulation in children. Biol Psychiatry 2006;60(9):991–7.

[14] Birmaher B, Axelson D, Strober M, et al. Clinical course of children and adolescents with bipolar spectrum disorders. Arch Gen Psychiatry 2006;63(2):175–83.

[15] Findling RL, Gracious BL, McNamara NK, et al. Rapid, continuous cycling and psychiatric co-morbidity in pediatric bipolar I disorder. Bipolar Disord 2001;3(4):202–10.

[16] Biederman J, Faraone S, Mick E, et al. Attention-deficit hyperactivity disorder and juvenile mania: an overlooked comorbidity? J Am Acad Child Adolesc Psychiatry 1996;35(8): 997–1008.

[17] Wozniak J, Biederman J, Kiely K, et al. Mania-like symptoms suggestive of childhood-onset bipolar disorder in clinically referred children. J Am Acad Child Adolesc Psychiatry 1995; 34(7):867–76.

[18] Tillman R, Geller B. Definitions of rapid, ultrarapid, and ultradian cycling and of episode duration in pediatric and adult bipolar disorders: a proposal to distinguish episodes from cycles. J Child Adolesc Psychopharmacol 2003;13(3):267–71.

[19] Butler SF, Arredondo DE, McCloskey V. Affective comorbidity in children and adolescents with attention deficit hyperactivity disorder. Ann Clin Psychiatry 1995;7(2):51–5.

[20] Fischer M, Barkley RA, Smallish L, et al. Young adult follow-up of hyperactive children: self-reported psychiatric disorders, comorbidity, and the role of childhood conduct problems and teen CD. J Abnorm Child Psychol 2002;30(5):463–75.

[21] Mannuzza S, Klein RG, Bessler A, et al. Adult outcome of hyperactive boys: educational achievement, occupational rank, and psychiatric status. Arch Gen Psychiatry 1993;50(7): 565–76.

[22] Rasmussen P, Gillberg C. Natural outcome of ADHD with developmental coordination disorder at age 22 years: a controlled, longitudinal, community-based study. J Am Acad Child Adolesc Psychiatry 2000;39(11):1424–31.

[23] Tillman R, Geller B. Controlled study of switching from attention-deficit/hyperactivity disorder to a prepubertal and early adolescent bipolar I disorder phenotype during 6-year prospective follow-up: rate, risk, and predictors. Dev Psychopathol 2006;18(4): 1037–53.

[24] Galanter CA, Pagar DL, Davies M, et al. ADHD and manic symptoms: diagnostic and treatment implications. Clin Neurosci Res 2005;5:283–94.

[25] Carlson GA, Loney J, Salisbury H, et al. Stimulant treatment in young boys with symptoms suggesting childhood mania: a report from a longitudinal study. J Child Adolesc Psychopharmacol 2000;10(3):175–84.

[26] Hazell PL, Carr V, Lewin TJ, et al. Manic symptoms in young males with ADHD predict functioning but not diagnosis after 6 years. J Am Acad Child Adolesc Psychiatry 2003;42: 552–60.

[27] Jaideep T, Reddy YC, Srinath S. Comorbidity of attention deficit hyperactivity disorder in juvenile bipolar disorder. Bipolar Disord 2006;8(2):182–7.

[28] Kowatch RA, Youngstrom EA, Danielyan A, et al. Review and meta-analysis of the phenomenology and clinical characteristics of mania in children and adolescents. Bipolar Disord 2005;7(6):483–96.

[29] Tillman R, Geller B, Bolhofner K, et al. Ages of onset and rates of syndromal and subsyndromal comorbid DSM-IV diagnoses in a prepubertal and early adolescent bipolar disorder phenotype. J Am Acad Child Adolesc Psychiatry 2003;42(12):1486–93.

[30] Faraone SV, Biederman J, Mennin D, et al. Attention-deficit hyperactivity disorder with bipolar disorder: a familial subtype? J Am Acad Child Adolesc Psychiatry 1997;36(10): 1378–87 [discussion: 1387–90].

[31] Perlis RH, Miyahara S, Marangell LB, et al. Long-term implications of early onset in bipolar disorder: data from the first 1000 participants in the systematic treatment enhancement program for bipolar disorder (STEP-BD). Biol Psychiatry 2004;55(9): 875–81.

[32] Masi G, Perugi G, Toni C, et al. Attention-deficit hyperactivity disorder: bipolar comorbidity in children and adolescents. Bipolar disorders 2006;8(4):373–81.

[33] Nierenberg AA, Miyahara S, Spencer T, et al. Clinical and diagnostic implications of life-time attention-deficit/hyperactivity disorder comorbidity in adults with bipolar disorder: data from the first 1000 STEP-BD participants. Biol Psychiatry 2005;57(11):1467–73.

[34] McClellan J, Kowatch R, Findling RL. Practice parameter for the assessment and treatment of children and adolescents with bipolar disorder. J Am Acad Child Adolesc Psychiatry 2007; 46(1):107–25.

[35] Geller B, Zimerman B, Williams M, et al. DSM-IV mania symptoms in a prepubertal and early adolescent bipolar disorder phenotype compared to attention-deficit hyperactive and normal controls. J Child Adolesc Psychopharmacol 2002;12(1):11–25.

[36] Owens JA. The ADHD and sleep conundrum: a review. J Dev Behav Pediatr 2005;26(4): 312–22.

[37] Young RC, Biggs JT, Ziegler VE, et al. A rating scale for mania: reliability, validity and sensitivity. Br J Psychiatry 1978;133:429–35.

[38] Pavuluri MN, Henry DB, Devineni B, et al. Child mania rating scale: development, reliability, and validity. J Am Acad Child Adolesc Psychiatry 2006;45(5):550–60.

[39] Youngstrom EA, Findling RL, Danielson CK, et al. Discriminative validity of parent report of hypomanic and depressive symptoms on the general behavior inventory. Psychol Assess 2001;13(2):267–76.

[40] Hirschfeld RM, Williams JB, Spitzer RL, et al. Development and validation of a screening instrument for bipolar spectrum disorder: the Mood Disorder Questionnaire. Am J Psychiatry 2000;157(11):1873–5.

[41] Wagner KD, Hirschfeld RM, Emslie GJ, et al. Validation of the mood disorder questionnaire for bipolar disorders in adolescents. J Clin Psychiatry 2006;67(5):827–30.

[42] Achenbach T. Manual for the Child Behavior Checklist/4—18 and 1991 profile. Burlington, VT: University of Vermont. Department of Psychiatry; 1991.

[43] Youngstrom E, Meyers O, Demeter C, et al. Comparing diagnostic checklists for pediatric bipolar disorder in academic and community mental health settings. Bipolar Disord 2005; 7(6):507–17.

[44] Youngstrom E, Meyers O, Youngstrom JK, et al. Diagnostic and measurement issues in the assessment of pediatric bipolar disorder: implications for understanding mood disorder across the life cycle. Dev Psychopathol 2006;18(4):989–1021.

[45] Volk HE, Todd RD. Does the child behavior checklist juvenile bipolar disorder phenotype identify bipolar disorder? Biol Psychiatry 2007;62(2):115–20.

[46] Scheffer RE, Kowatch RA, Carmody T, et al. Randomized, placebo-controlled trial of mixed amphetamine salts for symptoms of comorbid ADHD in pediatric bipolar disorder after mood stabilization with divalproex sodium. Am J Psychiatry 2005;162(1): 58–64.

[47] Biederman J, Mick E, Prince J, et al. Systematic chart review of the pharmacologic treatment of comorbid attention deficit hyperactivity disorder in youth with bipolar disorder. J Child Adolesc Psychopharmacol 1999;9(4):247–56.

[48] Galanter CA, Carlson GA, Jensen PS, et al. Response to methylphenidate in children with attention deficit hyperactivity disorder and manic symptoms in the multimodal treatment study of children with attention deficit hyperactivity disorder titration trial. J Child Adolesc Psychopharmacol 2003;13(2):123–36.

[49] Pappadopulos E, Woolston S, Chait A, et al. Pharmacotherapy of aggression in children and adolescents: efficacy and effect size. Journal of the Canadian Academy of Child and Adolescent Psychiatry 2006;15(1):27–39.

[50] Sarampote CS, Efron LA, Robb AS, et al. Can stimulant rebound mimic pediatric bipolar disorder? J Child Adolesc Psychopharmacol 2002;12(1):63–7.

[51] State RC, Frye MA, Altshuler LL, et al. Chart review of the impact of attention-deficit/hyperactivity disorder comorbidity on response to lithium or divalproex sodium in adolescent mania. J Clin Psychiatry 2004;65(8):1057–63.

[52] Masi G, Perugi G, Toni C, et al. Predictors of treatment nonresponse in bipolar children and adolescents with manic or mixed episodes. J Child Adolesc Psychopharmacol 2004;14(3): 395–404.

[53] Kafantaris V, Coletti DJ, Dicker R, et al. Are childhood psychiatric histories of bipolar adolescents associated with family history, psychosis, and response to lithium treatment? J Affect Disord 1998;51(2):153–64.

[54] Cherland E, Fitzpatrick R. Psychotic side effects of psychostimulants: a 5-year review. Can J Psychiatry 1999;44(8):811–3.

[55] Ross RG. Psychotic and manic-like symptoms during stimulant treatment of attention deficit hyperactivity disorder. Am J Psychiatry 2006;163(7):1149–52.

[56] Reichart CG, Nolen WA. Earlier onset of bipolar disorder in children by antidepressants or stimulants? An hypothesis. J Affect Disord 2004;78(1):81–4.

[57] Soutullo CA, DelBello MP, Ochsner JE, et al. Severity of bipolarity in hospitalized manic adolescents with history of stimulant or antidepressant treatment. J Affect Disord 2002; 70(3):323–7.

[58] DelBello MP, Soutullo CA, Hendricks W, et al. Prior stimulant treatment in adolescents with bipolar disorder: association with age at onset. Bipolar Disord 2001;3(2):53–7.

[59] Hillegers MH, Reichart CG, Wals M, et al. Five-year prospective outcome of psychopathology in the adolescent offspring of bipolar parents. Bipolar Disord 2005;7(4):344–50.

[60] Shaw JA, Egeland JA, Endicott J, et al. A 10-year prospective study of prodromal patterns for bipolar disorder among Amish youth. J Am Acad Child Adolesc Psychiatry 2005;44(11): 1104–11.

[61] Carlson GA, Weintraub S. Childhood behavior problems and bipolar disorder: relationship or coincidence? J Affect Disord 1993;28(3):143–53.

[62] Hirshfeld-Becker DR, Biederman J, Henin A, et al. Psychopathology in the young offspring of parents with bipolar disorder: a controlled pilot study. Psychiatry Res 2006;145(2-3):155–67.

[63] Chang KD, Steiner H, Ketter TA. Psychiatric phenomenology of child and adolescent bipolar offspring. J Am Acad Child Adolesc Psychiatry 2000;39(4):453–60.

[64] Faraone SV, Biederman J, Mennin D, et al. Bipolar and antisocial disorders among relatives of ADHD children: parsing familial subtypes of illness. Am J Med Genet 1998;81(1):108–16.

[65] Geller B, Tillman R, Bolhofner K, et al. Controlled, blindly rated, direct-interview family study of a prepubertal and early-adolescent bipolar I disorder phenotype: morbid risk, age at onset, and comorbidity. Arch Gen Psychiatry 2006;63(10):1130–8.

[66] Wozniak J, Biederman J, Mundy E, et al. A pilot family study of childhood-onset mania. J Am Acad Child Adolesc Psychiatry 1995;34(12):1577–83.

[67] Rende R, Birmaher B, Axelson D, et al. Childhood-onset bipolar disorder: evidence for increased familial loading of psychiatric illness. J Am Acad Child Adolesc Psychiatry 2007; 46(2):197–204.

[68] Hudziak JJ, Althoff RR, Derks EM, et al. Prevalence and genetic architecture of Child Behavior Checklist-juvenile bipolar disorder. Biol Psychiatry 2005;58(7):562–8.

[69] Feng J, Yan J, Michaud S, et al. Scanning of estrogen receptor alpha (ERalpha) and thyroid hormone receptor alpha (TRalpha) genes in patients with psychiatric diseases: four missense mutations identified in ERalpha gene. Am J Med Genet 2001;105(4):369–74.

[70] Cook EH Jr, Stein MA, Krasowski MD, et al. Association of attention-deficit disorder and the dopamine transporter gene. Am J Hum Genet 1995;56(4):993–8.

[71] Faraone SV, Perlis RH, Doyle AE, et al. Molecular genetics of attention-deficit/hyperactivity disorder. Biol Psychiatry 2005;57(11):1313–23.

[72] Kelsoe JR, Sadovnick AD, Kristbjarnarson H, et al. Possible locus for bipolar disorder near the dopamine transporter on chromosome 5. Am J Med Genet 1996;67(6):533–40.

[73] Greenwood TA, Schork NJ, Eskin E, et al. Identification of additional variants within the human dopamine transporter gene provides further evidence for an association with bipolar disorder in two independent samples. Mol Psychiatry 2006;11(2):125–33, 115.

[74] Kent L, Green E, Hawi Z, et al. Association of the paternally transmitted copy of common valine allele of the Val66Met polymorphism of the brain-derived neurotrophic factor (BDNF) gene with susceptibility to ADHD. Mol Psychiatry 2005;10(10):939–43.

[75] Geller B, Badner JA, Tillman R, et al. Linkage disequilibrium of the brain-derived neurotrophic factor Val66Met polymorphism in children with a prepubertal and early adolescent bipolar disorder phenotype. Am J Psychiatry 2004;161(9):1698–700.

[76] Kanazawa T, Glatt SJ, Kia-Keating B, et al. Meta-analysis reveals no association of the Val66Met polymorphism of brain-derived neurotrophic factor with either schizophrenia or bipolar disorder. Psychiatr Genet 2007;17(3):165–70.

[77] Mazei-Robison MS, Couch RS, Shelton RC, et al. Sequence variation in the human dopamine transporter gene in children with attention deficit hyperactivity disorder. Neuropharmacology 2005;49(6):724–36.

[78] Grunhage F, Schulze TG, Muller DJ, et al. Systematic screening for DNA sequence variation in the coding region of the human dopamine transporter gene (DAT1). Mol Psychiatry 2000;5(3):275–82.

[79] Rucklidge JJ. Impact of ADHD on the neurocognitive functioning of adolescents with bipolar disorder. Biol Psychiatry 2006;60(9):921–8.

[80] Dickstein DP, Garvey M, Pradella AG, et al. Neurologic examination abnormalities in children with bipolar disorder or attention-deficit/hyperactivity disorder. Biol Psychiatry 2005; 58(7):517–24.

[81] Pavuluri MN, Schenkel LS, Aryal S, et al. Neurocognitive function in unmedicated manic and medicated euthymic pediatric bipolar patients. Am J Psychiatry 2006;163(2):286–93.

[82] Shear PK, DelBello MP, Lee Rosenberg H, et al. Parental reports of executive dysfunction in adolescents with bipolar disorder. Child Neuropsychol 2002;8(4):285–95.

[83] Pavuluri MN, Henry DB, Nadimpalli SS, et al. Biological risk factors in pediatric bipolar disorder. Biol Psychiatry 2006;60(9):936–41.

[84] Rich BA, Vinton D, Grillon C, et al. An investigation of prepulse inhibition in pediatric bipolar disorder. Bipolar Disord 2005;7(2):198–203.

[85] Rich BA, Vinton DT, Roberson-Nay R, et al. Limbic hyperactivation during processing of neutral facial expressions in children with bipolar disorder. Proc Natl Acad Sci U S A 2006; 103(23):8900–5.

[86] Dickstein DP, Nelson EE, McClure EB, et al. Cognitive flexibility in phenotypes of pediatric bipolar disorder. J Am Acad Child Adolesc Psychiatry 2007;46(3):341–55.

[87] Lyoo IK, Lee HK, Jung JH, et al. White matter hyperintensities on magnetic resonance imaging of the brain in children with psychiatric disorders. Compr Psychiatry 2002;43(5): 361–8.

[88] Moore CM, Biederman J, Wozniak J, et al. Differences in brain chemistry in children and adolescents with attention deficit hyperactivity disorder with and without comorbid bipolar disorder: a proton magnetic resonance spectroscopy study. Am J Psychiatry 2006;163(2): 316–8.

[89] Adler CM, Delbello MP, Mills NP, et al. Comorbid ADHD is associated with altered patterns of neuronal activation in adolescents with bipolar disorder performing a simple attention task. Bipolar Disord 2005;7(6):577–88.

[90] Leibenluft E, Rich BA, Vinton DT, et al. Neural circuitry engaged during unsuccessful motor inhibition in pediatric bipolar disorder. Am J Psychiatry 2007;164(1):52–60.

[91] Greenhill LL, Pliszka S, Dulcan MK, et al. Summary of the practice parameter for the use of stimulant medications in the treatment of children, adolescents, and adults. J Am Acad Child Adolesc Psychiatry 2001;40(11):1352–5.

CHILD AND
ADOLESCENT
PSYCHIATRIC CLINICS
OF NORTH AMERICA

ELSEVIER
SAUNDERS

Child Adolesc Psychiatric Clin N Am
17 (2008) 347–366

Attention Deficit Hyperactivity Disorder in Preschool Children

Laurence L. Greenhill, MD[a],*, Kelly Posner, PhD[b],
Brigette S. Vaughan, APRN[c],
Christopher J. Kratochvil, MD[c]

[a]Department of Psychiatry, New York State Psychiatric Institute, Unit 78,
Columbia University, 1051 Riverside Drive, New York, NY 10032, USA
[b]Division of Child and Adolescent Psychiatry, Columbia University/New York State
Psychiatric Institute, 1051 Riverside Drive, New York, NY 10032, USA
[c]University of Nebraska Medical Center, 985581 Nebraska Medical Center,
42nd Street and Dewey Avenue, Omaha, NE, USA

Attention deficit hyperactivity disorder (ADHD) is a neurobehavioral disorder with an onset of symptoms before 7 years of age, often starting as early as the preschool years. This fact presents a dilemma for clinicians who then must balance the potential benefits of early identification and intervention with the risks for overidentification and potential treatment of preschool-aged children who do not have ADHD. Despite voluminous literature about ADHD in school-aged children and adolescents, much less is known about the presentation and identification of this disorder in preschoolers, the safest and most efficacious modalities of treatment, responsiveness to treatment, and ultimately their long-term outcomes.

Dr. Greenhill has received support from Celltech, Cephalon, Eli Lilly, Janssen, McNeil, Medeva, Novartis Corporation, Noven, Otsuka, Pfizer, Sanofi, Shire, Solvay, Somerset, and Thompson Advanced Therapeutics Communications. As part of an effort to help execute the FDA suicidality classification mandates, Dr. Posner has received funding from the FDA to develop and implement the suicidality classification system used in their child antidepressant safety analyses. This system was subsequently used in the adult antidepressant safety analyses. As part of an effort to help execute the FDA suicidality classification mandates, Dr. Posner has had research support from Abbott, Bristol Myers Squibb, Organon, Schwarz, GlaxoSmithKline, Eli Lilly, Johnson and Johnson, Wyeth Research, Sanofi-Aventis, Cephalon, Novartis, Shire Pharmaceuticals, Merck, Pfizer and Vivus. Dr. Kratochvil has received support from Cephalon, Eli Lilly, McNeil, Abbott, Pfizer, Shire, Somerset, and AstraZeneca.
    * Corresponding author.
    E-mail address: greenhil@child.cpmc.columbia.edu (L.L. Greenhill).

Medical and mental health service use is higher in children diagnosed with ADHD than those in the general population [1–3], and associated costs are also significantly higher, comparable with other chronic conditions such as asthma [3–5]. These findings are also true of preschoolers who have ADHD [6]. Very young children (1–3 years of age) who have ADHD have more chronic health conditions and high frequency of service use, with an average of 18 emergency room visits in 15 months [7]. Even so, many preschool children who have ADHD do not receive care for their ADHD. A community study of 320 preschoolers found only 19% of those who have a preschool-onset behavior disorder received services [8].

Prevalence of preschool-onset attention deficit hyperactivity disorder

Early onset of ADHD symptoms and associated impairment has been reported in community and clinical samples [9,10]. Although initial ADHD symptoms may be noticed as early as 3 years of age [11,12], the most common age of full ADHD diagnosis does not occur until 7 to 10 years of age [13]. Epidemiologic surveys of community samples have reported that 2% to 6% of preschoolers met full criteria for ADHD [12,14,15], somewhat lower than the worldwide 5.7% prevalence rates reported for ADHD in school-aged children [16–18].

Using the parent-rated Preschool Age Psychiatric Assessment (PAPA) [19], a semistructured diagnostic interview shown to be reliable and valid for assessing psychiatric disorders in preschoolers, 5.1% of 1073 preschoolers from a pediatric clinic met diagnostic criteria for ADHD, with 2.9% identified as having the hyperactive/impulsive subtype, 2.1% having the combined type, and only 0.1% meeting criteria for the primarily inattentive subtype [19]. Two additional studies reported that 59% to 86% of children aged 2 to 6 years referred to psychiatric clinics were reported to have at least some symptoms of the disorder [15,20].

Diagnostic validity

The validity of an ADHD diagnosis in the preschool years has often been questioned. The *Diagnostic and Statistical Manual of Mental Disorders, Fourth Edition* (DSM-IV) does not provide specific, developmentally adjusted ADHD criteria that apply to preschoolers. Rather, the same diagnostic criteria are applied to patients across the lifespan. The frequent use of pharmacotherapy in treating preschoolers, however, makes determining a valid diagnosis at this young age important [21]. Consequently, efforts have focused on sharpening the specificity of ADHD diagnostic criteria by using diagnostic tools, including the Preschool Age Psychiatric Assessment (PAPA), for children younger than 6 years. This task is particularly important because preschoolers referred for treatment of a wide variety of behavioral problems show the same symptoms on ADHD checklists as those observed for school-aged children with ADHD [22], and relying exclusively on symptom checklists may cause overidentification of ADHD [23].

Another question is whether early onset is associated with one specific subtype of ADHD [6]. In the DSM-IV field trials, 75% of the children who had ADHD who met DSM-IV criteria for the Hyperactive/Impulsive subtype were younger than 6 years [24]. The mean age for this group (5.7 years) was significantly lower than those identified as predominately Inattentive or Combined subtype. Parents, teachers, and clinicians rated these primarily hyperactive–impulsive children as severely impaired. However, this finding does not indicate that young children only present with hyperactivity, because all three subtypes of ADHD have been identified in children aged 4 to 6 [6,21]. Diagnoses were established by combining data from a structured diagnostic interview with the mother and teacher checklists. All subtypes differed significantly from controls in functional impairment in multiple domains. The primarily inattentive group was significantly older than the other two subtypes of ADHD [6], possibly suggesting that inattention is less apparent and not as impairing until school demands increase. However, a proportion of children diagnosed as preschoolers changed to another ADHD subtype over the next 8 years, questioning the stability and validity of ADHD subtyping in this population.

Impairment with attention deficit hyperactivity disorder

Current DSM-IV diagnostic criteria for ADHD require demonstration of impairment in a minimum of two settings [25]. Symptoms of ADHD in preschoolers produce significant impairment in a multitude of settings, including home, school, and during social functioning, even to the degree of impacting the child's safety [6,20,26]. Compared with same-aged controls, preschoolers who have ADHD are more often suspended from preschool or daycare (15% versus 0.8%) because of disruptive behavior (7.8% versus 0.4%) [27]. They also frequently experience more academic impairment and special education placements than classroom controls [6,21].

Rappley and colleagues [7] found that 1- to 3-year-olds identified with ADHD, even when treated with a psychostimulant, experienced physical injury during a 15-month follow-up period. This finding suggested that early onset of ADHD correlates with an increased risk for accidents or injuries. Children aged 4 to 6 years who have ADHD experience more unintentional injuries and accidental poisonings than their non-ADHD counterparts [6]. Similarly, school-aged children who have ADHD have more emergency department visits than their peers who do not have the disorder [28]. The highest rates of injury were seen in those children who have the hyperactive/impulsive subtype of ADHD [29]. Additionally, preschool boys who have ADHD and comorbid oppositional defiant disorder (ODD) have significantly higher rates of unintentional injury than comparison children [30].

Comorbidities

Just as with older children, preschool ADHD frequently co-occurs with other psychiatric disorders [31]. Young children who have ADHD have been shown to have increased rates of developmental delays and developmental coordination disorder [32]. Of preschoolers who had ADHD, 22% also had a language disorder [33]. High rates of language problems have also been reported in other preschool ADHD samples [7], along with under-achievement in reading and math [6]. Like their school-aged counterparts, preschoolers who have ADHD are also at risk for internalizing and externalizing disorders [15,31,34]. Wilens and colleagues [31] found that 74% of their clinically referred preschool sample had at least one other disorder. In a study of community-referred preschoolers assessed with the structured PAPA interview, 64% were identified as meeting criteria for at least one psychiatric comorbidity, most commonly conduct disorder and generalized anxiety disorder (35%), followed by ODD (6.8%), depression (5.2%), social phobia (1%), and separation anxiety disorder (0.9%) [27]. Wilens and colleagues [31] reported that nearly half of their preschoolers clinically referred for ADHD had a co-occurring mood disorder, with 26% meeting criteria for a diagnosis of bipolar disorder. These findings have not been reported in other samples, however, and may be partly the result of screening with the Kiddie Schedule for Affective Disorders and Schizophrenia (Kiddie-SADS) diagnostic interview, which is not validated for diagnosing mood disorders in children younger than 6 years [35]. Preschool children who have ADHD (ages 18–47 months) with parents who are psychiatrically ill are more likely to be identified with a comorbid affective disorder on the Diagnostic Classification of Mental Health and Developmental Disorders of Infancy and Early Childhood (0–3, 1994) [34].

Early ADHD symptom onset has been correlated with higher rates of parent-reported aggressive symptoms [36]. Additionally, 3-year-old preschoolers whose overactivity, poor attention, and disobedience were associated with peer problems (eg, not-liked, does not share) and aggressive-antisocial behavior (eg, destructive, tells lies, physically attacks, fights) were more likely to have persistent problems at follow-up compared with those who had ADHD symptoms and no peer relationship problems [37]. Preschoolers who have ADHD are at greater risk for later conduct disorder and ODD [38], exhibit more negative social behaviors, and fare worse on tests of preacademic skills than non-ADHD counterparts [26]. Teachers reported that preschoolers who had ADHD were harder to manage in the classroom and had more problems with social behavior and internalizing symptoms compared with non-ADHD counterparts [39].

Persistence of attention deficit hyperactivity disorder symptoms with preschool presentation

Longitudinal studies report that preschool-onset ADHD symptoms may persist over time [6,21,40]. ADHD symptoms identified in 3-year-olds remained in 50% of those children by 6 years of age, and 48% by 9 years of age [11], and the same children were more likely to meet diagnostic criteria at 13 years of age than comparisons [40].

Nearly all of the 255 4- to 6-year-olds who had ADHD followed up for 3 years by Lahey and colleagues [21] continued to meet criteria for one subtype of ADHD, although not necessarily the one that first presented. Parent, teacher, and clinician reports indicated ongoing impairment for these children over time. The persistence of academic, social, or behavioral problems found in teacher reports was particularly compelling, because different teachers, blinded to diagnosis, continued to describe impairment each year. Poor outcomes in later school years, including overall academic difficulties, poorer cognitive skills, and lower levels of reading ability in adolescence, were noted when children who had early-onset ADHD were seen at 12 years of age [41]. Ironically, the most common perceived barrier to parents seeking help for their preschooler's ADHD was a conviction that the symptoms would lessen over time without intervention.

Treatment of preschool attention deficit hyperactivity disorder

Stimulant treatment

Use of methylphenidate in children younger than 6 years who have attention deficit hyperactivity disorder

Despite a U.S. Food and Drug Administration (FDA) warning against its use in children younger than 6 years, methylphenidate has frequently been prescribed off-label for treating ADHD symptoms in preschoolers. As early as 1990, 34% of pediatricians and 15% of family practitioners reported prescribing stimulant medications to preschoolers who had ADHD [42]. This off-label use of methylphenidate increased between 1990 and 1995 [43], with a 49% increase between 2000 and 2003 for ADHD in children younger than 5 years [44]. An upsurge has also been documented in Europe [45,46]. Particularly concerning is the data from the Michigan Medicaid system, where 57% of 223 children aged 3 years or younger who were diagnosed with ADHD were treated with as many as 22 different medications in 30 different combinations, and monitored less than every 3 months [7]. Zuvekas and colleagues [47], however, reported that despite the rate of psychostimulant use in pediatric patients increasing from 2.7% to 2.9% between 1997 and 2002, the rate of use in the preschool-aged group remained stable.

Clinical trials of methylphenidate in preschool-aged children

Despite the well-documented efficacy of methylphenidate in the treatment of ADHD in school-aged children [45], controlled data concerning the safety and efficacy of stimulants in preschool children have been limited. Much of the early published literature is on school-aged children, offering clinicians limited guidance for selecting optimal pharmacotherapy and few dosing strategies specifically for preschoolers with ADHD. In the 6 decades since the development of methylphenidate, fewer than a dozen controlled studies of methylphenidate involving preschoolers have been published (Table 1).

Published trials of methylphenidate involving preschoolers vary in diagnostic standards, methods, duration, and findings. Because most of the studies omitted teacher ratings, they lacked the multiinformant approach required by DSM-IV for documenting impairment in more than one setting (DSM-IV, *Text Revision*) [25]. Until the National Institute of Mental Health (NIMH) Preschool ADHD Treatment Study (PATS), most trials were single-site crossover designs that did not control for carryover effects or test for period-by-treatment interactions, without baseline or placebo conditions. Methylphenidate doses did not exceed 0.6 mg/kg in the trials, a narrower range than the 0.3 to 1.0 mg/kg doses used in older children [48]. Additionally, doses of immediate-release methylphenidate were given once or twice daily, rather than the three-times-daily schedule often required to cover afternoon and evening times spent at home. The published trials were also limited in duration, lasting no longer than 7 weeks, and were therefore unable to provide data on the effects of stimulant exposure on growth and cognitive development over time, a current major research priority. Eight of the nine trials conducted from 1970 to 2001 showed treatment benefits with a greater variability in response than reported for school-aged children who had ADHD [49]. Results from one trial suggested that sadness and social withdrawal occured when in preschoolers taking stimulants [50].

PATS

PATS (Preschool ADHD Treatment Study), the NIMH-sponsored, six-site, randomized clinical trial, has recruited the largest sample of preschoolers with ADHD. Parent and teacher ratings of DSM-IV symptoms were obtained for 532 children, aged 3 to 5.5 years, who were referred and screened for participation in PATS [22]. Children selected for PATS had severe ADHD symptoms, and a wide variety of risky behaviors and injuries, including broken bones, concussions, leaning out of windows, running into traffic-filled streets, turning on the stove and stretching over burners, or spilling bleach all over their bodies. Minimum symptom severity and impairment levels were required for inclusion into PATS because the risk–benefit ratio associated with study treatment would be was more optimal for the children who were more significantly impaired. Comorbidity was frequent, with approximately 70% of subjects presenting with additional Axis 1 diagnoses consistent with the preschool developmental level,

Table 1
Placebo controlled methylphenidate trials in preschoolers before PATS

Study	N	Design/duration	Methylphenidate dose	Outcomes	Adverse events
Schliefer, et al [51]	26	Crossover 3 wk	Total daily dose 2.5–30 mg; mean dose 5 mg bid	Decreased hyperactivity at home, no significant change in school	Dysphoric, withdrawn
Conners [52]	59	Parallel 6 wk	Mean dose 11.8 mg	Statistically significant improvement	Well-tolerated
Cohen, et al [53]	24	Parallel 8 wk	30 mg	No drug effect	None
Barkley, et al [54]	18	Crossover 3 wk	0.15 or 0.5 mg/kg bid	No reliable effect on either dose during free play	
Barkley, et al [55]	27	Crossover 3 wk	0.15 or 0.5 mg/kg bid	Increased compliance and decreased off-task behavior on 0.5 mg/kg dose	
Mayes, et al [56]	14	ABA design 24 d	10 mg tid	71% response rate	AEs reported by 50% of subjects
Musten et al [57]; Firestone, et al [50]	31	Crossover 30 d	0.3 or 0.5 mg/kg bid	Improved attention, improved parent ratings of ADHD symptoms	Reported in 10% of subjects, generally not clinically significant, reports of sadness and social withdrawal.
Handen, et al [58]	11	Crossover 4 wk	0.3 or 0.6 mg/kg qd, bid, or tid	8 of 11 subjects responded to methylphenidate, significant improvement on activity level, compliance and on teacher ratings	Five reports of significant social withdrawal, especially at higher dose
Short, et al [59]	28	Crossover 3 wk	Best dose 5 mg, 10 mg, or 15 mg bid	82% of subjects improved on best dose	Decreased appetite

Abbreviations: ADHD, attention deficit hyperactivity disorder; AEs, adverse advents.

specifically ODD, communication disorders, and anxiety disorders. ADHD severity was correlated with the presence of internalizing symptoms and higher impairment scores [60].

Methylphenidate treatment of preschoolers in PATS

PATS examined the efficacy and safety of acute methylphenidate treatment in preschoolers and its effectiveness and tolerability over time. Its design included eight phases: (1) recruitment, screening, and enrollment; (2) a 10-week, uncontrolled, group parent training module; (3) baseline assessment of children who did not improve during parent training; (4) a 1-week, open-label, safety lead-in phase for exposure to all methylphenidate study doses; (5) a 5-week, random sequence, double-blind, crossover titration involving four doses of methylphenidate (1.25 mg, 2.5 mg, 5.0 mg, and 7.5 mg) and placebo, administered three times daily; (6) a 4-week, parallel design, placebo-controlled, double-blind, randomized trial of methylphenidate versus placebo; (7) a 40-week, open-label, maintenance phase; and (8) a 6-week, double-blind, placebo-controlled, discontinuation phase [61]. This design allowed for the collection of safety, tolerability, and dose-ranging data on methylphenidate for the treatment of ADHD in preschool-aged children.

The primary outcome results from the dose-ranging, double-blind, crossover titration trial showed that methylphenidate had short-term efficacy for reducing the symptoms of ADHD and that symptom reduction was proportional to dosage [62]. Methylphenidate doses ranged from 1.25 to 7.5 mg three times daily, with an average "best" methylphenidate total daily dose of 14 mg. The percentage of children at each "best dose" condition included 25% for those receiving 7.5 mg three times daily; 21% for 5 mg three times daily; 18% for 2.5 three times daily; 17% for 1.25 mg three times daily; 10% for placebo; and 5% experienced no response to any treatment condition. Effect sizes ranged from 0.16 to 0.72, with the largest effect size observed at the 7.5 mg three times daily dose [62]. Effect sizes were lower than those reported for methylphenidate in older children, which may have partially been reflective of dosing [62]. The mean best methylphenidate total daily dose for the entire group (14 mg/d) was significantly lower than the 30 mg/d reported for school-aged children in the Multimodal Treatment Study of Children with ADHD (MTA) [63].

The mean best dose in the PATS crossover trial was 23% lower than they later required in the in the 10-month open-treatment follow-on phase [64]. Of the 114 participants randomized into the parallel-design, best-dose versus placebo phase, only 21% of subjects taking methylphenidate and 13% of those taking placebo experienced remission [60], perhaps also reflective of the lower doses or a response varied by patient age.

Parents reported moderate to severe adverse events in 30% of participants. The most common adverse events cited were emotional outbursts, difficulty falling asleep, repetitive behaviors or thoughts, appetite decrease, and irritability [65]. In the titration phase, decreased appetite, trouble sleeping, and weight loss occurred more frequently with methylphenidate than placebo, and during maintenance treatment, appetite loss and trouble sleeping persisted with 11% discontinuinged because of adverse events. A significant decrease in growth rate was observed during 1 year of methylphenidate treatment in PATS, with children gaining less weight (-1.32 kg/y) and attaining less height (-1.38 cm/y) than predicted from their baseline measurements [66]. This finding, however, was consistent with observed growth rate reductions in school-aged children in MTA [67].

Preliminary pharmacokinetic data from PATS have yielded results suggesting that preschoolers may benefit from lower methylphenidate doses than those required by school-aged children who have ADHD. Wigal and colleagues [68] showed that the clearance of a single dose of methylphenidate in preschoolers takes longer than the same dose given to older, school-aged children ($P = .0002$). These preliminary findings suggest that preschoolers may experience response at lower methylphenidate doses and that starting at lower methylphenidate doses may improve tolerability for younger, smaller patients [68].

Secondary analysis showed possible predictors of treatment response using exploratory moderator analyses from the PATS crossover trial [69]. The most powerful predictor of treatment response was the number of comorbid conditions, with those responding best to methylphenidate having two or fewer co-occurring disorders. Children who had three or more comorbid psychiatric conditions did not show a response to methylphenidate. The highest methylphenidate effects sizes were found in those who had no or only one comorbid diagnosis (Cohen's $d = 0.89$ and 1.0, respectively), an effect comparable to that seen in the school-aged children who had ADHD treated with methylphenidate in MTA [63].

The potential effectiveness of stimulant treatment for reducing the impairments associated with ADHD was examined for the children randomized to either placebo or their best dose of methylphenidate in double-blind fashion during the 4-week parallel phase. Results showed that impairment ratings varied by informant and domain, not by medication [70]. This result was anticipated, however, because the very short treatment period of 4 weeks would not be expected to produce large improvements in social skills, parenting stress, or emotional status [60].

Examination of the 95 preschoolers who had ADHD who completed the 40-week maintenance phase showed that the significant decreases in ADHD symptoms were sustained, although the mean total daily dose of methylphenidate, regulated in an open-label fashion by the study clinicians, increased from 14 to 20 mg/d [64]. Of the 95 preschoolers entering the maintenance phase, 45 discontinued PATS; 7 for behavioral worsening, 7 for adverse events, 7 to switch to a long-acting stimulant preparation, 3 for inadequate benefit, and 21 for other reasons.

Nonstimulant treatment

Atomoxetine

No controlled studies of nonstimulant medications for young children who have ADHD have been completed. Kratochvil and colleagues [71] recently conducted a small open-label 8-week study of atomoxetine in 5- and 6-year-old children who had ADHD. In this study, 22 children who had ADHD were treated with flexibly dosed atomoxetine titrated to a maximum of 1.8 mg/kg per day. The group used a novel approach, having the pharmacotherapist provide parent education on behavioral management and ADHD at each pharmacotherapy session. A significant decrease was observed on the ADHD Rating Scale IV–Parent total score ($P < .001$) and the inattentive and hyperactive/impulsive subscale scores ($P < .001$ for both). The mean final daily dose of atomoxetine was approximately 1.25 mg/kg per day, which is in line with the typical target dose of 1.2 mg/kg per day. Mood lability was reported in more than half the subjects (n = 12, 54.5%), and 50% of subjects reported decreased appetite. No discontinuations occurred because of adverse events, although a mean 1.04 kg weight loss was observed for the group ($P < .001$). A larger randomized placebo-controlled trial of atomoxetine in 5- and 6-year-olds is underway and will provide additional information on the use of this nonstimulant medication. This study will be another step in making an appropriate risk–benefit analysis on the use of pharmacotherapy in an increasingly younger population.

Treatment follow-up studies

Although the literature has begun to unravel short-term issues, it provides less information on the developmental course of preschool-onset ADHD and how it differs from that of ADHD identified and treated in the elementary school years. The potential mediating effects of early treatment on the risk for later ADHD symptoms and potential future development of substance abuse or other psychiatric comorbidities warrants exploration, as does its effect on the developmental course of the disorder. Data on the long-term safety and tolerability of pharmacotherapy in young children are also needed.

Few studies have systematically assessed the continuity of ADHD symptoms in the context of long-term treatment. However, the studies conducted with school-aged children who have ADHD have shown an overall reduction in ADHD-related symptoms [72]. Most studies, however, suggest that methylphenidate treatment does not have an enduring effect on measures of academic performance for school-aged children who have ADHD [72], but whether early methylphenidate treatment before kindergarten would have a more positive impact is less clear.

The association of methylphenidate with growth rate reduction has been a long-standing concern for school-aged children [73,74], and preschoolers may be even more vulnerable to growth-related adverse effects. PATS suggested that reductions in weight velocity also occur when 1 year of methylphenidate treatment is administered to preschoolers who have ADHD [66]. Because ADHD treatment often lasts longer than 1 year, additional long-term data are needed. The effects of prolonged stimulant treatment on medical outcomes of cardiovascular, endocrine, and hepatic function [75] and tics [76] in school-aged children have been studied; however, they did not examine children who began treatment during the preschool years. The potential association of early pharmacotherapy exposure with development of other psychiatric disorders, such as affective disorders and substance abuse, must also be evaluated. Early treatment may minimize or prevent adverse events, such as accidents and injuries, in children who have ADHD but no studies have systematically evaluated this type of long-term safety.

The PATS group is conducting a 5-year follow-up of 202 of the 303 participants from the original study sample. The results will provide important information on the long-term stability of the ADHD symptoms, long-term impact of methylphenidate on growth in preschoolers, and tolerability of methylphenidate over time [60].

Psychosocial interventions and parental factors

Evidence for the efficacy of psychosocial interventions in school-aged children who have ADHD is weaker than that for psychopharmacologic treatments [77]. In fact, MTA showed that an intensive psychosocial intervention was less effective than a medication management strategy in school-aged children. When combined with medication treatment, behavioral intervention provided only negligible benefit on the core symptoms of ADHD in school-aged children who had ADHD [63]. However, behavioral parent training has strong empiric support for a positive outcome when applied to younger school-aged children [78].

Parenting variables impact behavioral outcomes of preschool-aged children who have ADHD [26,79], and the best parenting predictor of hyperactivity was maternal coping. Negative, inconsistent parental behavior and high levels of family adversity are associated with early-onset behavioral problems and are predictors of their persistence. Mothers of at-risk preschoolers exhibited more negative behavior and less encouragement with heightened situational demands [80]. Parents of preschoolers who had ADHD displayed twice as many controlling/negative management strategies as positive preventive strategies [39], and lax disciplinary practices, less-efficient parental coping, lower rates of father–child communication, and less synchronous mother–child interactions have been associated with ADHD in preschool-aged boys [81]. Interventions to improve parenting skills may therefore positively affect child behavior.

Sonuga-Barke and colleagues [82] conducted one of the few controlled investigations of parent training in the treatment of preschool ADHD (Table 2). Children in a community sample were randomized to either a home-based parent training intervention (n = 30), parent counseling and support therapy (n = 29), or a wait-list control group (n = 20).

Table 2
Controlled psychosocial intervention trials in preschoolers

Study	Age/grade	Presenting condition	N	Type of psychosocial intervention	Duration	Outcomes
Strayhorn and Weidman [83]; follow-up [94]	2–5 y	Child behavior problems; ADHD	96	Parent/child interaction training	–	Decreased ADHD and internalizing symptoms;
Pisterman [85]	3–6 y	ADHD	57	Parent training	12 sessions	Increased child compliance; no significant effect on inattentive symptoms
Barkley, et al [87]; follow-up	Kindergarten	Disruptive Behavior	158	Parent training/classroom training	1 y	No effect with parent training; increased teacher ratings of attention, self-control, and social skills and decreased aggression with classroom training; effects not sustained at 2-y follow-up
Cunningham, et al [92]	Preschool	Moderate to severe ADHD	261	COPE (Community Parent Education)	10 wk	Only 7.2% significant improvementon symptom measures
Sonuga-Barke, et al [82]	3 y	ADHD	78	Parent training/parent counseling and support/wait-list control	8 wk	Decreased ADHD symptoms; increased maternal sense of well- being

Bor, et al [86]	3–4 y	Co-occurring disruptive behavior with inattention and/or hyperactivity	87	Behavioral family intervention	15–17 wk + 1 y follow-up	Decreased behavior problems and observed negative behavior; similar effects observed at 1-y follow-up
Huang, et al [88]	3–6 y	ADHD and ODD symptoms	23	Parent training	10 wk	Decreased ADHD and ODD symptoms; improvement in at-home behaviors
Corrin [84]	4–8 y	ADHD	55	Group parent training and child group training	10 wk	Augmented efficacy of other psychosocial treatments; combination of both was more effective than child training alone in decreasing behavior problems and improving parent management

Abbreviations: ADHD, attention deficit hyperactivity disorder; ODD, oppositional defiant disorder.

ADHD symptoms were significantly reduced by the home-based parent training compared with the other two groups, with 53% of children in the parent training group showing clinically significant improvement. The maternal sense of well-being was also significantly improved with the home-based parent training intervention. In a related study of 96 children aged 2 to 5 years, parent–child interaction training also reduced ADHD and internalizing symptoms [83].

Parent training has also been shown to augment the efficacy of other psychological treatments in young children [84]. In a study of 55 families of 4- to 8-year-olds, a combination of group parent training and child group training was superior to the child intervention alone in improving child behavior and parental behavioral management ability. Both groups experienced significant improvement in child externalizing behaviors, social skills, child self-concept, parental stress, and parental efficacy. Pisterman and colleagues [85] found that parent training improved parental outcomes, although little change occurred in child symptomatology. Behavioral family intervention has been shown to lower levels of dysfunctional parenting and improve parental competence for parents of preschoolers [86]. Barkley and colleagues [87], however, compared a school-year–long parent-training program and classroom interventions in a group of 158 kindergarten children who had inattention and disruptive behavior. Although the classroom intervention yielded improvements on direct observation of classroom behavior and teacher ratings of in-class attention, aggression, self-control, and social skills, neither intervention reduced problem behaviors at home.

Preschool parent training interventions have been studied outside the United States and across cultures. A study of 23 Taiwanese families found that a 10-week parent training intervention significantly improved ADHD and ODD symptoms in preschoolers [88]. In an Australian sample of 87 preschoolers who had ADHD, a behavioral family intervention program was associated with significant reductions in parent-reported child behavior problems and directly observed negative behavior [86]. Gains were maintained at 1-year follow-up, with 80% continuing to show clinical improvement. In contrast, Shelton and colleagues [89] reported that the 2-year posttreatment follow-up evidenced no enduring benefits.

Consistent with American Academy of Pediatrics [90] and American Academy of Child and Adolescent Psychiatry [91] recommendations for treating ADHD in young children, PATS preschoolers were eligible for medication treatment only if they showed no significant improvement in ADHD symptoms after a 10-week parent training program (Community Parent Education model [92]). Of the 261 subjects who completed parent training, only 7.2% showed significant improvement; however, the high ADHD symptom severity in these preschoolers may have been less responsive to psychosocial intervention alone.

The efficacy of parent training on preschool ADHD can be compromised by parental psychopathology. High levels and severity of maternal ADHD, for example, have been shown to limit the effectiveness of parent training interventions for preschoolers who have ADHD [93]. This effect remained after controlling for other aspects of maternal mental health and child functioning. Maternal depression [39] and ADHD in the parents also interferes with successful implementation of parent training interventions. Treating parental psychopathology is required to maximize the potential benefit from parent training programs [93].

Summary

Preschool ADHD is an impairing behavioral disorder, and it co-occurs with other serious psychiatric disorders. Early identification of ADHD and intervention may potentially minimize or prevent adverse outcomes and future pathology. Although data from studies of school-aged children have guided the use of stimulants in preschoolers, the limited safety and efficacy information on the short- and long-term effects of these medications in young children makes initiating pharmacotherapy a difficult decision for clinicians. The studies presented in this article suggest that methylphenidate is a moderately effective short-term treatment for preschoolers who have ADHD. Data evaluating dose-range parameters of extended-release formulations and the long-term impact of early medication treatment are needed to further inform clinical practice. Additional research on psychosocial interventions, including parent training and school-based interventions, is needed to determine which children may most likely benefit from them, how they compare with stimulant treatment, and the potential augmentative effect they may have when combined with pharmacotherapy. In general, understanding of this chronic and impairing disorder in preschoolers is growing and research into treatment options is encouraging. Much more research is needed to determine the most appropriate intervention for treating preschoolers who have ADHD.

References

[1] Bussing R, Zima BT, Perwien AR, et al. Children in special education programs: attention deficit hyperactivity disorder, use of services, and unmet needs. Am J Public Health 1998; 88(6):880–6.

[2] Cornelius JR, Pringle J, Jernigan J, et al. Correlates of mental health service utilization and unmet need among a sample of male adolescents. Addict Behav 2001;26(1):11–9.

[3] Leibson CL, Katusic SK, Barbaresi WJ, et al. Use and costs of medical care for children and adolescents with and without attention-deficit/hyperactivity disorder. JAMA 2001;285(1): 60–6.

[4] Kelleher KJ, McInerny TK, Gardner WP, et al. Increasing identification of psychosocial problems: 1979–1996. Pediatrics 2000;105:1313–21.

[5] Chan E, Zhan C, Homer CJ. Health care use and costs for children with attention-deficit/ hyperactivity disorder: national estimates from the medical expenditure panel survey. Arch Pediatr Adolesc Med 2002;156(5):504–11.

[6] Lahey BB, Pelham WE, Stein MA, et al. Validity of DSM-IV attention-deficit/hyperactivity disorder for younger children. J Am Acad Child Adolesc Psychiatry 1998;37(7):695–702.

[7] Rappley MD, Mullan PB, Alvarez FJ, et al. Diagnosis of attention-deficit/hyperactivity disorder and use of psychotropic medication in very young children. Arch Pediatr Adolesc Med 1999;153(10):1039–45.

[8] Pavuluri MN, Luk SL, McGee R. Help-seeking for behavior problems by parents of preschool children: a community study. J Am Acad Child Adolesc Psychiatry 1996;35(2): 215–22.

[9] Applegate B, Lahey BB, Hart EL, et al. Validity of the age-of-onset criterion for ADHD: a report from the DSM-IV field trials. J Am Acad Child Adolesc Psychiatry 1997;36(9):1211–21.

[10] Palfrey JS, Levine MD, Walker DK, et al. The emergence of attention deficits in early childhood: a prospective study. J Dev Behav Pediatr 1985;6(6):339–48.

[11] Campbell SB, Ewing LJ. Follow-up of hard-to-manage preschoolers: adjustment at age 9 and predictors of continuing symptoms. J Child Psychol Psychiatry 1990;31(6):871–89.

[12] Lavigne JV, Gibbons RD, Christoffel KK, et al. Prevalence rates and correlates of psychiatric disorders among preschool children. J Am Acad Child Adolesc Psychiatry 1996;35(2): 204–14.

[13] Richters JE, Arnold LE, Jensen PS, et al. NIMH collaborative multisite multimodal treatment study of children with ADHD: I. Background and rationale. J Am Acad Child Adolesc Psychiatry 1995;34(8):987–1000.

[14] Angold A, Erkanli A, Egger HL, et al. Stimulant treatment for children: a community perspective. J Am Acad Child Adolesc Psychiatry 2000;39(8):975–84 [discussion: 984–94].

[15] Keenan K, Wakschlag LS. More than the terrible twos: the nature and severity of behavior problems in clinic-referred preschool children. J Abnorm Child Psychol 2000;28(1):33–46.

[16] Barbaresi W, Katusic S, Colligan R, et al. How common is attention-deficit/hyperactivity disorder? Towards resolution of the controversy: results from a population-based study. Acta Paediatr Suppl 2004;93(445):55–9.

[17] Costello EJ, Angold A, Burns BJ, et al. The Great Smoky Mountains Study of Youth. Goals, design, methods, and the prevalence of DSM-III-R disorders. Arch Gen Psychiatry 1996; 53(12):1129–36.

[18] Polanczyk G, de Lima MS, Horta BL, et al. The worldwide prevalence of ADHD: a systematic review and metaregression analysis. Am J Psychiatry 2007;164(6):942–8.

[19] Egger HL, Angold A. The preschool age psychiatric assessment (PAPA): a structured parent interview for diagnosing psychiatric disorders in preschool children. In: DelCarmen-Wiggins R, Carter A, editors. Handbook of infant, toddler, and preschool mental assessment. New York: Oxford University Press; 2004.

[20] Wilens TE, Biederman J, Brown S, et al. Patterns of psychopathology and dysfunction in clinically referred preschoolers. J Dev Behav Pediatr 2002;23(1 Suppl):S31–6.

[21] Lahey BB, Pelham WE, Loney J, et al. Three-year predictive validity of DSM-IV attention deficit hyperactivity disorder in children diagnosed at 4-6 years of age. Am J Psychiatry 2004; 161(11):2014–20.

[22] Hardy KK, Kollins SH, Murray DW, et al. Factor structure of parent- and teacher-rated ADHD symptoms in preschoolers in the preschoolers with ADHD treatment study (PATS). J Child Adolesc Psychopharmacol 2007;17(5):621–34.

[23] Gimpel GA, Kuhn BR. Maternal report of attention deficit hyperactivity disorder symptoms in preschool children. Child Care Health Dev 2000;26(3):163–76 [discussion: 169–76].

[24] Lahey BB, Applegate B, McBurnett K, et al. DSM-IV field trials for attention deficit hyperactivity disorder in children and adolescents. Am J Psychiatry 1994;151(11):1673–85.

[25] American Psychiatric Association. Diagnostic and statistical manual of mental disorders. 4th edition. [text revision]. Washington, DC: American Psychiatric Association; 2000.

[26] DuPaul GJ, McGoey KE, Eckert TL, et al. Preschool children with attention-deficit/hyperactivity disorder: impairments in behavioral, social, and school functioning. J Am Acad Child Adolesc Psychiatry 2001;40(5):508–15.

[27] Angold A, Egger HL. Preschool psychopathlogy: lessons for the lifespan. Journal of Child Psychology and Psychiatry 2007;48(10):961–6.

[28] DiScala C, Lescohier I, Barthel M, et al. Injuries to children with attention deficit hyperactivity disorder. Pediatrics 1998;102(6):1415–21.

[29] Byrne JM, Bawden HN, Beattie T, et al. Risk for injury in preschoolers: relationship to attention deficit hyperactivity disorder. Child Neuropsychol 2003;9(2):142–51.

[30] Schwebel DC, Speltz ML, Jones K, et al. Unintentional injury in preschool boys with and without early onset of disruptive behavior. J Pediatr Psychol 2002;27(8):727–37.

[31] Wilens TE, Biederman J, Brown S, et al. Psychiatric comorbidity and functioning in clinically referred preschool children and school-age youths with ADHD. J Am Acad Child Adolesc Psychiatry 2002;41(3):262–8.

[32] Kadesjo B, Gillberg C. Attention deficits and clumsiness in Swedish 7-year-old children. Dev Med Child Neurol 1998;40(12):796–804.

[33] Posner K, Melvin GA, Murray DW, et al. Clinical presentation of ADHD in preschool children: preschoolers with ADHD treatment study (PATS). J Child Adolesc Psychopharmacol 2007;17(5):547–62.

[34] Thomas JM, Guskin KA. Disruptive behavior in young children: what does it mean? J Am Acad Child Adolesc Psychiatry 2001;40(1):44–51.

[35] McClellan JM, Speltz ML. Psychiatric diagnosis in preschool children. J Am Acad Child Adolesc Psychiatry 2003;42(2):127–8 [author reply: 128–30].

[36] Connor DF, Edwards G, Fletcher KE, et al. Correlates of comorbid psychopathology in children with ADHD. J Am Acad Child Adolesc Psychiatry 2003;42(2):193–200.

[37] Campbell SB. Parent-referred problem three-year-olds: developmental changes in symptoms. J Child Psychol Psychiatry 1987;28(6):835–45.

[38] Shelton TL, Barkley RA, Crosswait C, et al. Psychiatric and psychological morbidity as a function of adaptive disability in preschool children with aggressive and hyperactive-impulsive-inattentive behavior. J Abnorm Child Psychol 1998;26(6):475–94.

[39] Cunningham CE, Boyle MH. Preschoolers at risk for attention-deficit hyperactivity disorder and oppositional defiant disorder: family, parenting, and behavioral correlates. J Abnorm Child Psychol 2002;30(6):555–69.

[40] Pierce EW, Ewing LJ, Campbell SB. Diagnostic status and symptomatic behavior of hard-to-manage preschool children in middle childhood and early adolescence. J Clin Child Psychol 1999;28(1):44–57.

[41] McGee R, Prior M, Willams S, et al. The long-term significance of teacher-rated hyperactivity and reading ability in childhood: findings from two longitudinal studies. J Child Psychol Psychiatry 2002;43(8):1004–17.

[42] Wolraich ML, Lindgren S, Stromquist A, et al. Stimulant medication use by primary care physicians in the treatment of attention deficit hyperactivity disorder. Pediatrics 1990;86(1):95–101.

[43] Zito JM, Safer DJ, dosReis S, et al. Trends in the prescribing of psychotropic medications to preschoolers. JAMA 2000;283(8):1025–30.

[44] Greenhill LL. Drug Trend Report 2004. New York: Medco Health Solutions Inc.; 2004.

[45] Greenhill LL. The use of psychotropic medication in preschoolers: indications, safety, and efficacy. Can J Psychiatry 1998;43(6):576–81.

[46] Rappley MD, Eneli IU, Mullan PB, et al. Patterns of psychotropic medication use in very young children with attention-deficit hyperactivity disorder. J Dev Behav Pediatr 2002; 23(1):23–30.

[47] Zuvekas SH, Vitiello B, Norquist GS. Recent trends in stimulant medication use among U.S. children. Am J Psychiatry 2006;163(4):579–85.

[48] Arnold LE, Abikoff HB, Cantwell DP, et al. National Institute of Mental Health Collaborative Multimodal Treatment Study of Children with ADHD (the MTA). Design challenges and choices. Arch Gen Psychiatry 1997;54(9):865–70.

[49] Connor DF. Preschool attention deficit hyperactivity disorder: a review of prevalence, diagnosis, neurobiology, and stimulant treatment. J Dev Behav Pediatr 2002;23(1 Suppl):S1–9.

[50] Firestone P, Musten LM, Pisterman S, et al. Short-term side effects of stimulant medication are increased in preschool children with attention-deficit/hyperactivity disorder: a double-blind placebo-controlled study. J Child Adolesc Psychopharmacol 1998;8(1):13–25.

[51] Schleifer M, Weiss G, Cohen N, et al. Hyperactivity in preschoolers and the effect of methylphenidate. Am J Orthopsychiatry 1975;45(1):38–50.

[52] Conners CK. Controlled trial of methylphenidate in preschool children with minimal brain dysfunction. Journal of Mental Heath 1975;4:61–74.

[53] Cohen NJ, Sullivan J, Minde K, et al. Evaluation of the relative effectiveness of methylphenidate and cognitive behavior modification in the treatment of kindergarten-aged hyperactive children. J Abnorm Child Psychol 1981;9(1):43–54.

[54] Barkley RA, Karlsson J, Strzelecki E, et al. Effects of age and Ritalin dosage on the mother-child interactions of hyperactive children. J Consult Clin Psychol 1984;52(5):750–8.

[55] Barkley RA. The effects of methylphenidate on the interactions of preschool ADHD children with their mothers. J Am Acad Child Adolesc Psychiatry 1988;27(3):336–41.

[56] Mayes SD, Crites DL, Bixler EO, et al. Methylphenidate and ADHD: influence of age, IQ and neurodevelopmental status. Dev Med Child Neurol 1994;36(12):1099–107.

[57] Musten LM, Firestone P, Pisterman S, et al. Effects of methylphenidate on preschool children with ADHD: cognitive and behavioral functions. J Am Acad Child Adolesc Psychiatry 1997;36(10):1407–15.

[58] Handen BL, Feldman HM, Lurier A, et al. Efficacy of methylphenidate among preschool children with developmental disabilities and ADHD. J Am Acad Child Adolesc Psychiatry 1999;38(7):805–12.

[59] Short EJ, Manos MJ, Findling RL, et al. A prospective study of stimulant response in preschool children: insights from ROC analyses. J Am Acad Child Adolesc Psychiatry 2004;43(3):251–9.

[60] Riddle MA. Commentary by an academic child and adolescent psychiatrist. J Child Adolesc Psychopharmacol 2007;17(3):300–2.

[61] Kollins S, Greenhill L, Swanson J, et al. Rationale, design, and methods of the Preschool ADHD Treatment Study (PATS). J Am Acad Child Adolesc Psychiatry 2006;45(11): 1275–83.

[62] Greenhill L, Kollins S, Abikoff H, et al. Efficacy and safety of immediate-release methylphenidate treatment for preschoolers with ADHD. J Am Acad Child Adolesc Psychiatry 2006; 45(11):1284–93.

[63] MTA Cooperative Group. A 14-month randomized clinical trial of treatment strategies for attention-deficit/hyperactivity disorder. The MTA Cooperative Group. Multimodal Treatment Study of Children with ADHD. Arch Gen Psychiatry 1999;56(12):1073–86.

[64] Vitiello B, Abikoff H, Chuang SZ, et al. Effectiveness of methylphenidate in the 10-month continuation phase of the Preschoolers with ADHD Treatment Study (PATS). J Child Adolesc Psychopharmacol 2007;17(5):593–604.

[65] Wigal T, Greenhill L, Chuang S, et al. Safety and tolerability of methylphenidate in preschool children with ADHD. J Am Acad Child Adolesc Psychiatry 2006;45(11):1294–303.

[66] Swanson J, Greenhill L, Wigal T, et al. Stimulant-related reductions of growth rates in the PATS. J Am Acad Child Adolesc Psychiatry 2006;45(11):1304–13.

[67] National Institute of Mental Health Multimodal Treatment Study of ADHD follow-up: changes in effectiveness and growth after the end of treatment. Pediatrics 2004;113(4): 762–9.

[68] Wigal SB, Gupta S, Greenhill L, et al. Pharmacokinetics of methylphenidate in preschoolers with attention-deficit/hyperactivity disorder. J Child Adolesc Psychopharmacol 2007;17(2): 153–64.

[69] Ghuman JK, Riddle MA, Vitiello B, et al. Comorbidity moderates response to methylphenidate in the Preschoolers with Attention-Deficit/Hyperactivity Disorder Treatment Study (PATS). J Child Adolesc Psychopharmacol 2007;17(5):563–80.

[70] Abikoff H, Vitiello B, Riddle M, et al. Methylphenidate effects on functional outcomes in the Preschoolers with ADHD Treatment Study (PATS). J Child Adolesc Psychopharmacol 2007;17(5):581–92.

[71] Kratochvil CJ, Vaughan BS, Mayfield-Jorgensen ML, et al. A pilot study of atomoxetine in young children with attention-deficit/hyperactivity disorder. J Child Adolesc Psychopharmacol 2007;17(2):175–85.

[72] Schachar R, Jadad AR, Gauld M, et al. Attention-deficit hyperactivity disorder: critical appraisal of extended treatment studies. Can J Psychiatry 2002;47(4):337–48.

[73] Joshi SV. ADHD, growth deficits, and relationships to psychostimulant use. Pediatr Rev 2002;23(2):67–8 [discussion: 67–8].

[74] Safer D, Allen R, Barr E. Growth rebound after termination of stimulant drugs. J Pediatr 1975;86:113–6.

[75] Satterfield JH, Schell AM, Barb SD. Potential risk of prolonged administration of stimulant medication for hyperactive children. J Dev Behav Pediatr 1980;1(3):102–7.

[76] Gadow KD, Sverd J, Sprafkin J, et al. Long-term methylphenidate therapy in children with comorbid attention-deficit hyperactivity disorder and chronic multiple tic disorder. Arch Gen Psychiatry 1999;56(4):330–6.

[77] Diagnosis and treatment of attention deficit hyperactivity disorder (ADHD). NIH Consens Statement 1998;16(2):1–37.

[78] Pelham WE Jr, Wheeler T, Chronis A. Empirically supported psychosocial treatments for attention deficit hyperactivity disorder. J Clin Child Psychol 1998;27(2):190–205.

[79] Campbell SB. Behavior problems in preschool children: a review of recent research. J Child Psychol Psychiatry 1995;36(1):113–49.

[80] Marks DJ, Burwid OG, Santra A, et al. Neuropsychological correlates of ADHD symptoms in preschoolers. Neuropsychology 2005;19(4):446–55.

[81] Keown LJ, Woodward LJ. Early parent-child relations and family functioning of preschool boys with pervasive hyperactivity. J Abnorm Child Psychol 2002;30(6):541–53.

[82] Sonuga-Barke EJ, Daley D, Thompson M, et al. Parent-based therapies for preschool attention-deficit/hyperactivity disorder: a randomized, controlled trial with a community sample. J Am Acad Child Adolesc Psychiatry 2001;40(4):402–8.

[83] Strayhorn JM, Weidman C. Reduction of attention deficit and internalizing symptoms in preschoolers through parent-child interaction training. J Am Acad Child Adolesc Psychiatry 1989;28(6):888–96.

[84] Corrin EG. Child group training versus parent and child group training for young children with ADHD. Dissertation Abstracts International: Section B: The Sciences & Engineering. Vol. 64; 2004.

[85] Pisterman S, Firestone P, McGrath P, et al. The role of parent training in treatment of preschoolers with ADDH. Am J Orthopsychiatry 1992;62(3):397–408.

[86] Bor W, Sanders MR, Markie-Dadds C. The effects of the triple p-positive parenting program on preschool children with co-occurring disruptive behavior and attentional/hyperactive difficulties. J Abnorm Child Psychol 2002;30(6):571–87.

[87] Barkley RA, Shelton TL, Crosswait C, et al. Multi-method psycho-educational intervention for preschool children with disruptive behavior: preliminary results at post-treatment. J Child Psychol Psychiatry 2000;41(3):319–32.

[88] Huang HL, Chao CC, Tu CC, et al. Behavioral parent training for Taiwanese parents of children with attention-deficit/hyperactivity disorder. Psychiatry Clin Neurosci 2003;57(3): 275–81.

[89] Shelton TL, Barkley RA, Crosswait C, et al. Multimethod psychoeducational intervention for preschool children with disruptive behavior: two-year post-treatment follow-up. J Abnorm Child Psychol 2000;28(3):253–66.

[90] American Academy of Pediatrics. Clinical practice guideline: treatment of the school-aged child with attention-deficit/hyperactivity disorder. J Pediatr 2001;108(4):1033–44.

[91] American Academy of Child and Adolescent Psychiatry. Practice parameters for the assessment and treatment of children, adolescents, and adults with attention-deficit/hyperactivity disorder. J Am Acad Child Adolesc Psychiatry 1997;36:85S–125S.

[92] Cunningham CE, Boyle M, Offord D, et al. Tri-ministry study: correlates of school-based parenting course utilization. J Consult Clin Psychol 2000;68(5):928–33.

[93] Sonuga-Barke EJ, Daley D, Thompson M. Does maternal ADHD reduce the effectiveness of parent training for preschool children's ADHD? J Am Acad Child Adolesc Psychiatry 2002; 41(6):696–702.

[94] Strayhorn JM, Weidman CS. Follow-up one year after parent-child interaction training: effects on behavior of preschool children. J Am Acad Child Adolesc Psychiatry 1991; 30(1):138–43.

ELSEVIER
SAUNDERS

Child Adolesc Psychiatric Clin N Am
17 (2008) 367–384

CHILD AND
ADOLESCENT
PSYCHIATRIC CLINICS
OF NORTH AMERICA

Executive Dysfunction and Delay Aversion in Attention Deficit Hyperactivity Disorder: Nosologic and Diagnostic Implications

Edmund J.S. Sonuga-Barke, PhD[a,b,c,*],
Joseph A. Sergeant, PhD[d], Joel Nigg, PhD[e],
Erik Willcutt, PhD[f]

[a]School of Psychology, Institute for Disorder on Impulse and Attention,
University of Southampton, Highfield, Southampton SO17 1BJ, UK
[b]Child Study Center, New York University, New York, NY 10016, USA
[c]Social, Genetic, Developmental Psychiatry Centre, Institute of Psychiatry,
University of London, London SE5 8AF, UK
[d]Department of Neuropsychology, Clinical Neuropsychology, Vrije Unviersiteit Amsterdam,
Van der Boechorstraat 1, 1081 Amsterdam, Netherlands
[e]Department of Psychology, Michigan State University, 300 Spartan Way,
202B Psychology Building, East Lansing, MI 48824-1116, USA
[f]Department of Psychology, University of Colorado, Muenzinger D244,
345 UCB, Boulder, CO 80309, USA

The questions at the core of this article are twofold: (1) do neuropsychological markers of underlying pathophysiology have value in the diagnosis of attention deficit hyperactivity disorder (ADHD) and (2) if not, under what conditions would they? These two questions are particularly relevant now as revisions of the *Diagnostic and Statistical Manual of Mental Disorders* (DSM) and ICD classifications of mental disorders are considered [1–3]. Can value be added to diagnostic criteria in these revised manuals by grounding them in laboratory tests arguably less prone to reporter effects,

Potential conflicts of interest: Dr. Sonuga-Barke is a consultant, serves on the speakers' bureau, and is an advisory board member for UCB Pharma; an advisory board member for Shire; and is on the speaker panel for and received a research grant from Janssen-Cilag. Dr. Sergeant serves on the advisory board for Lilly, received a research grant from and is an advisory board member for Shire. Drs. Nigg and Willcutt have no potential conflicts to report.

* Corresponding author. School of Psychology, University of Southampton, Highfield, Southampton SO17 1BJ, UK.
E-mail address: ejb3@soton.ac.uk (E.J.S. Sonuga-Barke).

childpsych.theclinics.com

or will they remain rooted in the phenomenology of the subjective perception (although obtained with objectively scored cutoffs) of symptoms and associated impairment? The answer to this question depends entirely on the state of the science of ADHD. This article reviews evidence in relation to two mechanisms within two separate domains of functioning. One is primarily cognitive, namely executive function (EF) deficits, and the other is primarily motivational, namely delay aversion (DAv). This article does not include all potential neuropsychological markers. Potential markers in other areas of interest, such as millisecond timing deficits [4], state regulation failures [5], intra-individual fluctuations in performance over time [6], and altered sensitivity to stimulation [7], are not addressed, although each represents a construct of some potential value as a diagnostic marker for future taxonomic systems. This article rather presents a selective review of perhaps the two most promising, or at least the two most-studied, markers in terms of their empiric basis in the literature. If the evidence does not support the inclusion of these classes of markers in the revised DSM systems, then it will unlikely do so for others at this juncture.

Executive function deficits in attention deficit hyperactivity disorder

Definition and theory

The concept of EF has been difficult to define definitively and continues to evolve. A generally accepted conception is that it represents a class of higher-order cognitive abilities that are associated with the activity of the prefrontal cortex and one of several functionally segregated but neuroanatomically proximate brain circuits connecting cortical foci, basal ganglia, and thalamic nuclei [8]. This circuit (ie, the executive circuit) links the prefrontal cortex to the dorsal neostriatum (preferentially the caudate nucleus) with reciprocal excitatory connections back up to cortical regions through the dorsomedial sections of the thalamus. EF has been defined as "ability to maintain an appropriate problem-solving set for attainment of a future goal" [9].

Whether EF reflects a unitary process, or rather the accumulation of several lower order processes only, is still undecided. Component processes may involve response inhibition, set shifting, and working memory updating [10], among others [11]. Response suppression and working memory are perhaps the two critical elements of EF most studied in relation to ADHD. These operations depend on a function more commonly referred to now as *cognitive control*, which refers to the ability to exert top-down control (ie, what is observed in neuroimaging to correspond with prefrontal activation in conjunction with suppression of activation in posterior cortex or subcortical regions) to overcome stimulus triggers or affect arousal to achieve a goal end point held in working memory [12,13].

Control, however, must be activated. This activation also requires bottom-up signaling about current events and their match to expectations from subcortical circuits, especially in striatum and cerebellum [14]. Most

EF tasks used to assess impairment determine whether a control operation has failed but do not sort out whether it failed because of ineffective top-down processing or bottom-up signaling that should have recruited the top-down activity. Experimental paradigms developed in the cognitive neurosciences have now begun to map these control operations with considerable precision to particular regions of prefrontal cortex, and their intersection with attentional functions in dorsal and ventral networks in parietal cortex. Many of these paradigms, validated through functional neuroimaging data, have not been examined extensively in relation to ADHD or in large enough samples to evaluate their potential clinical usefulness. Thus, a major gap at this stage is that the literature available for meta-analyses [15] still relies primarily on clinical measures developed for detecting brain damage and not for assessing subtle problems in cognitive control theorized to exist in ADHD. More recent and potentially more sensitive measures have not been heavily studied. Therefore, whether maximal effect sizes have been measured with the existing clinical measures is unclear.

Furthermore, developmental dynamics are crucial because the brain circuits implicated in EF develop throughout childhood and adolescence, gaining increasing specialization as myelination and pruning of circuitry unfolds [16–20]. These processes mature at varying rates in different cortical and subcortical areas, with the regions of prefrontal cortex that are most important for cognitive control completing synaptic specialization the latest [21,22].

Recently, ADHD has been seen primarily as a disorder of dysregulation of cognition, action, and cognitive–energetic state associated with the disruption of neurocognitive control, or in other words, an EF deficit disorder broadly defined [23]. Although nonexecutive processes have been implicated in the disorder [24], the boldest models could be called strong executive dysfunction models because they view brain-behavior relations as fully mediated by neuropsychological deficits in EF. In the most influential model of this sort, Barkley [25] provided a detailed account suggesting that the general pattern of executive impairment associated with ADHD is grounded in more-specific early appearing deficits in response inhibition. Response inhibition refers to the ability to inhibit an inappropriate prepotent or dominant response in favor of a more appropriate alternative (ie, referring to top-down control). It is now known to rely on a region in the right inferior frontal gyrus [26] and associated subcortical regions. In Barkley's [25] model, establishing an inhibition faculty was regarded as a necessary precondition for the development of a broad range of regulatory and executive competencies.

From a clinical standpoint, the concept of EF, as currently used, may seem both abstract and poorly delimited. Clinicians who feel comfortable using concepts related to either general intelligence or specific cognitive functions (eg, short-term memory) may nevertheless have difficulty with the concept of EF. Furthermore, although broadly implicated in a range of disorders (eg, ADHD, autism, conduct disorder, schizophrenia), EF deficits at this stage seem to lack the disease specificity needed to be of practical value in the therapeutic setting. The clinical research goal is therefore to better define the boundaries of the concept, and the interaction and overlap among its subcomponents, such as inhibition, planning, and working memory, and other aspects of cognition, and then to determine EF's specific relevance to ADHD as opposed to other disorders. This article provides an account of progress toward these goals.

Empirical evidence for executive function deficits
in attention deficit hyperactivity disorder

Barkley's [25] seminal model made strong claims, many of which have yet to be really tested, about the interplay of cognitive control and other abilities. However, it provides a useful starting point because it is currently the most fully articulated cognitive model of the mechanisms in ADHD. Although not stated by Barkley, who previously pointed out that EF problems are not universal in ADHD [27], many researchers have implicitly assumed a unitary theory of ADHD in which EF deficits, if they are core to the disorder, should also be identifiable in all cases of ADHD. This supposition is almost certainly wrong, as clinical practice and recent literature have shown.

Data from neuroimaging and psychopharmacologic studies (structural and functional) provide some circumstantial evidence for the EF deficit model of ADHD at the group level. Structural studies suggest volumetric anomalies in the dorsolateral prefrontal and anterior cingulate cortex [28] at effect sizes similar to those seen in behavioral literature (equivalent to approximately a 10% reduction in volume in key regions at the group level). In addition, functional studies show hypofrontality [29], sometimes with large effect sizes. However, effects are not specific to what are assumed to be the executive brain circuits [30], suggesting that more refined and comprehensive conceptualization of the nature of neural dysfunction is needed.

The evidence from clinical neuropsychological data supports the view that EF deficits, although found in some, perhaps many, individuals among groups of children and adults who have ADHD, are not a necessary feature of ADHD and therefore do not have diagnostic value for the DSM-defined syndrome [3]. Two key recent publications, one a meta-analysis [15] and the other an examination of EF deficits in a large sample of children who have ADHD assessed across multiple EF domains using a broad-based battery of tasks [14], amplify this point. The meta-analysis showed only moderate pooled effect size estimates (eg, Cohen's d < .7) for even the most discriminating measures used to date (eg, inhibitory control and working memory).

The second had two key findings. First, only a subpopulation of children who had ADHD had putative clinically significant impairment on any one executive task (ie, they had worse scores than 90% of controls on that task). The most discriminating tasks (again tapping inhibitory control) identified approximately 50% of children who had ADHD as impaired. Second, a pattern of severe and pervasive impairment (as might be predicted by a model of general collapse of EF) was present in only a minority of ADHD cases (ie, only approximately 10% of ADHD cases displayed impairment on four or more different EF measures), although this may be partly because of measurement weaknesses on some tasks.

A more recent review of the literature by Sergeant and colleagues [3] raised additional questions. First, children and (to a lesser extent) adults who have ADHD [31] can be distinguished from individuals who undergo typical development on many clinical EF measures at the group level. However, considerable variation exists between measures in how much they discriminate. This variation could be from artifact (eg, differential reliability, excessive task-specific variance) or real differences in signal regarding core problems. Friedman and colleagues [10] showed that a latent variable approach to EF may yield more reliable measures that relate more strongly to measures of ADHD. Although previous studies reported small correlations among individual EF tasks and ADHD symptoms ($r = 0.1–0.3$) [32], these authors reported stronger relations between teacher ratings of attention problems and a latent trait measure of response inhibition. This latent variable approach has been used little with ADHD, although Nigg and colleagues [33] found approximately the same effect sizes as cited in Willcutt and colleagues [15] using a latent variable approach across EF domains.

As Sergeant and colleagues [3] noted, the largest effects are observed for spatial working memory [34], with moderate discrimination on response inhibition [15]. All of these effects, however, were at approximately $d = 1.0$ or smaller, which is nowhere near adequate for clinically relevant sensitivity or specificity [27].

Second, Sergeant and colleagues [3] raised the question of the cognitive specificity of the EF effects in ADHD. For example, case-control differences in general intelligence quotient are substantial, as are differences on other non-EF measures. Poor ADHD performance on EF tasks may simply be an epiphenomenon of some other more basic problem [24,35]. In contrast, the ability to integrate multiple low level functions may be the core of EF problems in ADHD and so will not be identified through studies of modular functions alone. Answering this conundrum requires testing of more advanced process models of cognition than have typically been operationalized in ADHD research.

Third, how should the apparent lack of clinical specificity of EF deficits to ADHD be understood? Pennington and Ozonoff [11] identified key domains of EF, such as response inhibition and planning, that seemed to be specific to ADHD. However, evidence exists of EF effects in conduct disorder [36,37] and in high-functioning autism [38,39]; these seem to hold when ADHD is covaried. Of course, both disorders are heavily comorbid with ADHD (nearly all children who have conduct disorder also meet criteria for ADHD, as do at least half of children who have HFA). What is the correct statistical or developmental understanding of this nonspecificity? Does EF lead to different disorders under different contexts? Is EF a "gateway" deficit that can emanate in multiple outcomes? Or is ADHD an early stage of conduct disorder, and autism in some cases a severe form of ADHD? Alternatively, and on the more prosaic side, is EF simply an epiphenomenon of many disorders? These fundamental nosologic questions have barely been examined. Additional studies are needed with direct comparisons in which distinct components of EF are compared across different clinical and subclinical comorbidities.

Fourth, Sergeant and colleagues [3] pointed out that small—although not necessarily clinically relevant—differences exist between (some) ADHD subtypes. Most studies could not differentiate ADHD-I (predominantly inattentive type) from ADHD-C (combined type) (Refs. [40–43]), although this may be because of reliance on DSM-IV criteria, which do not strongly separate the groups clinically (ie, children who are hyperactive but shy of cutoff for combined type are typically placed in the "primarily inattentive" group, this problem is beyond the scope of this article). Better discrimination was found in the review by Sergeant and colleagues [3] of ADHD predominantly hyperactive–impulsive type versus ADHD inattentive type. This finding would be consistent with the idea that EF is related primarily to inattentive rather than hyperactive–impulsive symptoms. Nevertheless, the effect sizes for these comparisons remain small, suggesting that ADHD subtypes are not currently optimized to identify groups with differences in cognitive mechanism related to EF.

In summary, EF deficits are associated with ADHD but are not a necessary condition of its diagnosis. ADHD is most likely neuropsychologically heterogeneous. Thus, many children who have ADHD undoubtedly do not have a clinically observable EF deficit. Furthermore, children who have other disorders and those who have none also display deficits on EF tasks [38], suggesting that EF interacts with other predisposing factors to contribute to ADHD, that more refined analysis of component operations is needed, or that EF is a gateway problem that exposes children to risk for more disorders than ADHD, depending on other factors.

Delay aversion in attention deficit hyperactivity disorder

Definition and theory

Renewed interest has recently been shown in the role of motivational dysfunction in ADHD, partly because EF deficits do not fully explain the disorder [44]. A need exists to discover what processes mediate the underlying causes of ADHD in children unimpaired by executive dysfunction if EF deficits occur in only some children who have ADHD. Motivational dysfunction represents a plausible candidate.

Luman and colleagues [45] recently reviewed this literature and considered a range of motivational hypotheses implicating different parameters and processes in ADHD. The most striking result of their review was the largely inconclusive nature of the empiric research in relation to motivational dysfunction in ADHD. With possibly one exception, the database—when taken as a whole—provides no conclusive evidence of motivational dysfunction in ADHD. Instead, overall results suggest that effects of motivational factors are often not restricted to children who have ADHD, with similar effects often seen in unaffected children. Interestingly, several studies present examples of new, promising, but largely unexplored, avenues of enquiry [46–48].

The DAv hypothesis may represent an exception to this generally disappointing picture. The concept of DAv has evolved since its introduction in the early 1990s [49]. It is now probably best regarded as an integrated motivational framework whereby the established preference of immediate over delayed rewards by children who have ADHD is just one expression of a broader motivational style. According to the most recent accounts [49], DAv has several key elements.

First, it is grounded in the neurocircuitry of catecholamine-modulated brain reward circuits [50,51]. These circuits are functionally segregated from the executive circuits described earlier and link the ventral striatum (in particular the nucleus accumbens) to frontal regions (especially the anterior cingulate and orbitofrontal cortex), reciprocated by way of the ventral pallidum and related structures through the thalamus. The amygdala is also implicated in this system, possibly playing a role in defining the motivational significance of incentives [52]. Dopamine is again a key neuromodulator [53]. This circuit is specifically implicated in signaling rewards, coding incentive value, and regulating other behavioral processes involved in the maintenance of responding under conditions of delayed rewards [50].

Second, DAv is driven by fundamental impairments in the neural signaling of delayed rewards that lead to steeper discounting of delayed rewards associated with failures to choose future rewards, a feature emphasized in an alternative but related model of ADHD mechanism suggested by Sagvolden and colleagues [54].

Third, DAv is compounded by a pattern of delay-related negative affect acquired during development as the delay-impaired child learns to associate delay settings with censure and failure [55]. This pattern leads to a motivation to escape or avoid delay. In combination with the prior point, then, choosing small immediate rewards over large delayed rewards is controlled by two components: an unconditional preference for immediacy linked to deficits in signaling future rewards, and the escape or avoidance of acquired negative affect associated with delay. These components combine to create a marked preference for immediacy over delay [56].

Fourth, DAv is expressed in various settings in different ways as a function of whether delay can be escaped or must be tolerated and modified [57]. When a choice is available, children who have DAv will choose small immediate over large delayed rewards. However, when no choice is available and delay is imposed, DAv is hypothesized to be expressed as increased activity, inattention, or frustration, especially when this imposition of delay is unexpected.

Empirical evidence for delay aversion in attention deficit hyperactivity disorder

Choosing small immediate over large delayed rewards on simple laboratory choice tasks is regarded as the signal indicator of DAv, although this choice could be made because of several mechanisms, including poor EF. The evidence in relation to this concept has recently been reviewed [2]. Individuals who have ADHD can be satisfactorily differentiated from controls in their choices of small immediate over large delayed rewards with pooled effect sizes (Hedge's g) for one type of task—the Maudsley Index of Delay Aversion [58]—of 0.57 (625 individuals who had ADHD versus 349 controls; with 57% and 74% preference for the large reward, respectively [56,58–60]), and for another—The Choice Delay Task [48]—of 0.71 (230 individuals who had ADHD versus 409 controls; with 42% and 61% mean preference for the large reward, respectively [49,61–64]) (E. Willcutt, personal communication, 2006).

These effect sizes are similar to the more discriminating tasks reported in the meta-analysis of EF deficits in ADHD by Willcutt and colleagues [15] and the meta-analysis of working memory in ADHD reported by Martinussen and colleagues [34], both of which ranged from $d = 0.6$ to 0.8, except for spatial working memory, which was approximately $d = 1.0$. Thus, the DAv effects, like the EF effects, are too small to be clinically diagnostic of DSM-defined cases but may pertain to a meaningful subgroup. The notion that the choice of immediate small over large delayed rewards is the result of two processes is also supported by a recent large-scale study examining the effects of pre- and post-reward delay on choice for delayed rewards [56]. Children who had ADHD chose the immediate reward more than controls under both conditions, but this preference was greater when no postreward delay was present and overall delay could be avoided. Data from several sources also support DAv in ADHD as a broad-based motivational style. For instance, children who have ADHD respond inappropriately to the unexpected imposition of delay [65] and extinction of reward [66]; prematurely disengage from long and challenging tasks [67]; show more activity than controls during delay [68]; are biased toward task responses associated with immediate rewards [69]; are unusually vigilant to environmental delay-related cues [70]; prefer reward immediacy to high reward rate or task ease [71]; discount future hypothetical rewards (although one report provides a countercase for this finding [72]); and are differentially affected by slow event rates/sparse schedules [73,74]. However, these effects are at the group level, not individual diagnostic effects.

In summary, DAv seems to be an associate of ADHD, not only when narrowly defined in terms of preference for small immediate over large delayed reward but also when defined in terms of a broader motivational style. However, like EF deficits, DAv is only moderately associated with ADHD and therefore, like EF deficits, is likely to affect only a subgroup of ADHD cases. Compared with the studies undertaken in EF deficits, little or no study has been undertaken of the clinical specificity or the links to current clinical subtypes (however, one study provides evidence of specificity vis-a-vis high functioning autistic children [59]). Currently no published imaging studies evaluate the role of ventral/dorsal dysregulation in relation DAv. However, a recent study by Scheres and colleagues [75] suggests hypoactivation in the ventral striatum in ADHD in response to cues for reward. More studies of this nature are crucial for validating the broader claims of the DAv hypothesis.

The relationship between delay aversion and executive function deficits in attention deficit hyperactivity disorder: additive and/or synergistic effects

Based on the earlier analysis and review, both DAv and EF deficits are neurobiologically plausible and empirically supported impairments in ADHD. Each may represent a mechanism-based pathway that can result in ADHD. However, each probably affects only a subset of children who have ADHD as this disorder is currently defined. To understand the implication of this heterogeneity for ADHD nosology and diagnosis, the relationship between DAv and EF deficits must be established. Perhaps they are two different manifestations of the same underlying pathophysiology shared by the same subset of children who have ADHD. For instance, DAv therefore may really only be an alternative manifestation of the inhibitory problems, part of EF deficits, described earlier. On the other hand, they may be distinct impairments with little overlap other than that which would occur by chance, mirroring the functional segregation of the neural circuitry of the executive and reward systems that is hypothesized to be at their core [76–78]. Perhaps they are independent but related processes that act additively or interactively to produce ADHD.

Solanto and colleagues [62] were the first to address this issue through administering an EF (stop-signal task) and DAv measure (choice delay task) to a group of children who had ADHD. They found that although the key indictors of the two tasks (stop-signal reaction time and proportion of large delayed choices) were largely uncorrelated, they both were associated with ADHD. This pattern of associations meant that four distinct groups of children could be identified using a cutoff of worse than 90% of the control group [33]: 23% had only an inhibitory deficit; 15% had DAv only; 23% showed both characteristics; and 39% had neither deficit. DAv and EF deficits seemed to be dissociable constructs implicated in ADHD but often affecting a different subpopulation of cases. The independent association of EF and DAv has since been replicated [79,80], extended to other motivational systems such as the "hot" cognition involved in decision making [48], and validated in animal models of impulsiveness and aggression [81].

Although initially the distinction between EF deficits and DAv may seem too subtle and esoteric to be of clinical value, the data described earlier highlight the possible potential for differentiating groups of children based on different neuropsychological impairment profiles. This possibility recently motivated the development of several proposed multiple pathway/process models, including models of specific distinct origins [82,83]. Most relevant to this article, however, is the dual-pathway hypothesis concerning mechanisms in ADHD [55,57,84]. The dual-pathway model states that alterations within the EF circuit modulated by mesocortical dopamine and the reward circuit modulated by mesolimbic dopamine constitute more or less discrete neuropsychological bases for dissociable psychological processes leading to EF deficits and DAv, respectively. In turn, Sonuga-Barke [84] hypothesized that cognitive control problems may contribute to inattentive symptoms, and motivational problems to hyperactive impulsive symptoms. Preliminary data support that supposition [85]. Clinically, this model would be consistent with the idea that different neuropsychological subtypes would be subsumed under the overall ADHD umbrella.

Nonetheless, simple models, such as proposed in the dual-pathway hypothesis, are clearly inadequate to fully account for the heterogeneity and complexity of ADHD. First, although in initial models the two pathways were presented as independent factors acting additively [84], more recent accounts have recognized the likelihood of synergistic interactions between motivational and cognitive factors [44,55,57]. These synergies could have a developmental or biologic basis. For instance, during development DAv can create the context for the development of EF deficits, because this motivational style limits the opportunity for children to consolidate the EF skills required to exploit time on extended tasks. Alternatively, as Barkley [25] argued, weakness in EF could result in expression of motivational problems because of lack of top-down control.

Synergies between EF and motivational factors are also likely at the neurobiologic level [44]. Haber [86] argued that nonreciprocal cascading basal ganglia circuits allow cross-talk among the segregated frontostriatal loops that allow the transfer of information from motivational, to cognitive, to motor programs. These neurobiologic synergies could be crucial for understanding the relationship between motivation and cognition in ADHD, although they remain speculative.

Second, and perhaps more importantly, a substantial minority of children who have ADHD seem to be unaffected by either DAv or EF impairments. Identifying the basis for ADHD in these cases is an important goal of future research. Are these patients misdiagnosed, expressing difficulty adapting to a difficult context but lacking an internal dysfunction as required in the DSM-type models of psychopathology [87]? Or do they have yet another cognitive impairment such as state dysregulation or temporal information processing deficits? Studies underway in the authors' laboratories will clarify that question.

Do markers of executive function deficits and delay aversion have diagnostic value for attention deficit hyperactivity disorder?

So should neuropsychological markers of ADHD pathophysiology be incorporated into future diagnostic systems, and if so, how? This issue has been studied most comprehensively for EF, but the case is likely to be very similar for DAv and probably for other future candidate mechanisms. With EF deficits, heterogeneity within ADHD and their overlap across ADHD and other disorders means that tests of EF will inevitably lack the specificity required for diagnostic markers of ADHD if it continues to be defined solely on the basis of the current behavioral criteria [88], adding little in terms of diagnostic efficiency to current symptom-based approaches.

However, the field–trial approach of evaluating incremental validity of individual symptoms has not been implemented with cognitive measures, and therefore the empiric question remains whether they will provide added value regarding an external criterion, such as identifying impaired children. Such studies seem important. Biederman and colleagues [89] noted that even though children who had ADHD with and without EF problems had similar levels of ADHD symptoms, those who had EF problems had worse academic outcomes. Biederman and colleagues [90] found the same thing in adults who had ADHD. Stavro and colleagues [91] showed that EF overlapped with symptoms of inattention (but not hyperactivity) as a route to functional impairment in adults who had ADHD. Therefore, further examination of the clinical usefulness of EF measures in value-added prediction of impairment and other clinical indicators seems warranted.

Similarly, although DAv, seen either as a choice of small immediate over large delayed reward or as a more broadly based motivational style, seems to be a promising marker of motivational dysfunction in ADHD, like EF deficits, it is only moderately associated with ADHD but is not a necessary basis for ADHD, with only a minority of cases affected. However, its clinical usefulness as a marker of outcome, treatment response, or other clinical indicators remains largely untested.

Therefore, neither DAv or EF deficits are a diagnostic marker of ADHD as it is currently conceptualized. Their clinical usefulness in providing value-added information on impairment, outcome, or treatment response remains largely untested.

Regarding taxonomy, the next important thing to recognize is that although cognitive and motivational factors will inevitably interact at many levels [14], DAv and EF deficits seem to be partially dissociable in their relationship to ADHD (ie, some children show one and not the other characteristic), with each having predictive power independent of the other. At the same time, other patterns of impairment, such as deficits in millisecond timing [4] or impairments in fundamental non-EF deficits [24], may mark something distinctive about the psychopathophysiology of other subgroups of children who have ADHD unaffected by either EF deficits and DAv.

One strategy worth exploring is to combine different measures of dissociable constructs, such as DAv and EF, to try to maximize the predictive/diagnostic power of tests. When Solanto and colleagues [62] used this strategy, they saw a substantial increase in both specificity and sensitivity. Adding markers of other constructs independently associated with ADHD could only improve this picture. What is crucial from a clinical perspective, however, and is currently unknown, is the extent to which such an approach would be equally successful in differentiating between ADHD and different disorders. Little is known about the differential diagnostic credentials of DAv, but the review described earlier in relation to EF is not encouraging [3].

Therefore, if the neuropsychology of ADHD may not differentiate ADHD from other clinical conditions in the consulting room, what is its value? For one thing, these behavioral findings have already guided neuroimaging and genetic work and continue to influence understanding of the mechanisms of current and proposed treatments. Furthermore, and crucial to the authors' argument, including markers of key domains of dysfunction or impairment in diagnostic systems, such as EF deficits and DAv, could help parse the heterogeneity of the disorder and therefore be crucial in the future refinement of ADHD nosology. This strategy may have clinical payoffs with regard to characterizing subgroups, which could lead to important developments in diagnosing and assessing ADHD and help provide more tailored interventions guided to the needs of individual children. However, establishing the efficacy of tailored intervention is challenging [92] and remains speculative.

Exactly how this result is achieved will depend on how the relationship between domains of impairment and clinical symptoms is conceptualized. This relationship has been typically considered in deterministic and mechanistic terms. That is, the underlying EF or DAv impairment is seen as directly mediating the link between alternations in brain structure and symptomatic expression as captured, for instance, in the dual-pathway model of ADHD [50] and other multicomponent models [82,93]. The assumption is that these causal pathways give rise to psychopathophysiologic subtypes of ADHD, for example, a DAv ADHD subtype and an EF deficit subtype of ADHD. In turn, these mechanistic subtypes might lead to distinct etiologies, as outlined in detail by Nigg [82], which could then suggest specific treatment interventions and prognosis. The results of a recent study by Thorell [80] showing that EF deficits, but not DAv, is associated with the failures to develop preacademic skills illustrates this possibility nicely.

An alternative and less-narrowly drawn way of conceptualizing the relationship between ADHD symptoms and psychopathophysiology is in terms of dissociable but overlapping impairment dimensions (eg, DAv and EF deficits) operating at a different conceptual level to symptom-based definitions of syndromes (eg, ADHD, conduct disorder, autism) in a way that allows for the nonexclusive mapping of different impairment dimensions and syndromes. In this model, no causal role is specified for the impairment in relation to any particular condition. In clinical terms, the overlap at these different levels then might be characterized in terms of complicating clinical features rather than subtypes. In this sense, DAv or EF deficits may be considered comorbidities affecting subgroups of children who have ADHD and those who also have other disorders rather than subtypes.

Whichever way DAv and EF deficits (subtypes or comorbidities) are considered, a practical way may exist to move forward in relation to psychopathophysiological diagnostic markers. A new axis within diagnostic manuals may be useful for specifying key pathophysiological dimensions associated with ADHD that may be significant for characterizing and treating children who have ADHD at an individual level but for whom insufficient evidence exists for establishing new diagnostic categories or subtypes. This axis would usefully include reference to both cognitive and motivational markers.

Summary

The study of the neuropsychology of ADHD and its broader pathophysiology has the potential to greatly influence the nosology and eventually the diagnosis of ADHD. However, the apparent heterogeneity of ADHD at the neuropsychological level and the overlap shown with other disorders means that, as currently conceived, no individual neuropsychological markers exist that would add to diagnostic efficiency, if the goal is to identify the behavioral syndrome defined by DSM-IV. However, other goals may be as worthy. Some objectives to be addressed in future research include the following:

- Establish the stability of neuropsychological markers, such as DAv and EF deficits, as dysfunctional traits over time and context,
- Determine population norms for neuropsychological markers and establish algorithms for clinical thresholds,
- Identify the most diagnostically efficient and cost-effective test measures for neuropsychological markers,
- Test the relationship between different disorders and neuropsychological markers,
- Gauge the clinical significance of neuropsychological markers (incremental validity beyond behavioral symptoms, comorbidity, long-term outcome, and treatment response) and how it varies according to disorder type,
- Validate neuropsychological markers by studying their functional neuroanatomy.

Work is underway in many laboratories, and the future is likely to bring further insights. What is important at this stage is to recognize the potential in considering this level of analysis along with behavioral features in defining the disorder over time.

References

[1] Stefanatos GA, Baron IS. Attention-deficit/hyperactivity disorder: a neuropsychological perspective towards DSM-V. Neuropsychol Rev 2007;17:5–38.

[2] Sonuga-Barke EJS. What role, if any, should markers of motivational dysfunction play in the diagnosis of attention deficit hyperactivity disorder? In: Shaffer D, Leibenluft E, Rohde LA, et al, editors. Externalizing disorders of childhood: refining the research agenda for DSM-V. Arlington (VA): American Psychiatric Association, in press.

[3] Sergeant JA, Willcutt E, Nigg J. How clinically functional are executive function measures of ADHD? In: Shaffer D, Leibenluft E, Rohde LA, et al, editors. Externalizing disorders of childhood: refining the research agenda for DSM-V. Arlington (VA): American Psychiatric Association, in press.

[4] Toplak ME, Dockstader C, Tannock R. Temporal information processing in ADHD: findings to date and new methods. J Neurosci Methods 2006;151(1):15–29.

[5] Sergeant JA. Modeling attention-deficit/hyperactivity disorder: a critical appraisal of the cognitive-energetic model. Biol Psychiatry 2005;57:1248–55.

[6] Sonuga-Barke EJ, Castellanos FX. Spontaneous attentional fluctuations in impaired states and pathological conditions: a neurobiological hypothesis. Neurosci Biobehav Rev 2007; 31(7):977–86.

[7] Söderlund G, Sikström S, Smart A. Listen to the noise: noise is beneficial for cognitive performance in ADHD. J Child Psychol Psychiatry 2007;48(8):840–7.

[8] Tekin S, Cummings JL. Frontal-subcortical neuronal circuits and clinical neuropsychiatry—an update. J Psychosom Res 2002;53:647–54.

[9] Welsh MC, Pennington BF. Assessing frontal lobe functioning in children: views from developmental psychology. Dev Neuropsychol 1988;4(3):199–230.

[10] Friedman NP, Miyake A, Corley RP, et al. Not all EFs are related to intelligence. Psychol Sci 2006;17:172–9.

[11] Pennington BF, Ozonoff S. Executive functions and developmental psychopathology. J Child Psychol Psychiatry 1996;37:51–87.

[12] Herwig U, Baumgartner T, Kaffenberger T, et al. Modulation of anticipatory emotion and perception processing by cognitive control. Neuroimage 2007;37(2):652–62.

[13] Sohn MH, Albert MV, Jung K, et al. Anticipation of conflict monitoring in the anterior cingulate cortex and the prefrontal cortex. Proc Natl Acad Sci U S A 2007;104(25): 10330–4 [epub].

[14] Nigg JT, Casey BJ. An integrative theory of attention-deficit/hyperactivity disorder based on the cognitive and affective neurosciences. Dev Psychopathol 2005;17:785–806.

[15] Willcutt EG, Doyle AE, Nigg JT, et al. Validity of the executive function theory of attention-deficit/hyperactivity disorder: a meta-analytic review. Biol Psychiatry 2005;57:1336–46.

[16] Benes FM. Brain development, VII. Human brain growth spans decades. Am J Psychiatry 1998;155(11):1489.

[17] Sowell ER, Trauner DA, Gamst A, et al. Development of cortical and subcortical brain structures in childhood and adolescence: a structural MRI study. Dev Med Child Neurol 2002;44(1):4–16.

[18] Sowell ER, Thompson PM, Holmes CJ, et al. Localizing age-related changes in brain structure between childhood and adolescence using statistical parametric mapping. Neuroimage 1999;9(6 Pt 1):587–97.

[19] Rubia K, Smith AB, Woolley J, et al. Progressive increase of frontostriatal brain activation from childhood to adulthood during event-related tasks of cognitive control. Hum Brain Mapp 2006;27(12):973–93.

[20] Durston S, Davidson MC, Tottenham N, et al. A shift from diffuse to focal cortical activity with development. Dev Sci 2006;9(1):1–8.

[21] Casey BJ, Tottenham N, Liston C, et al. Imaging the developing brain: what have we learned about cognitive development? Trends Cogn Sci 2005;9(3):104–10.

[22] Huttonlocher PR, Dabholkar AS. Regional differences in synaptogenesis in human cerebral cortex. J Comp Neurol 1997;387(2):167–78.

[23] Nigg JT. Neuropsychological theory and findings in ADHD: the state of the field and salient challenges for the coming decade. Biol Psychiatry 2005;57:1424–35.

[24] Rhodes SM, Coghill DR, Matthews K. Neuropsychological functioning in stimulant-naive boys with hyperkinetic disorder. Psychol Med 2005;35:1109–20.

[25] Barkley RA. Behavioral inhibition, sustained attention, and executive functions: constructing a unifying theory of ADHD. Psychol Bull 1997;121:65–94.

[26] Aron AR, Robbins TW, Poldrack RA. Inhibition and the right inferior frontal cortex. Trends Cogn Sci 2004;8(4):170–7.

[27] Grodzinsky GM, Barkley RA. Predictive power of frontal lobe tests in the diagnosis of attention deficit hyperactivity disorder. Clin Neuropsychol 1999;13:12–21.

[28] Seidman L, Valera E, Makris N. Structural brain imaging of attention-deficit/hyperactivity disorder. Biol Psychiatry 2006;57(11):1263–72.

[29] Dickstein SG, Bannon K, Castellanos FX, et al. The neural correlates of attention deficit hyperactivity disorder: an ALE meta-analysis. J Child Psychol Psychiatry 2006;47(10): 1051–62.

[30] Taylor EA, Sonuga-Barke EJS. Attention deficit hyperactivity disorder: a developmental lifespan perspective. In: Rutter M, Taylor E, Stevenson J, et al, editors. Chapter in Rutter's Child & Adolescent Psychiatry. 5th edition, in press.

[31] Hervey AS, Epstein JN, Curry JF. Neuropsychology of adults with attention-deficit/ hyperactivity disorder: a meta-analytic review. Neuropsychology 2004;18:485–503.

[32] Nigg JT, Hinshaw SP, Carte ET, et al. Neuropsychological correlates of childhood attention-deficit/hyperactivity disorder: explainable by comorbid disruptive behavior or reading problems? J Abnorm Psychol 1998;107:468–80.

[33] Nigg JT, Stavro G, Ettenhofer M, et al. Executive functions and ADHD in adults: evidence for selective effects on ADHD symptom domains. J Abnorm Psychol 2005;114:706–17.

[34] Martinussen R, Hayden J, Hogg-Johnson S, et al. A meta-analysis of working memory impairments in children with attention-deficit/hyperactivity disorder. J Am Acad Child Adolesc Psychiatry 2005;44:377–84.

[35] Marks DJ, Berwid OG, Santra A, et al. Neuropsychological correlates of ADHD symptoms in preschoolers. Neuropsychology 2005;19(4):446–55.

[36] Morgan AB, Lilienfeld SO. A meta-analytic review of the relation between antisocial behavior and neuropsychological measures of executive function. Clin Psychol Rev 2000; 20(1):113–36.

[37] Oosterlaan J, Logan GD, Sergeant JA. Response inhibition in AD/HD, CD, co-morbid AD/ HD + CD, anxious, and control children: a meta-analysis of studies with the stop task. J Child Psychol Psychiatry 1998;39:411–25.

[38] Geurts HM, Vertie S, Oosterlaan J, et al. How specific are executive functioning deficits in attention deficit hyperactivity disorder and autism? J Child Psychol Psychiatry 2004;45: 836–54.

[39] Happé F, Booth R, Charlton R, et al. Executive function deficits in autism spectrum disorders and attention-deficit/hyperactivity disorder: examining profiles across domains and ages. Brain Cogn 2006;61:25–39.

[40] Hinshaw SP, Carte ET, Sami N, et al. Preadolescent girls with attention-deficit/hyperactivity disorder: II. Neuropsychological performance in relation to subtypes and individual classification. J Consult Clin Psychol 2002;70:1099–111.

[41] Riccio CA, Homack S, Pissitola-Jarratt K, et al. Differences in academic and executive function domains among children with ADHD predominantly inattentive and combined types. Arch Clin Neuropsychol 2006;21:657–67.

[42] Nigg JT, Blaskey LG, Huag-Pollock CL, et al. Neuropsychological executive functions and DSM-IV ADHD subtypes. J Am Acad Child Adolesc Psychiatry 2002;41:59–66.

[43] O'Driscoll GA, Depatie L, Holahan AL, et al. Executive functions and methylphenidate response in subtypes of attention-deficit/hyperactivity disorder. Biol Psychiatry 2005;57: 1452–60.

[44] Castellanos FX, Sonuga-Barke EJS, Milham MP, et al. Characterizing cognition in ADHD: beyond executive dysfunction. Trends Cogn Sci 2006;10:117–23.

[45] Luman M, Oosterlaan J, Sergeant JA. The impact of reinforcement contingencies on AD/HD: a review and theoretical appraisal. Clin Psychol Rev 2005;25:183–213.

[46] Kollins SH, Lane SD, Shapiro SK. Experimental analysis of childhood psychopathology: a laboratory matching analysis of the behavior of children diagnosed with attention-deficit hyperactivity disorder. Psychol Rec 1997;47:25–44.

[47] Tripp G, Alsop B. Sensitivity to reward frequency in boys with attention deficit hyperactivity disorder. J Clin Child Psychol 1999;28:366–75.

[48] Toplak ME, Jain U, Tannock R. Executive and motivational processes in adolescents with attention-deficit-hyperactivity disorder (ADHD). Behav Brain Funct 2005;1:8.

[49] Sonuga-Barke EJS, Taylor E, Sembi S, et al. Hyperactivity and delay aversion—1. The effect of delay on choice. J Child Psychol Psychiatry 1992;33:387–98.

[50] Cardinal RN, Pennicott DR, Sugathapala CL, et al. Impulsive choice induced in rats by lesions of the nucleus accumbens core. Science 2001;292:2499–501.

[51] Wade TR, de Wit H, Richards JB. Effects of dopaminergic drugs on delayed reward as a measure of impulsive behaviour in rats. Psychopharmacology (Berl) 2000;150:90–101.

[52] Robins TW, Everitt BJ. Neurobehavioural mechanisms of reward and motivation. Curr Opin Neurobiol 1996;6(2):228–36.

[53] Wightman RM, Robinson DL. Transient changes in mesolimbic dopamine and their association with 'reward'. J Neurochem 2002;82:721–35.

[54] Sagvolden T, Johansen EB, Aase H, et al. A dynamic developmental theory of attention-deficit/hyperactivity disorder (ADHD) predominantly hyperactive/impulsive and combined subtypes. Behav Brain Sci 2005;28:397.

[55] Sonuga-Barke EJS. The dual pathway model of AD/HD: an elaboration of neuro-developmental characteristics. Neurosci Biobehav Rev 2003;27:593–604.

[56] Marco R, Schlotz W, Melia A, et al. Delay aversion in ADHD: a large scale assessment of the impact of pre- and post-reward delay on choice behaviour. Presented at the 1st International ADHD Congress. Würzburg (Germany), June 3–5, 2007.

[57] Sonuga-Barke EJS. Causal Models of ADHD: from simple single deficits to multiple developmental pathways. Biol Psychiatry 2005;57:1231–8.

[58] Kuntsi J, Oosterlaan J, Stevenson J. Psychological mechanisms in hyperactivity: I response inhibition deficit, working memory impairment, delay aversion, or something else? J Child Psychol Psychiatry 2001;42:199–210.

[59] Antrop I, Stock P, Verte S, et al. ADHD and delay aversion: the influence of non-temporal stimulation on choice for delayed rewards. J Child Psychol Psychiatry 2006;47:1152–8.

[60] Bitsakou P. Neuropsychological Heterogeneity in ADHD. PhD Thesis University of Southampton. 2007.

[61] Schweitzer JB, Sulzer-Azaroff B. Self-control in boys with attention-deficit hyperactivity disorder—effects of added stimulation and time. J Child Psychol Psychiatry 1995;36:671–86.

[62] Solanto M, Abikoff H, Sonuga-Barke EJS, et al. The ecological validity of measures related to impulsiveness in AD/HD. J Abnorm Child Psychol 2001;29:215–28.

[63] Hoerger ML, Mace FC. A computerized test of self-control predicts classroom behavior. J Appl Behav Anal 2006;39:147–59.

[64] Dalen L, Sonuga-Barke EJS, Hall M, et al. Inhibitory deficits, delay aversion and preschool ADHD: implications for the dual pathway model. Neural Plast 2004;11:1–12.

[65] Bitsakou P, Antrop I, Wiersema JR, et al. probing the limits of delay intolerance: preliminary young adult data from the delay frustration task (DeFT). J Neurosci Methods 2006;151:38–44.

[66] Sagvolden T, Aase H, Zeiner P, et al. Altered reinforcement mechanisms in attention-deficit/hyperactivity disorder. Behav Brain Res 1998;94:61–71.

[67] Scime M, Norvilitis JM. Task performance and response to frustration in children with attention deficit hyperactivity disorder. Psychol Sch 2006;43:377–86.

[68] Antrop I, Roeyers H, Van Oost P, et al. Stimulation seeking and hyperactivity in children with ADHD. J Child Psychol Psychiatry 2003;41(2):225–31.

[69] Tripp G, Alsop B. Sensitivity to reward delay in children with attention deficit hyperactivity disorder (ADHD). J Child Psychol Psychiatry 2001;42:691–8.

[70] Sonuga-Barke EJS, De Houwer J, De Ruiter K, et al. AD/HD and the capture of attention by briefly exposed delay-related cues: evidence from a conditioning paradigm. J Child Psychol Psychiatry 2004;45:274–83.

[71] Neef NA, Marckel J, Ferreri SJ, et al. Behavioral assessment of impulsivity: a comparison of children with and without attention deficit hyperactivity disorder. J Appl Behav Anal 2005; 38(1):23–37.

[72] Scheres A, Dijkstra M, Ainslie E, et al. Temporal and probabilistic discounting of rewards in children and adolescents: effects of age and ADHD symptoms. Neuropsychologia 2006; 44(11):2092–103.

[73] Wiersema R, van der Meere J, Roeyers H, et al. Event rate and event-related potentials in ADHD. J Child Psychol Psychiatry 2006;47:560–7.

[74] Aase H, Sagvolden T. Infrequent, but not frequent, reinforcers produce more variable responding and deficient sustained attention in young children with attention-deficit/hyperactivity disorder (ADHD). J Child Psychol Psychiatry 2006;47:457–71.

[75] Scheres A, Milham MP, Knutson B, et al. Ventral striatal hyporesponsiveness during reward anticipation in attention-deficit/hyperactivity disorder. Biol Psychiatry 2007;61(5):720–4.

[76] Cardinal RN. Neural systems implicated in delayed and probabilistic reinforcement. Neural Netw 2006;19:1277–301.

[77] Cardinal RN, Winstanley CA, Robbins TW, et al. Limbic corticostriatal systems and delayed reinforcement. Ann N Y Acad Sci 2004;1021:33–50.

[78] Winstanley CA, Eagle DM, Robbins TW. Behavioral models of impulsivity in relation to ADHD: translation between clinical and preclinical studies. Clin Psychol Rev 2006;26: 379–95.

[79] Sonuga-Barke EJS, Dalen L, Remington RER. Do delay aversion and inhibitory deficits make distinct contributions to pre-school AD/HD? J Am Acad Child Adolesc Psychiatry 2003;42:1335–42.

[80] Thorell L. Do delay aversion and executive function deficits make distinct contributions to the functional impact of ADHD symptoms: a study of early academic skill deficits. J Child Psychol Psychiatry, in press.

[81] Van den Bergh F, Spronk M, Ferreira L, et al. Relationship of delay aversion and response inhibition to extinction learning, aggression, and sexual behaviour. Behav Brain Res 2006; 175:75–81.

[82] Nigg JT. What causes ADHD? Toward a multi-path model for understanding what goes wrong and why. New York: Guilford Press; 2006.

[83] Swanson JM, Kinsbourne M, Nigg J, et al. Etiologic subtypes of attention-deficit/hyperactivity disorder: brain imaging, molecular genetic and environmental factors and the dopamine hypothesis. Neuropsychol Rev 2007;17(1):39–59.

[84] Sonuga-Barke EJS. Psychological heterogeneity in AD/HD: a dual pathway model of behaviour and cognition. Behav Brain Res 2002;130:29–36.

[85] Martel MM, Nigg JT. Child ADHD and personality/temperament traits of reactive and effortful control, resiliency, and emotionality. J Child Psychol Psychiatry 2006;47:1175–83.

[86] Haber SN. The primate basal ganglia: parallel and integrative networks. J Chem Neuroanat 2004;26(4):317–30.

[87] Wakefield JC. When is development disordered? Developmental psychopathology and the harmful dysfunction analysis of mental disorder. Dev Psychopathol 1997;9(2):269–90.

[88] Nutt DJ, Fone K, Asherson P, et al. Evidence-based guidelines for management of attention-deficit/hyperactivity disorder in adolescents in transition to adult services and in

adults: recommendations from the British association for psychopharmacology. J Psychopharmacol 2007;21:10–41.

[89] Biederman J, Monuteaux MC, Doyle AE, et al. Impact of executive function deficits and attention-deficit/hyperactivity disorder (ADHD) on academic outcomes in children. J Consult Clin Psychol 2004;72(5):757–66.

[90] Biederman J, Petty C, Fried R, et al. Impact of psychometrically defined deficits of executive functioning in adults with attention deficit hyperactivity disorder. Am J Psychiatry 2006; 163(10):1730–8.

[91] Stavro GM, Ettenhofer ML, Nigg JT. Executive functions and adaptive functioning in young adult attention-deficit/hyperactivity disorder. J Int Neuropsychol Soc 2007;13(2): 324–34.

[92] Abikoff H. Tailored psychosocial treatments for ADHD: the search for a good fit. J Clin Child Psychol 2001;30(1):122–5.

[93] Pennington BF. From single to multiple deficit models of developmental disorders. Cognition 2006;101(2):385–413.

CHILD AND
ADOLESCENT
PSYCHIATRIC CLINICS
OF NORTH AMERICA

Child Adolesc Psychiatric Clin N Am
17 (2008) 385–404

Neuroimaging of Attention Deficit Hyperactivity Disorder: Can New Imaging Findings Be Integrated in Clinical Practice?

George Bush, MD[a,b,c,d],*

[a]Department of Psychiatry, Harvard Medical School,
25 Shattuck Street, Boston, MA 02115, USA
[b]Psychiatric Neuroscience Division, Department of Psychiatry,
Massachusetts General Hospital, 55 Fruit Street, Boston, MA 02114, USA
[c]MIT/HMS/MGH Athinoula A. Martinos Center for Functional
and Structural Biomedical Imaging (Massachusetts Institute of Technology,
Harvard Medical School and Massachusetts General Hospital), MGH–East,
CNY 2614, Building 149, Thirteenth Street, Charlestown, MA 02129, USA
[d]Clinical and Research Program in Pediatric Psychopharmacology,
Massachusetts General Hospital, Boston, MA 02114, USA

Neuroimaging research has provided a great deal of exciting new data on the neurobiology of attention deficit hyperactivity disorder (ADHD) and the neural effects of medications used to treat the disorder. Rapid technologic advances in neuroimaging, genetics, and neurochemical research techniques have converged with cognitive neuroscience and neuropsychologic

This review was produced without direct support or compensation. Indirect support has been provided to the author for ADHD-related work within the past decade in the form of grant or general support by the National Institute of Mental Health, the National Science Foundation, the Mental Illness and Neuroscience Discovery (MIND) Institute, the National Alliance for Research on Schizophrenia and Depression (NARSAD), the Johnson and Johnson Center for the Study of Psychopathology, the Center for Functional Neuroimaging Technologies (P41RR14075), McNeil Pharmaceuticals, Pfizer Pharmaceuticals, and Eli Lilly and Company. The author has or has had in the past a relationship with one or more organizations listed as follows: former advisory board member and speaker's honoraria from Eli Lilly and Company and Novartis Pharmaceuticals; and has received speaker's honoraria from Shire U.S. Inc., Janssen Pharmaceuticals, Johnson & Johnson, and McNeil Pharmaceuticals. The author does not now and has not at any time had a financial interest in any of these entities.
* Massachusetts General Hospital-East, Psychiatric Neuroscience Program, MGH–East, CNY 2614, Building 149, Thirteenth Street, Charlestown, MA 02129.
E-mail address: geo@nmr.mgh.harvard.edu

findings to implicate dysfunction of frontostriatal structures (dorsal anterior midcingulate cortex, dorsolateral prefrontal cortex, caudate, and putamen) as likely contributing to the pathophysiology of ADHD, and several reports have helped elucidate the mechanism of action of stimulant medications. Although these developments are promising, they also create confusion over the possible usefulness of imaging techniques as an aid to clinical decision-making. Specifically they present challenges for the clinician as to how best to integrate this burgeoning literature and to determine when and how, if at all, to incorporate these new brain imaging capabilities into clinical practice.

Although currently there are no accepted uses for imaging in diagnosing ADHD (other than ruling out identifiable medical/neurologic conditions that may mimic ADHD), this article: (1) provides a context within which to understand the potential future role of imaging in clinical practice; (2) discusses the inter-relationship of clinical diagnostic controversies with imaging research; (3) briefly overviews the main imaging techniques used to study ADHD and highlights some major recent advances that exemplify the current state of imaging capabilities; (4) identifies issues and complexities facing psychiatric neuroimaging research in general and highlights disorder-specific challenges of ADHD research; and (5) suggests guidelines for possible future clinical uses of imaging in ADHD. It is not intended as a comprehensive review or meta-analysis of imaging of ADHD, which can be found elsewhere [1–12], but rather as a primer to aid clinicians and non-imaging ADHD researchers in understanding the relevant complexities of ADHD imaging and possible future applications to clinical practice.

> *Eight-year-old Johnny can't wait to climb into the sleek, space-age scanner. His mother—who has been concerned about his poor school performance, disruptive classroom behavior, and difficulties keeping friends—tries to give him one more kiss on the forehead, but he excitedly pulls away and hops up onto the scanner bed. The imaging tech gives mom a reassuring smile, slides Johnny into the large magnet, and shows Johnny how to work the video game buttons that keep him occupied during the scan. Twenty minutes later (all too short for Johnny), it's time for him to come out again. His child psychiatrist enters the adjoining consultation room and there explains to mom what the brightly-colored blobs on the incredibly realistic, seemingly 3-dimensional images of Johnny's brain mean. No, there are no tumors, but compared with the International Pediatric Brain Database (IPBD), Johnny's brain is 3.5% smaller than other boys his age, his cingulate cortex and caudate are smaller than normal, and his cortical attention network is underactive. Combining that with the PET scan results from earlier that morning, his diagnosis of ADHD, combined type, is confirmed, and the child psychiatrist explains to mom why a certain pattern of colored blobs on the scan indicates Johnny is more likely to respond to one medication than another. Reassured, mom smiles, and they all go back to the office to review the treatment plan.*

Of course, this scenario sounds wonderful, and (were it reality), represents an ideal situation for patient, parent, and clinician alike. Given the frequent reports of new advances in brain imaging, many of which appear in the mainstream media, it even seems tantalizingly close to what might be possible in our current state-of-the-art facilities. The question is, though, just how far off is this vision from our current or near-future capabilities? This article provides a concise overview of ADHD imaging research potentially relevant to the clinical care of patients who have ADHD and offers guidance for the clinician to help determine when (at some time in the future) that imaging might finally be deemed acceptable and appropriate as an aid in clinical decision-making.

As detailed elsewhere in this issue, ADHD is a psychiatric disorder characterized by developmentally inappropriate symptoms of inattention, impulsivity, and motor restlessness [13]. Affecting approximately 5% of school-age children and frequently persisting into adulthood [14–16], ADHD is a source of great morbidity across the lifespan. Convergent data from neuroimaging, neuropsychologic, genetics, and neurochemical studies have implicated frontostriatal network abnormalities as the likely cause of ADHD [1–11,17,18], (see articles by Castellanos and Tannock, elsewhere in this issue). Although there is no currently accepted diagnostic imaging test for ADHD, can this rapidly growing database of information on the pathophysiology of ADHD and the biologic effects of medications used to treat it soon be translated into a protocol that would be useful in clinical practice?

Is the goal worthwhile?

Using brain imaging to study the pathophysiology of ADHD (which is already being done with multiple current imaging technologies) is intrinsically important, but it is another matter to attempt to translate that type of research (which can be done using group-averaged brain data) into the development of a clinically useful diagnostic imaging test for ADHD (which would require, by definition, the capability to reliably identify unique imaging biomarkers of ADHD in single subjects and would entail a large expenditure of time, effort, and money to properly validate). Before even beginning to discuss the technical challenges of such an endeavor, it is essential to ask whether pursuing the development of such a clinical imaging test is justified (ie, presupposing that such a diagnostic imaging test is eventually feasible—would it be worthwhile?). Imaging would entail a higher upfront cost that must be justified (shown to have added value above clinical diagnosis alone). To be clear, for the purposes of discussion, such a test would not be used as a screening test (as screening would be done much more quickly and cheaply by way of history and questionnaire). Such a test would instead be used in combination with clinical assessment, but with enough testing could conceivably one day be elevated to the status of gold standard (acceptable proof in and of itself that a patient has the disorder in question).

There are many reasons that developing a diagnostic imaging test would be important. Such a test would simultaneously reduce overdiagnosis and underdiagnosis. Both goals are clinically important, because overdiagnosis leads to unnecessary exposure to medications and time-consuming behavioral treatment, with their additional costs, and underdiagnosis (and subsequent nontreatment) leads to increased functional, social, and occupational impairment and increased morbidity and mortality. Aside from the important alleviation of suffering and avoidance of unnecessary risk for individuals, ADHD's long-term economic burden to society is not trivial. If, as estimated, approximately 5% to 8% of children and 3% to 4% of adults have ADHD [15,19,20], and in light of the fact treatment lasts years and often decades, a diagnostic imaging test could be highly cost-effective, saving patients and society enormous amounts of money by eliminating unnecessary testing and treatment in some, and by targeting treatment appropriately in those who have ADHD. These long-term savings along with reducing indirect costs of ADHD by helping to decrease motor vehicle accidents and substance abuse [21,22] would more than justify the initial costs of imaging. An imaging-confirmed diagnosis would identify those who need treatment and possibly assist clinicians in monitoring treatment response and could help in refining treatment decisions based on subtyping of ADHD. Such a test would spare those patients ruled out for ADHD the risks and expense of unnecessary treatments and in these cases could help lead clinicians to identify other medical or neurologic disorders that mimic ADHD.

Furthermore, identification of an imaging biomarker for ADHD can improve treatment studies by refined case definition. Similarly, objective case definition can improve and facilitate cross-cultural studies, helping to address longstanding questions about differences in prevalence rates among different countries. Such a test would improve genetic studies by way of better case identification and by reducing variability/noise from analysis. An imaging-based diagnostic test would clearly benefit pharmaceutical development by potentially helping to identify new drug targets and by providing improved outcome measures. Imaging of ADHD could indirectly assist with the understanding of other disorders that also involve attention problems (schizophrenia, depression, and learning disorders) and could more directly improve the clinical treatment and research of patients who have complex cases involving comorbid conditions, such as ADHD in the presence of bipolar disorder or learning disabilities.

Finally, for the individual an imaging test could help with treatment compliance if the patient sees tangible evidence (on a brain scan) that he or she has ADHD and can be shown that the treatment selected is having an observable effect. Moreover, such an objective measure may reduce stigma if one can identify a neurobiologic causation and can therefore show that the patient is not simply "lazy" or unmotivated. For many reasons, the quest to develop a diagnostic imaging test is thus clearly justified.

Inter-relationship with clinical diagnostic issues

Before attempting to develop a diagnostic imaging test for ADHD, it is also essential to define what specifically such a test would be designed to identify, and herein lies one of the first major challenges. It must be recalled that at present the diagnosis ADHD is clinically defined, generally requiring the presence of developmentally inappropriate symptoms of inattention, impulsivity, and motor restlessness [13]. But as discussed elsewhere in this issue and in detail by McGough and Barkley [23], without an established neurobiologic pathophysiology, controversy remains as to how to best define ADHD clinically. In DSM-IV [13], three subtypes are recognized: inattentive, hyperactive–impulsive, and combined (reflecting a combination of the other two types). Symptoms must be observed early in life (before age 7 years), pervasive across situations, and chronic. The increasing identification of adults who have ADHD, however, and the inclusion of the diagnosis of ADHD, not otherwise specified, in DSM-IV [13] suggest that there may be multiple processes leading to ADHD, with different time courses and etiologies. This does not even involve consideration of alternate diagnostic schemes, such as the Wender Utah Criteria [24], which among other things emphasizes hyperactivity, thereby excluding the inattentive subtype of ADHD, and introduces potential confounds with the inclusion of "irritability" and "hot temper" as part of the formulation; or ICD-10 criteria [25], which are used more often in European studies. This review makes no value judgments on the validity of these and other diagnostic schemes, but merely raises these few points to illustrate that it must be recognized early on that there is a continual push–pull of clinical and neuroimaging findings that mutually influence one another and profoundly shape the conceptualization of what ADHD is and encompasses. The identification of the neural substrates underlying the proposed existence of ADHD subtypes is certainly a question that can be approached empirically using brain imaging, but the issue is complex. Similarly, data need to be viewed within a developmental context to determine if ADHD identified in youth is the same as that seen in adults, and consideration needs to be made for parsing out ADHD's overlap with comorbid conditions.

Brief review of different imaging modalities

In this section, the main functional imaging techniques currently used to study ADHD are introduced. This review does not discuss structural scanning techniques, such as morphometric (volumetric) studies, cortical thickness studies, or diffusion tensor (white matter tract tracing) techniques. Although these are all invaluable research tools, the small effect sizes typically observed in these studies make it highly unlikely that they could, on their own, become clinically useful (and even if they did, most of the same issues faced by functional imaging would apply to a structural imaging test).

Functional imaging studies (regardless of technique) can be broadly divided into studies of: (1) pathophysiology, (2) treatment effects, and (3) potential tests to aid clinical diagnosis. Generally, functional imaging studies have been designed using group-averaging statistical analytic techniques (ie, because of the usually limited power to detect reliable and robust results in individuals, analysis strategies have relied on reconstructing image data in a standardized anatomic space (eg, Talairach and Tournoux [26]) and comparing the results within a group-averaged sample of ADHD subjects with that of a healthy or psychiatrically-impaired control group). Such group-averaged designs can be useful in studying pathophysiology and medication effects, but are inadequate to assist in clinical diagnostic decision-making (which by definition requires the ability to reliably distinguish normal from abnormal at the individual subject level).

Radioactivity-based techniques

Single photon emission computed tomography (SPECT) and photon emission tomography (PET) were among the earliest functional imaging studies used. SPECT involves the injection or inhalation of radiopharmaceuticals (eg, xenon-133, iodine-123, or techitium-99m) that then distribute throughout the body and brain and emit single photon radiation (typically gamma rays) as they decay. More active brain areas receive greater blood flow, and thus greater amounts of the radioactive tracer, which is then detected with the SPECT camera. PET works similarly (ie, it also uses injected or inhaled radiopharmaceuticals, typically oxygen-15, carbon-11, or fluorine-18). As these decay they emit positrons, which are detected by the PET camera. Some PET methods are blood flow-dependent, whereas others measure cerebral metabolism rates. SPECT and PET have generally been supplanted by functional MRI (fMRI) for functional studies, because fMRI offers superior spatial and temporal resolution, and SPECT and PET's use of radiopharmaceuticals makes it ethically difficult to justify their use in healthy volunteers, especially children [27]. Both SPECT and PET, however, still have their important niche uses, because they can use radioligands for receptor characterization to measure dopamine transporter levels and to quantify extracellular dopamine [3,28–31], and it is possible that one day one of these types of uses could be translated into a clinically useful test.

Functional MRI

The newest of the major functional imaging methods, fMRI presents several advantages for functional studies over SPECT and PET. It is noninvasive (no injections or inhalations are needed) and does not require subjects to be exposed to ionizing radiation. Subjects (including children) can thus be scanned repeatedly, facilitating longitudinal, developmental, and drug studies. This ability to repeatedly scan the same subject also permits progressive "functional dissections" within the same subject (ie, the same subject can be scanned on different occasions using many different tasks, permitting researchers to probe different brain structures and networks). fMRI has superior spatial and temporal resolution, and tasks can be performed in either a blocked format or an event-related manner, allowing greater flexibility in task design. Also, newer arterial spin labeling techniques can and have been used to scan subjects in resting states and can provide absolute measures of regional cerebral blood flow [32–35]. Higher field strength magnets coupled with specialized cognitive activation tasks are able to produce reliable and robust results in individual subjects, which has enabled characterization of drug effects in single subjects and analyses of intersubject variability [36]. For these reasons, fMRI has become the dominant imaging modality used by cognitive neuroscientists and psychiatric functional imaging researchers and may potentially be able to be developed into a clinically useful imaging test.

Magnetic resonance spectroscopy

Magnetic resonance spectroscopy (MRS) is a noninvasive, MRI-based method for quantifying various neurochemicals, including putative markers for neuronal integrity, myelin breakdown, and others. In the small number of studies published to date [1,37–43], MRS has shown some early promise in identifying neurochemical abnormalities associated with ADHD. Although these MRS findings are preliminary, require group-averaging, often contain small samples with comorbidities, and are regionally limited, they do offer the promise of being able to noninvasively quantify biologically relevant neurometabolites. MRS is thus a technique deserving further exploration for usefulness in understanding ADHD pathophysiology and treatment and for a possible role in the clinical arena.

Electrophysiology studies

Electrophysiologic methods, including quantitative electroencephalograms (QEEG) and event-related potentials (ERPs) have been used in a large number of ADHD studies (for reviews, see [44–48]). QEEG generally involves computer-assisted spectral analysis of the EEG signal with relative and absolute quantification of alpha, beta, theta, and delta frequencies, and sometimes measures of coherence. The generators of these signals, however, are not localized to specific neural structures with any precision. Some proponents of QEEG have argued that it can distinguish patients who have ADHD from control subjects [45], with ADHD supposedly being characterized by "theta excess" and "alpha slowing." The same review, however, later stated that "theta excess" or "abnormal alpha" is associated with dementia, schizophrenia, mood disorders, obsessive–compulsive disorder, specific developmental learning disorders, alcoholic intoxication, chronic alcoholism, mild to severe head injury, and postconcussion syndrome. Similarly, others have argued that a higher theta:beta ratio is associated with

ADHD, while simultaneously noting that this same pattern occurs in other psychiatric disorders [46]. Such nonspecificity renders QEEG clinically unproven.

ERPs are different from QEEG. They are measured using multielectrode arrays placed over the scalp and represent the averaged electrical response of the brain over many trials [49–51]. ERPs main problems are limited spatial resolution and the "inverse problem" (ie, there are no unique solutions when determining the position of sources within the head, making it extremely difficult to localize brain activity with certainty). ERPs do possess millisecond temporal resolution, however, and efforts to combine modalities (eg, using fMRI to spatially constrain source models and then ERPs to test the electrical activity within the identified nodes) may eventually be applied to ADHD research with success. There are no reports, however, that have successfully used ERPs to distinguish patients who have ADHD from healthy control subjects and other patients who have psychiatric disorders at the single subject level, so like the other imaging methods, ERPs are not deemed clinically useful at this time.

Functional imaging findings in attention deficit hyperactivity disorder

It is far beyond the purpose and scope of this article to provide even a cursory review of imaging results related to ADHD. For this the interested reader is referred to other reviews [1,4–9,12]. A couple of illustrative examples, however, help to show possible future avenues of research.

One such type of diagnostic test using fMRI might use cognitive activation task strategies. Examples of these might be the Multi-Source Interference Task (MSIT, [36,52,53]), Stroop and Stroop-like tasks [54–56], stop-signal or go/no-go tasks [57–59], or continuous performance tasks [60]. Akin to a cardiac stress test, these imaging tests use a cognitive/attention task or tasks to activate brain regions under conditions of engagement within the task to assess the functional integrity of the cortical structures supporting attention or response inhibition in neuropsychiatric disorders like ADHD. An ideal functional neuroimaging-based diagnostic test of this type should possess many of the following characteristics. (1) It must produce reliable and robust activation of the cortical regions of interest (ROI) within healthy individuals. (2) It should be hypothesis-driven (that is, pre-existing evidence should support a mechanism explaining why the task would be expected to recruit the ROI). (3) It should include the collection of concomitant imaging and performance data (reaction times and accuracy). (4) Testing procedures must be standardized. (5) The task instructions should be easy to learn and retain so that the task can be performed by subjects who have impaired attention or cognition (eg, ADHD or schizophrenia) and by subjects across a wide age spectrum (to enable developmental studies in children and studies of elderly subjects). (6) It should not require an excessive time commitment, because children and elderly subjects tend to tire more easily than young adults. (7) It should not be language-specific (to allow cross-cultural studies). (8) Performance data should vary within a narrow range in healthy volunteers. (9) Imaging and performance data should be related. (10) Imaging and performance data should show temporal stability (ie, they should display sufficient test–retest reliability to permit longitudinal and treatment studies). (11) Imaging and perfor-mance data should be sensitive to changes with successful treatment. (12) Results should be disorder-specific.

Many of the currently used cognitive activation tasks (with currently available imaging methods) do not meet even the first cut for translation into a diagnostically useful task, because they do not reliably activate brain ROIs in single subjects. It is not fair to even expect this from them, however, for although they might produce reliable group-averaged data, they were designed to test groups, not to have the power to produce activation in single subjects. Although the MSIT may be more likely to one day meet the diagnostic test criteria, having been specifically designed with many of the ideal diagnostic features in mind [53] and having already demonstrated ability to activate the cingulo-frontal-parietal cognitive/attention network in approximately 95% of more than 100 subjects tested (Fig. 1) [52], the MSIT is far from being validated as a diagnostic test. Studies are underway using the MSIT to directly compare patients who have ADHD with healthy control subjects, and follow-up studies are planned to also include other disorders, such as schizophrenia and depression, but there is no prospective, large-scale study that would provide sufficient data for calculation of sensi-tivity, specificity, or other measures of diagnostic accuracy. At this point in time, there are no adequately validated functional diagnostic imaging tests.

Another promising but controversial avenue of investigation involves the quantification of striatal dopamine transporter (DAT). DAT is responsible for presynaptic reuptake of dopamine, and it has been shown that methylphenidate blocks DAT and increases extracellular dopamine [3,7,30,31,61]. Also, significant for a potentially useful diagnostic test, it has recently been shown that Altropane (a carbon-11 agent) and PET have demonstrated ability to image drug effects in single subjects (Fig. 2) [29]. Although initial reports found a large (up to 70%) increase in striatal DAT in patients who have ADHD [62], however, subsequent reports using different ligands and techniques have found lesser effect sizes, and in some cases, even lower DAT in patients who have ADHD [3,31]. The compari-sons of ligands and techniques used in these different studies are far beyond the scope of this article, but suffice it to say that although the approach in general is extremely promising in helping understand the pathophysiology of ADHD and the mechanism of action of treatments for ADHD, the pro-cess of attempting to translate such exciting and pioneering work into a clin-ically useful diagnostic imaging task has only begun.

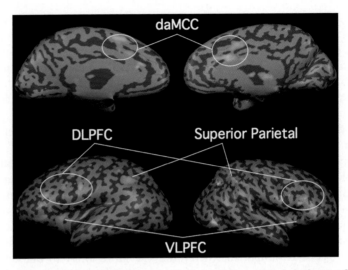

Fig. 1. Typical single subject fMRI response during MSIT. A typical single scan fMRI response during the MSIT is shown for an individual subject in the inflated view format (*light gray, gyri; dark gray, sulci*). Note the robust bilateral activation ($P < 10^{-4}$) in the cingulo-frontal-parietal cortical/attention network (daMCC, DLPFC, and superior parietal cortex). Additional activity is often seen, as here, in ventrolateral prefrontal cortex (VLPFC). The dorsal anterior midcingulate cortex (daMCC) lying on the medial surface of the frontal lobe maintains strong connections to dorsolateral prefrontal cortex (DLPFC), parietal cortex, and striatum. The daMCC is believed to play critical roles in complex and effortful cognitive processing, target detection, response selection and inhibition, error detection, performance monitoring, and motivation (see [74,75] for reviews). Particularly relevant to ADHD, it is believed to modulate reward-based decision-making [75,76]. Dysfunction of daMCC thus could lead to all of the cardinal signs of ADHD (inattention, impulsivity, and hyperactivity) and could explain the seeming paradoxic ability of patients who have ADHD to perform normally on some tasks (when motivated) but to show deficient performance when the task is not deemed salient. Numerous imaging studies have reported functional hypoactivity of daMCC [12,36], recent reports of structural and biochemical abnormalities of daMCC have been published [41,77–79], and methylphenidate has been shown to increase activity of daMCC [36]. That daMCC and the cingulo-frontal-parietal cortical/attention network can reliably be imaged in single subjects is promising, but much work needs to be done before using the MSIT as part of a clinical diagnostic imaging test for ADHD. (*Reproduced from* Bush G, Shin LM. The multi-source interference task: an fMRI task that reliably activates the cingulo-frontal-parietal cognitive/attention network in individual subjects. Nat Protoc 2006;1:308–13; with permission.)

Diagnostic imaging test issues

The next two sections discuss issues related to the development of diagnostic imaging tests. The first section addresses general concepts that apply to most proposed diagnostic imaging tests of psychiatric disorders. The second section highlights issues that may be more specific to the development of a possible ADHD diagnostic test.

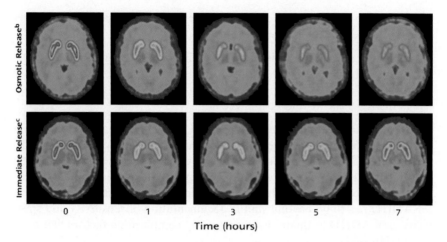

Time (hours)

Fig. 2. Serial PET brain images showing striatal dopamine transporter receptor occupancy after receipt of a single dose of immediate-release or osmotic-release methylphenidate in two healthy subjects. (*A*) Dopamine transporter receptor occupancy in the striatum of two individual healthy adults was assessed by measuring binding of a carbon-11-labeled imaging agent (Altropane). Red color indicates greater binding of Altropane to presynaptic DAT; yellow indicates lesser binding by Altropane caused by displacement by methylphenidate. (*B*) Subject took long-acting osmotic release oral system methylphenidate. Significant drug effect is still observed at 7 h. (*C*) Subject took short-acting immediate release methylphenidate. Striatal DAT occupancy returns more quickly toward baseline level in hours 3 through 7. The technique exemplifies the capability to quantify drug effects with dynamic range within single subjects. (*Reproduced from* Spencer TJ, Biederman J, Ciccone PE, et al. PET study examining pharmacokinetics, detection and likeability, and dopamine transporter receptor occupancy of short- and long-acting oral methylphenidate. Am J Psychiatry 2006;163(3):387–95; with permission.)

General issues

As stated, there is currently no accepted role for functional imaging in guiding clinical diagnosis or therapeutic decision-making. Despite the exciting preliminary advances that have been made in understanding pathophysiology and drug treatment mechanisms, none of the imaging modalities has been fully validated in the peer-reviewed literature as a proven method for reliably distinguishing patients who have ADHD from normal control subjects, distinguishing patients who have ADHD from other subjects who have other psychiatric or neurologic comorbidities, identifying subtypes of ADHD, or predicting treatment response at the level of the individual subject. To achieve full validation, what are some of the main benchmarks that would need to be met?

First, of paramount importance, it must be recognized that the exciting potential for brain imaging and the complexity of the technology underlying it must in large part be ignored when evaluating whether a test based on an imaging technique would be worthwhile diagnostically. The only real questions to be answered are the exact same ones that must be asked of any type of diagnostic laboratory test:

1. How well does the test identify the condition of interest (here, ADHD)?
2. How well does the test distinguish the condition from other similar disorders?
3. Is the test feasible and cost-effective?

More formally, any proper validation of a proposed diagnostic imaging test would have to include peer-reviewed published data (collected in dedicated testing performed in large samples of carefully characterized subjects) that quantifies and meets or exceeds the appropriate and acceptable benchmarks. As shown, such validation of any proposed diagnostic imaging test for ADHD has to go beyond simple documentation of sensitivity and specificity, and ADHD evaluations present many complicating factors that need to be addressed.

Briefly, diagnostic testing validation requires at the least quantification of sensitivity and specificity. To calculate these measures, the proposed test results are compared in binary fashion (ie, test result positive versus negative) to the gold standard (the procedure or test that unambiguously defines the pathology, such as a biopsy or direct surgical inspection in the case of tumor). Herein lies the first problem—as seen, there is no gold standard for ADHD, which, in the absence of defined pathophysiology, remains a clinical diagnosis whose criteria are fluid and still a matter of debate. For the sake of further discussion, here one could choose to accept the latest DSM-IV diagnosis as a proxy gold standard, but admittedly must recall in the end that this is not a true gold standard. Sensitivity of the diagnostic test indicates the proportion of true positives the test identifies (as compared with the gold standard), whereas specificity refers to the proportion of true negatives correctly identified. Although both of these values are important to know, they do not provide sufficient information about the diagnostic accuracy of the test, because in clinical practice, one is more interested in approaching the problem from the other direction (ie, one would be given the scan result of "normal" or "abnormal" scan, and would therefore need to know how well that scan result reflected the presence or absence of ADHD).

This information is expressed in the form of predictive values [63]. The positive predictive value of an imaging test is the proportion of patients who have positive scans that are correctly diagnosed, whereas the negative predictive value of an imaging test is the proportion of patients who have negative scans that are correctly diagnosed. These predictive values are not absolute but relative, and their estimates can be heavily influenced by the prevalence of the abnormality. Another important characteristic to know is the likelihood ratio (sensitivity/1-specificity), which reflects the certainty about a positive diagnosis [63,64].

Another complicating factor is that the preceding evaluations are performed on discrete (yes/no or positive/negative) data. In reality, imaging data are most likely going to be continuous data (eg, percent fMRI signal change or dopamine transporter binding). In these cases, it is highly unlikely that two completely separable distributions of data exist (one for ADHD, one for healthy subjects), but rather that the two sample distributions overlap and therefore a cutoff needs to be set for distinguishing a positive from a negative result. In these types of cases, receiver operating characteristic (ROC) plots (which plot sensitivities versus the inverse of specificities) can be useful in selecting an appropriate cutoff value and comparing one or more measurements [65]. Similarly, although some forms of diagnostic imaging tests may be amenable to "expert interpretation," for the most part this approach should be minimized, and even in these cases, empiric data with strict and explicit criteria must be provided and independently replicable. Also, "expert interpretation" methodologies still provide quantitative diagnostic accuracy information and test–retest reliability measures and are subject to rigorous standardization. There should be no acceptance of a claim that is pinned solely on "specialized knowledge" without the support of fully independent replication. Certainly specialized training and clinical imaging expertise are required for the interpretation of any diagnostic imaging test (because this is the current model for much of neuroradiology)—but any such claims should not be accepted until there is consensus agreement that such claims are adequately supported by proof of technique from unbiased, independent replications.

This list is far from exhaustive—there are many more general issues that are important to address before being able to fully evaluate diagnostic accuracy. What is the effect size (ie, the magnitude of the mean differences between the ADHD and healthy populations, taking into account the degree of variance in the samples)? What is the diagnostic specificity with respect to other disorders that may produce test results that overlap with ADHD? What is the test–retest reliability within a particular imaging center or the variability between readers or between imaging centers? For fuller discussion of these and other issues beyond the scope of this article, the interested reader is referred to a concise statement of standards for reporting studies of diagnostic accuracy [66], but the short list of general issues alone provided here should already provide pause for consideration before accepting claims that a diagnostic test for ADHD has been developed.

Attention deficit hyperactivity disorder-specific issues and technologic challenges

Beyond the more general issues discussed, there are myriad complicating factors that face psychiatric neuroimagers in general, and more specifically, related to the imaging of ADHD. A brief sampling of such factors is offered here:

1. Any tests using specific tasks (cognitive interference tasks, target detection, vigilance tasks, response inhibition, working memory tasks) may

be useful, but it must be recalled that each tests only a specific cognitive domain and does not provide a comprehensive picture of patients who have ADHD. It may be that a battery of tests could and will be used, but this approach is complex and requires cooperative patients, which may be difficult in ADHD populations, especially in young children who have ADHD.

2. Some resting state or dopaminergic tests may be confounded, because controversy exists surrounding the definition of whether or not the healthy brain has a "default resting state" or how to determine in a simple way if a subject is "mentally resting" (and this is then compounded by the likelihood that patients who have ADHD may have increased activity or variability at "rest") [67,68].

3. It is well known that dopaminergic firing can change rapidly (on a trial-by-trial basis), and that dopaminergic cells show tonic firing (longer term stable) and phasic firing (which changes on a second-by-second basis). It may be that these temporal effects could produce disparate findings in some dopaminergic studies.

4. There is the high likelihood that ADHD may represent a syndrome that can be caused by or associated with multiple causes (one group may have dopaminergic, noradrenergic, serotonergic, or cholinergic abnormalities), whereas there may be others who have genetic-based structural abnormalities, and still others with disordered cortico-cortical connections), all of which may have differing imaging profiles.

5. A similar accounting must be made for phenomenologic subtypes of ADHD, because it is likely that inattentive, hyperactive, and combined subtypes have distinct features when imaged.

6. Studies involving task performance must take into account the effects of variable performance on imaging data on mean differences between groups and on trial-to-trial variability within individual runs for a subject [68,69].

7. Related to performance and as discussed at length previously [1], error detection systems in the brain can have a profound impact on brain imaging results and must be accounted for using sophisticated data analysis techniques.

8. ADHD imaging in particular must address developmental issues. How does normal development affect age-defined norms? Is ADHD a unitary concept that remains the same throughout one's lifespan, or are there age-related adjustments?

9. Anatomic variability of brain structures makes region definition complex. Further complicating this fact are suggestions that ADHD brains show greater degrees of anatomic variability than healthy brains [36]. Such variability needs to be quantified and accounted for.

10. Laterality effects must be addressed. Most brain structures are bilateral, but what implications does this have for a test result? How are data to be interpreted if effects are normal range on one side and abnormal on

the other? Are only right- or left-sided results clinically meaningful? Should data be averaged to provide one single data point for bilateral structures? Does handedness affect results?

11. There are many potential confounds (anxiety, substance abuse, effects of other medications, caffeine, IQ) that can be controlled in a research study but that may affect results and interpretation in the real world.

12. There are likely to be potential confounds from differential effects of motivational status. Reward and decision-making systems involve many of the same structures implicated in ADHD (cingulate, dorsolateral prefrontal cortex, striatum), and it is hard to imagine that this effect is easily addressed for all subjects.

13. Medication status is another issue that must be paid attention. Although wash-out procedures adequate to produce nearly complete elimination of the medications can validly be used in some studies, the long-term effects of medications are not yet known and represent a potential confound [70]. Medication-naive normative data are needed, and the effects of varying wash-out periods for medications commonly used in patients who have ADHD need to be considered.

14. Finally, all this assumes that the clinician is dealing with an honest patient who has a lack of malfeasance or potential for secondary gain. In the real world, competitive forces and attempts at secondary gains (test accommodations, disability payments, desire to obtain legal source of amphetamines) are certain to lead some patients to attempt to affect test results in some way, and procedures must be in place to guard against this.

Guidelines for considering imaging for clinical purposes

In just a few short decades, functional imaging has made great strides in helping to elucidate the pathophysiology of ADHD and the mechanism of action of the stimulant medications that are the mainstay of ADHD treatment. The veritable explosion of cognitive neuroscience work on the brain's attention, affective, motor, and motivation systems, combined with the rapid pace of technologic advances, has promised to make the next few decades exciting times for ADHD researchers. As has been shown, however, there remains a huge amount of work to be done to translate these early successes into a clinically useful diagnostic imaging test. Although the requirements may seem daunting, they can likely eventually be met with perseverance, patience, and time. That said, there can be no short cuts, and imaging researchers and clinicians alike need to ensure that sufficient proof of diagnostic accuracy and reliability are proven before accepting a proposed methodology.

Until a proposed diagnostic test is fully validated (ie, has satisfactorily met the criteria listed, including publication and independent replication in peer-reviewed journals and widespread acceptance in the field), there can be no ethical use of functional imaging outside of the research realm—especially any type of invasive research or technique that exposes children to ionizing radiation—because there is no accepted, identified benefit, only unnecessary risk and unjustified additional cost. Any such imaging must only be performed in a research context with the oversight of an established human subjects committee or investigational review board. Any other use at this time would be unethical.

The eventual development of a diagnostic imaging test for ADHD would be a wonderful advance, but it would not be a panacea, nor should it replace clinical judgment. Clinicians would be advised as always to first take a careful history, perform a physical examination, obtain relevant blood tests, and then consider whether imaging would tangibly guide diagnostic decision-making or treatment. The differential diagnosis for ADHD is large [71], and although it is agreed that functional imaging is not currently useful for confirming a diagnosis of ADHD [72,73], in certain cases with an index of suspicion (eg, atypical presentation, abnormal neurologic findings, abrupt change in behavior/personality), structural MRI can presently be recommended to rule out disorders mimicking ADHD.

It is hoped that one day, just as a chest radiograph can be useful in guiding treatment decisions by distinguishing between pneumonia and bronchitis, a validated ADHD imaging test could be used as an adjunct to a comprehensive clinical evaluation of ADHD. Until then it must be remembered that colorful brain images can be dramatic, and this fact (when combined with brain imaging's highly technical nature) can unfortunately lead to a situation with potential for misinterpretation or worse—outright misuse and deliberate exploitation. Efforts to push forward the technology need to be matched with equal vigor in protecting patients from unproven methods. In particular, we must clearly define for ourselves and our patients the acceptable uses of imaging and ensure that these techniques are properly validated and integrated with clinical evaluation.

Acknowledgments

The author wishes to thank Joseph Biederman, Tom Spencer, Jennifer Space, and the MGH Pediatric Psychopharmacology Clinic staff.

References

[1] Bush G, Valera EM, Seidman LJ. Functional neuroimaging of attention-deficit/hyperactivity disorder: a review and suggested future directions. Biol Psychiatry 2005;57(11):1273–84.

[2] Seidman LJ, Valera EM, Bush G. Brain function and structure in adults with attention-deficit/hyperactivity disorder. Psychiatr Clin North Am 2004;27(2):323–47.

[3] Spencer TJ, Biederman J, Madras BK, et al. In vivo neuroreceptor imaging in attention-deficit/hyperactivity disorder: a focus on the dopamine transporter. Biol Psychiatry 2005; 57(11):1293–300.

[4] Durston S. A review of the biological bases of ADHD: what have we learned from imaging studies? Ment Retard Dev Disabil Res Rev 2003;9(3):184–95.

[5] Giedd JN, Blumenthal J, Molloy E, et al. Brain imaging of attention deficit/hyperactivity disorder. Ann N Y Acad Sci 2001;931:33–49.

[6] Dickstein SG, Bannon K, Xavier Castellanos F, et al. The neural correlates of attention deficit hyperactivity disorder: an ALE meta-analysis. J Child Psychol Psychiatry 2006;47(10): 1051–62.

[7] Swanson JM, Kinsbourne M, Nigg J, et al. Etiologic subtypes of attention-deficit/hyperactivity disorder: brain imaging, molecular genetic and environmental factors and the dopamine hypothesis. Neuropsychol Rev 2007;17(1):39–59.

[8] Casey BJ, Nigg JT, Durston S. New potential leads in the biology and treatment of attention deficit-hyperactivity disorder. Curr Opin Neurol 2007;20(2):119–24.

[9] Nigg JT, Casey BJ. An integrative theory of attention-deficit/ hyperactivity disorder based on the cognitive and affective neurosciences. Dev Psychopathol 2005;17(3): 785–806.

[10] Seidman LJ, Valera EM, Makris N. Structural brain imaging of attention-deficit/hyperactivity disorder. Biol Psychiatry 2005;57(11):1263–72.

[11] Valera EM, Faraone SV, Murray KE, et al. Meta-analysis of structural imaging findings in attention-deficit/hyperactivity disorder. Biol Psychiatry 2007;61(12):1361–9.

[12] Bush G. Dorsal anterior midcingulate cortex: roles in normal cognition and disruption in attention-deficit/hyperactivity disorder. In: Vogt BA, editor. Cingulate neurobiology and disease. Oxford, UK: Oxford University Press; in press.

[13] Association AP. Diagnostic and statistical manual of mental disorders. 4th edition. Washington, DC: American Psychiatric Press; 1994.

[14] Biederman J. Attention-deficit/hyperactivity disorder: a life-span perspective. J Clin Psychiatry 1998;59(Suppl 7):4–16.

[15] Faraone SV, Biederman J, Mick E. The age-dependent decline of attention deficit hyperactivity disorder: a meta-analysis of follow-up studies. Psychol Med 2006;36(2):159–65.

[16] Faraone SV, Biederman J, Spencer T, et al. Attention-deficit/hyperactivity disorder in adults: an overview. Biol Psychiatry 2000;48(1):9–20.

[17] Arnsten AF. Stimulants: therapeutic actions in ADHD. Neuropsychopharmacology 2006; 31(11):2376–83.

[18] Biederman J, Faraone SV. Current concepts on the neurobiology of attention-deficit/hyperactivity disorder. J Atten Disord 2002;6(Suppl 1):S7–16.

[19] Faraone SV, Sergeant J, Gillberg C, et al. The worldwide prevalence of ADHD: is it an American condition? World Psychiatry 2003;2(2):104–13.

[20] Faraone SV, Biederman J. What is the prevalence of adult ADHD? Results of a population screen of 966 adults. J Atten Disord 2005;9(2):384–91.

[21] Biederman J. Impact of comorbidity in adults with attention-deficit/hyperactivity disorder. J Clin Psychiatry 2004;65(Suppl 3):3–7.

[22] Wilens TE, Faraone SV, Biederman J. Attention-deficit/hyperactivity disorder in adults. JAMA 2004;292(5):619–23.

[23] McGough JJ, Barkley RA. Diagnostic controversies in adult attention deficit hyperactivity disorder. Am J Psychiatry 2004;161(11):1948–56.

[24] Wender PH. Attention-deficit hyperactivity disorder in adults. New York: Oxford University Press; 1995.

[25] Organization WH. ICD-10 Classification of mental and behavioural disorders: diagnostic research criteria. Geneva (Switzerland): World Health Organization; 1992.

[26] Talairach J, Tournoux P. Co-planar stereotaxic atlas of the human brain. New York: Thieme Medical Publishers; 1988.

[27] Castellanos FX. Proceed, with caution: SPECT cerebral blood flow studies of children and adolescents with attention deficit hyperactivity disorder. J Nucl Med 2002;43(12): 1630–3.

[28] Madras BK, Xie Z, Lin Z, et al. Modafinil occupies dopamine and norepinephrine transporters in vivo and modulates the transporters and trace amine activity in vitro. J Pharmacol Exp Ther 2006;319:561–9.

[29] Spencer TJ, Biederman J, Ciccone PE, et al. PET study examining pharmacokinetics, detection and likeability, and dopamine transporter receptor occupancy of short- and long-acting oral methylphenidate. Am J Psychiatry 2006;163(3):387–95.

[30] Volkow ND, Wang GJ, Fowler JS, et al. Imaging the effects of methylphenidate on brain dopamine: new model on its therapeutic actions for attention-deficit/hyperactivity disorder. Biol Psychiatry 2005;57(11):1410–5.

[31] Volkow ND, Wang GJ, Newcorn J, et al. Brain dopamine transporter levels in treatment and drug naive adults with ADHD. Neuroimage 2007;34(3):1182–90.

[32] Detre JA, Wang J. Technical aspects and utility of fMRI using BOLD and ASL. Clin Neurophysiol 2002;113(5):621–34.

[33] Aguirre GK, Detre JA, Wang J. Perfusion fMRI for functional neuroimaging. Int Rev Neurobiol 2005;66:213–36.

[34] Kim J, Whyte J, Wang J, et al. Continuous ASL perfusion fMRI investigation of higher cognition: quantification of tonic CBF changes during sustained attention and working memory tasks. Neuroimage 2006;31(1):376–85.

[35] Wang Z, Wang J, Connick TJ, et al. Continuous ASL (CASL) perfusion MRI with an array coil and parallel imaging at 3T. Magn Reson Med 2005;54(3):732–7.

[36] Bush G, Spencer TJ, Holmes J, et al. Functional magnetic resonance imaging of methylphenidate and placebo in attention-deficit/hyperactivity disorder during the Multi-Source Interference Task. Arch Gen Psychiatry, in press.

[37] Carrey N, MacMaster FP, Fogel J, et al. Metabolite changes resulting from treatment in children with ADHD: a 1H-MRS study. Clin Neuropharmacol 2003;26(4):218–21.

[38] Courvoisie H, Hooper SR, Fine C, et al. Neurometabolic functioning and neuropsychological correlates in children with ADHD-H: preliminary findings. J Neuropsychiatry Clin Neurosci 2004;16(1):63–9.

[39] Jin Z, Zang YF, Zeng YW, et al. Striatal neuronal loss or dysfunction and choline rise in children with attention-deficit hyperactivity disorder: a 1H-magnetic resonance spectroscopy study. Neurosci Lett 2001;315(1–2):45–8.

[40] MacMaster FP, Carrey N, Sparkes S, et al. Proton spectroscopy in medication-free pediatric attention-deficit/hyperactivity disorder. Biol Psychiatry 2003;53(2):184–7.

[41] Perlov E, Philipsen A, Hesslinger B, et al. Reduced cingulate glutamate/glutamine-to-creatine ratios in adult patients with attention deficit/hyperactivity disorder—a magnet resonance spectroscopy study. J Psychiatr Res 2007;41:934–41.

[42] Sun L, Jin Z, Zang YF, et al. Differences between attention-deficit disorder with and without hyperactivity: a 1H-magnetic resonance spectroscopy study. Brain Dev 2005;27(5):340–4.

[43] Yeo RA, Hill DE, Campbell RA, et al. Proton magnetic resonance spectroscopy investigation of the right frontal lobe in children with attention-deficit/hyperactivity disorder. J Am Acad Child Adolesc Psychiatry 2003;42(3):303–10.

[44] Loo SK, Barkley RA. Clinical utility of EEG in attention deficit hyperactivity disorder. Appl Neuropsychol 2005;12(2):64–76.

[45] Hughes JR, John ER. Conventional and quantitative electroencephalography in psychiatry. J Neuropsychiatry Clin Neurosci 1999;11:190–208.

[46] Snyder SM, Hall JR. A meta-analysis of quantitative EEG power associated with attention-deficit hyperactivity disorder. J Clin Neurophysiol 2006;23(5):440–55.

[47] Chabot RJ, di Michele F, Prichep L. The role of quantitative electroencephalography in child and adolescent psychiatric disorders. Child Adolesc Psychiatr Clin N Am 2005; 14(1):21–53, v–vi.

[48] Barry RJ, Clarke AR, Johnstone SJ. A review of electrophysiology in attention-deficit/hyperactivity disorder: I. Qualitative and quantitative electroencephalography. Clin Neurophysiol 2003;114(2):171–83.

[49] Barry RJ, Johnstone SJ, Clarke AR. A review of electrophysiology in attention-deficit/hyperactivity disorder: II. Event-related potentials. Clin Neurophysiol 2003;114(2):184–98.

[50] Tannock R. Attention deficit hyperactivity disorder: advances in cognitive, neurobiological, and genetic research. J Child Psychol Psychiatry 1998;39(1):65–99.

[51] Liotti M, Pliszka SR, Perez R, et al. Abnormal brain activity related to performance monitoring and error detection in children with ADHD. Cortex 2005;41(3):377–88.

[52] Bush G, Shin LM. The multi-source interference task: an fMRI task that reliably activates the cingulo-frontal-parietal cognitive/attention network in individual subjects. Nat Protoc 2006;1:308–13.

[53] Bush G, Shin LM, Holmes J, et al. The multi-source interference task: validation study with fMRI in individual subjects. Mol Psychiatry 2003;8:60–70.

[54] Bush G, Frazier JA, Rauch SL, et al. Anterior cingulate cortex dysfunction in attention-deficit/hyperactivity disorder revealed by fMRI and the counting Stroop. Biol Psychiatry 1999;45(12):1542–52.

[55] Smith AB, Taylor E, Brammer M, et al. Task-specific hypoactivation in prefrontal and temporoparietal brain regions during motor inhibition and task switching in medication-naive children and adolescents with attention deficit hyperactivity disorder. Am J Psychiatry 2006;163(6):1044–51.

[56] Zang YF, Jin Z, Weng XC, et al. Functional MRI in attention-deficit hyperactivity disorder: evidence for hypofrontality. Brain Dev 2005;27(8):544–50.

[57] Aron AR, Dowson JH, Sahakian BJ, et al. Methylphenidate improves response inhibition in adults with attention-deficit/hyperactivity disorder. Biol Psychiatry 2003;54(12):1465–8.

[58] Vaidya CJ, Austin G, Kirkorian G, et al. Selective effects of methylphenidate in attention deficit hyperactivity disorder: a functional magnetic resonance study. Proc Natl Acad Sci U S A 1998;95(24):14494–9.

[59] Durston S, Tottenham NT, Thomas KM, et al. Differential patterns of striatal activation in young children with and without ADHD. Biol Psychiatry 2003;53(10):871–8.

[60] Valera EM, Faraone SV, Biederman J, et al. Functional neuroanatomy of working memory in adults with attention-deficit/hyperactivity disorder. Biol Psychiatry 2005;57(5):439–47.

[61] Volkow ND, Fowler JS, Wang G, et al. Mechanism of action of methylphenidate: insights from PET imaging studies. J Atten Disord 2002;6(Suppl 1):S31–43.

[62] Dougherty DD, Bonab AA, Spencer TJ, et al. Dopamine transporter density in patients with attention deficit hyperactivity disorder. Lancet 1999;354(9196):2132–3.

[63] Altman DG, Bland JM. Diagnostic tests 2: predictive values. BMJ 1994;309(6947):102.

[64] Deeks JJ, Altman DG. Diagnostic tests 4: likelihood ratios. BMJ 2004;329(7458):168–9.

[65] Altman DG, Bland JM. Diagnostic tests 3: receiver operating characteristic plots. BMJ 1994; 309(6948):188.

[66] Bossuyt PM, Reitsma JB, Bruns DE, et al. Towards complete and accurate reporting of studies of diagnostic accuracy: the STARD initiative. BMJ 2003;326(7379):41–4.

[67] Raichle ME, MacLeod AM, Snyder AZ, et al. A default mode of brain function. Proc Natl Acad Sci U S A 2001;98(2):676–82.

[68] Sonuga-Barke EJ, Castellanos FX. Spontaneous attentional fluctuations in impaired states and pathological conditions: a neurobiological hypothesis. Neurosci Biobehav Rev 2007;31: 977–86.

[69] Castellanos FX, Sonuga-Barke EJ, Scheres A, et al. Varieties of attention-deficit/hyperactivity disorder-related intra-individual variability. Biol Psychiatry 2005;57(11):1416–23.

[70] Langleben DD, Acton PD, Austin G, et al. Effects of methylphenidate discontinuation on cerebral blood flow in prepubescent boys with attention deficit hyperactivity disorder. J Nucl Med 2002;43(12):1624–9.

[71] Pearl PL, Weiss RE, Stein MA. Medical mimics. Medical and neurological conditions simulating ADHD. Ann N Y Acad Sci 2001;931:97–112.

[72] Flaherty LT, Arroyo W, Chatoor I, et al. Brain imaging and child and adolescent psychiatry with special emphasis on SPECT. 2005. p. 1–11.

[73] Zametkin A, Schroth E, Faden D. The role of brain imaging in the diagnosis and management of ADHD. ADHD Report 2005;13(5):11–4.

[74] Bush G, Luu P, Posner MI. Cognitive and emotional influences in anterior cingulate cortex. Trends Cogn Sci 2000;4(6):215–22.

[75] Bush G, Vogt BA, Holmes J, et al. Dorsal anterior cingulate cortex: a role in reward-based decision making. Proc Natl Acad Sci U S A 2002;99(1):523–8.

[76] Williams ZM, Bush G, Rauch SL, et al. Human anterior cingulate neurons and the integration of monetary reward with motor responses. Nat Neurosci 2004;7(12):1370–5.

[77] Makris N, Biederman J, Valera EM, et al. Cortical thinning of the attention and executive function networks in adults with attention-deficit/hyperactivity disorder. Cereb Cortex 2007;17(6):1364–75.

[78] Seidman LJ, Valera EM, Makris N, et al. Dorsolateral prefrontal and anterior cingulate cortex volumetric abnormalities in adults with attention-deficit/hyperactivity disorder identified by magnetic resonance imaging. Biol Psychiatry 2006;60:1071–80.

[79] Shaw P, Lerch J, Greenstein D, et al. Longitudinal mapping of cortical thickness and clinical outcome in children and adolescents with attention-deficit/hyperactivity disorder. Arch Gen Psychiatry 2006;63(5):540–9.

ELSEVIER
SAUNDERS

Child Adolesc Psychiatric Clin N Am
17 (2008) 405–420

CHILD AND
ADOLESCENT
PSYCHIATRIC CLINICS
OF NORTH AMERICA

Is There a Need to Reformulate Attention Deficit Hyperactivity Disorder Criteria in Future Nosologic Classifications?

Luis Augusto Rohde, MD, PhD

*ADHD Outpatient Program, Division of Child and Adolescent Psychiatry,
Hospital de Clínicas de Porto Alegre, Federal University of Rio Grande do Sul,
Rua Ramiro Barcelos 2350, Room 2201A, Porto Alegre, RS, 90035-003 Brazil*

The development of classification systems in psychiatry has been a complex task. In clinical settings, these classification systems help communication about disorders among professionals and between them and their patients. In addition, a diagnosis based on these nosologic systems has a central role for mental health insurance policies. There is a recent interest in research opportunities for improving the nosology of attention deficit hyperactivity disorder (ADHD) in future classification systems like the DSM-V and the ICD-11. This article addresses the following issues: (1) Do differences between DSM-IV and ICD-10 criteria for ADHD/hyperkinetic disorder (HD) have any clinical and research impact? (2) Should ADHD criteria be modified to capture a more dimensional perspective that provides a better understanding for the disorder? (3) Do new classification systems for ADHD need to be more developmental sensitive? (4) Should different criteria or thresholds according to gender be incorporated?

Potential conflict of interest: The ADHD Outpatient Program receives research support from the following pharmaceutical companies: Bristol-Myers Squibb, Eli-Lilly and Company, Janssen-Cilag, and Novartis. Professor Rohde is on the speakers' bureau or is a consultant for the same companies and is on the advisory board for Eli Lilly and Company.

Funding sources: This work was partially supported by research grants from Conselho Nacional de Desenvolvimento Científico e Tecnológico (CNPq, Brazil) (Grant MCT/CNPq 02/2006 - Universal), Hospital de Clinicas de Porto Alegre.

A previous version of this manuscript was presented in the Eunethydis meeting (ADHD European Consortium), October 2006, Bruges, Belgium. The opinions expressed here reflect solely the personal view of the author.

E-mail address: lrohde@terra.com.br

(5) Are we ready to include any biologic marker for ADHD in new classification systems? (6) Do we need more data on validity for different aspects of the ADHD criteria? (7) Are the proposed subtypes valid? (8) Is age-of-onset of symptoms or impairment a valid criterion for ADHD?

Traditionally, several medical fields have assumed a framework known as causalism in the understanding of diseases and in the development of nosologic classifications. That is, a true disease should be associated with a discrete and unique cause [1].

Previous initiatives of refining psychiatric classifications, however, relied on the so-called "descriptivism" framework [1]. In this framework, a set of relative cohesive clinical characteristics are defined and tested in field trials. The rationale behind this approach is that we do not know which are the exact causes for most mental disorders, although currently there is a certain degree of agreement that they are determined by complex interactions between genes and environmental factors [2]. Ultimately the set of criteria should differentiate a group of patients who have some specific characteristics. More than 30 years ago, Robins and Guze [3] proposed a strategy for assessing the validity of diagnostic constructs in psychiatric disorders that has been used in several investigations. They suggested that a group of symptoms would differentiate a group of patients, generating a valid diagnosis if the group of symptoms determines a specific clinical presentation and is associated with a clear pattern of family history, course, specific laboratory findings, and response to treatment. Regarding psychiatric disorders of childhood and adolescence, Jensen and colleagues [4] adapted the strategy, including the following eight criteria: clinical phenomenology; demographic, psychosocial, and biologic factors; family genetics and environmental factors; natural history; and intervention response.

Recently the American Psychiatric Association prepared a research agenda for the DSM-V [5]. Two key issues are: (1) to move toward a more unified DSM/ICD classification and (2) to study the validity of disorders, linking them to pathophysiology whenever possible. In the same direction, the World Health Organization is joining a group of experts from different cultures to define priorities for mental disorders in the ICD-11.

Why should clinicians care about classification systems in psychiatry? In clinical environments, mental health professionals see specific patients. On the other side, classification systems anchor their criteria in research involving groups of subjects. Not always, individuals behave or express emotions according to means and standard deviations. These nosologic systems, however, provide evidence-based criteria for the establishment of reliable and valid diagnoses. A reliable and valid diagnosis of a mental disorder is clinically important, because it allows a better communication among clinicians and between them and their patients [6]. The possibility of having a diagnosis sometimes provides relief for the patient and their family (eg, a child who has an ADHD diagnosis might understand that his or her school failure is not related to laziness or lack of intelligence). In addition, diagnoses based in well-established systems are increasingly a central aspect in mental health insurance policies worldwide. Clinicians are thus requested to assess if their patients fulfill criteria according to these systems.

Several aspects should be tested regarding reliability and validity of a mental health diagnosis from a classification system before it would be ready to be incorporated in clinical settings. An extensive discussion on this topic for child psychiatry is far beyond the scope of this article and can be found in the excellent article by Volkmar and colleagues [6]. In sum, diagnoses derived from a classification system must present internal consistency, test–retest and inter-rater reliability, face, construct, predictive, and concurrent validity [6].

There is recent interest in research opportunities for improving the nosology of ADHD in future classification systems like the DSM-V and the ICD-11. Potential modifications in ADHD criteria have thus been the target of ongoing debate in recent editorials in psychiatric journals [7,8].

From a historical perspective, what is now recognized as ADHD was described in the second edition of the DSM-II as "the hyperkinetic reaction of childhood" in 1968. After that, operational criteria for the syndrome were provided in DSM-III [9]. In this classification system, attention deficit disorder (ADD) was categorized according to whether or not hyperactivity was present. Inattention and hyperactivity were thus represented in two separate domains, and it was possible to derive an ADHD diagnosis based on the presence of enough symptoms in only one dimension. In the next two revisions of the DSM, different conceptualizations of the disorder were proposed. DSM-III-R grouped these symptoms in a unique domain, along with impulsivity [10]. More recently the DSM-IV listed inattentive and hyperactivity–impulsivity symptoms in separate domains. It is possible to derive a diagnosis of ADHD according to DSM-IV based on the presence of symptoms in one or both domains, resulting in three possible subtypes. The symptoms must be associated with functional impairment in at least two settings, and some symptoms associated with functional impairment must have been present before the age of 7 years [11].

The list of ADHD symptoms is similar in the DSM-IV and the ICD-10, although the latter uses a different nomenclature—hyperkinetic disorder (HD) [12]. Differences are more related to the way the diagnosis is formulated. The ICD-10 requires a minimum number of symptoms in all three dimensions (inattention, overactivity, and impulsivity) and the presence of each symptom in at least two different settings. Furthermore, the ICD-10 has mood, anxiety, and developmental disorders as exclusion diagnoses. The DSM-IV and DSM-III-R allow the establishment of an ADHD diagnosis in the presence of mood and anxiety disorders, but not in that of pervasive developmental disorders (PDD). These differences are related to the fact the ICD-10 is conceptually a more restrictive classification system than the DSM-IV. In addition, ICD-10 allows combinations of disorders instead of treating them as comorbidities (eg, hyperkinetic conduct disorder).

The main objective of this article is thus to provide a selective review of the literature addressing areas that might need some modifications in criteria for ADHD in future nosologic classification.

Do differences between DSM-IV and ICD-10 criteria for attention deficit hyperactivity disorder–hyperkinetic disorder have any clinical and research impact?

Not surprisingly, several investigations using DSM-IV and ICD-10 in clinical and community samples clearly documented that higher prevalence rates of ADHD were generated using DSM-IV than ICD-10 criteria [13].

Recently the author's conducted a comprehensive systematic review on ADHD/HD prevalence during childhood and adolescence, providing an estimated pooled prevalence for the disorder. In addition, the author's applied meta-regression analyses to evaluate the role of methodologic characteristics on the variability of results. After a broad review and a rigorous analysis of articles, the author's included 102 studies comprising 171,756 subjects from all world regions. The aggregated prevalence of ADHD/HD based on all studies was 5.29% (95% CI, 5.01–5.56). Furthermore, adjusting for methodologic issues, estimates from North America and Europe were not significantly different. Differences between studies regarding the diagnostic criteria used (DSM-III, DSM-III-R, DSM-IV, or ICD-10), source of information (best-estimate procedure, parents, "and rule," "or rule," teachers, or subjects), and requirement or not of impairment for the diagnosis were associated with significant variability of results [14].

Santosh and colleagues [15] also documented in reanalyses of the data from the MTA that defining cases according to ICD-10 would result in a group of patients more prone to respond to psychopharmacologic interventions than did selecting patients based on DSM-IV criteria.

Although HD cases defined by ICD-10 criteria might have a high degree of similarity with those cases fulfilling DSM-IV criteria for ADHD combined type [16], the kind of data discussed above suggests that differences between these two classification systems have a clear impact on ADHD epidemiology and response to psychopharmacologic interventions. Ultimately the use of two classification systems imposes difficulties in interpreting cross-cultural studies and a logistic problem of needing training in different systems.

It thus makes perfect sense that a key nosologic issue for future revisions of the classification systems would be the search for an even more unified conceptualization of ADHD between the ICD and the DSM.

Should attention deficit hyperactivity disorder criteria be modified to capture a more dimensional perspective that provides a better understanding for the disorder?

There is a long debate in the literature about whether ADHD is better conceptualized as a categoric or a dimensional disorder [17]. Recently

Haslam and colleagues [18] conducted an investigation with almost 3000 children and adolescents from an epidemiologic sample in Australia using two modern taxometric procedures—MAXEIG and MAMBAC—documenting that ADHD construct is better modeled dimensionally in children and adolescents.

Even assuming a dimensional construct for ADHD, however, there is a clear need of categoric decisions for pragmatic reasons in clinical settings. In this case, it seems logical to choose an external validator to help in the decision as to where to establish an artificial cutoff point. The most-used strategy is to use impairment or need for treatment as the external validator [18]. This kind of situation is also common in other medical fields such as cardiology, in which there is a need to determine a cutoff point in a latent dimensional construct (level of blood pressure) to establish the diagnosis of hypertension, identifying those at risk in outcome.

Do new classification systems need to be more developmental-sensitive for the attention deficit hyperactivity disorder diagnosis?

One of the major criticisms for DSM-IV/ICD-10 classification of child and adolescent psychiatric disorders was always that the proposed criteria do not take into account a development perspective [6].

This is especially important for ADHD, because DSM-IV field trials were conducted with samples composed mainly of children with only some adolescents and no adults [19]. For instance, several investigations have suggested the decline of hyperactive symptoms during adolescence [20]. There is thus no reason to believe that the same threshold for symptoms of hyperactivity should be required throughout the life cycle.

In the same direction, Kooij and colleagues [21] evaluated the presence of ADHD symptoms in a sample of 1813 primary-care adult patients from The Netherlands. Inattentive and hyperactivity symptoms were significantly associated with psychosocial impairment. Subjects with four or more inattentive or hyperactive–impulsive symptoms were significantly more impaired than subjects with two, one, and without symptoms. The prevalence of ADHD was 1.0% (95% CI, 0.6–1.6) for a cutoff of six symptoms, and 2.5% (95% CI, 1.9–3.4) for a cutoff of four symptoms, with the requirement of the presence of all three core symptoms during childhood.

Clinically the issue of different ADHD symptomatic profiles during the life cycle is even more relevant. The level of preponderance among the three core components of the disorder—inattention, hyperactivity, and impulsivity—clearly varies from preschool years to adolescence. Clinicians dealing with the diagnosis of ADHD in childhood and adolescence thus should have a solid knowledge of child development. In addition, there are emerging new data suggesting that some inattention problems and executive functioning impairments are the key residual symptoms in adults who have ADHD [22]. Although the issue of diagnosis of ADHD in adults is beyond the scope of this article, one of the most important improvements in ADHD classification in future nosographic systems should be derived from huge international studies with community samples to validate adult ADHD clinical profiles suggested in small clinical studies [23,24].

Is there a need for different attention deficit hyperactivity disorder criteria according to gender?

Most data from ADHD investigations was obtained from samples with a huge preponderance of males. There are several investigations documenting that the patterns of ADHD type and comorbidity might be different in females compared with males [25]. For example, females tend to have a higher ratio of ADHD inattentive type/combined type than males, which might be associated with lower referral to treatment [26].

More recently Waschbusch and King [27] assessed behavior ratings reported by mothers and teachers regarding a sample of 1491 elementary school children. They documented that a subgroup of girls with only subthreshold symptoms but important impairment would be left out of the ADHD diagnosis when using standard DSM-IV thresholds. Defining gender-specific thresholds, however, would include these females in the diagnostic category.

Again, impact of gender issues is also relevant for diagnosis in other medical specialties. For instance, coronary artery disease in women might have a completely different clinical picture than the one frequently found in men. In addition, some diagnostic tools like exercise testing might have different performance requirements according to gender [28].

This is an area, investigation of community female samples at different ages, in which much more research is needed to generate new data, helping nosologic classifications to be more in tune with gender issues.

Are we ready to incorporate any biologic marker for attention deficit hyperactivity disorder in new classification systems?

Since the publication of the DSM-IV in 1994, there was an enormous amount of new data published suggesting that ADHD is best conceptualized as a neurobiologic disorder (see the article by Kieling and colleagues, elsewhere in this issue) [29,30]. Much debate still exists, however, as to whether there would be worth in including any molecular genetic, neuropsychologic, neurophysiologic, or neuroimaging marker in future classification systems for ADHD.

The discussion addressing some of these specific issues can be found in the articles by Bush, Faraone, and Sergeant and colleagues, elsewhere in this issue. For the scope of this article, it is important to discuss what would be minimal conditions to accept any biologic markers as relevant for the diagnostic process.

Again, the criteria proposed by Robins and Guze [3] for assessing the validity of diagnostic constructs in psychiatric disorders might serve as

a starting point. Adapting this proposal for the discussion here, ideally a biologic marker to be included in the classification system, would have to improve
the nosology in several if not all the domains mentioned. In other words, it
should (1) determine a more phenotypically homogeneous group of patients;
(2) be associated with specific demographic and psychosocial factors; (3) be
highly heritable; (4) be associated with a more homogeneous course of symptoms; and (5) determine a specific pattern of response to treatment.

ADHD is an extremely heterogeneous disorder. For instance, there is
sufficient evidence to understand the genetic vulnerability for ADHD as
determined by several genes of small effect [31]. Each of them would thus
explain a small fraction of the variability of symptoms in a given population.
In other words, despite the massive amount of data documenting a genetic
predisposition for the disorder [32], the presence of no single polymorphism
at any gene would seem to have sufficient positive or negative predictive
value to deal with all heterogeneity of the ADHD phenotype.

Regarding neuroimaging, there is some convergence on structural neuroimaging findings suggesting lower volumes in the whole brain and in specific
areas in subjects who have ADHD compared with non-ADHD control
subjects [33,34]. In addition, there is an impressive amount of evidence
suggesting the involvement of specific prefrontal areas and their connections
with striatum and other subcortical structures and the involvement of cerebellar areas in the pathophysiology of the disorder [35]. There is, however,
a huge variability across studies for the exact location of dysfunctions, and
lateralization among others. The same applies to findings from functional
neuroimaging [36]. Differences on neuroimaging findings probably reflect
not only the heterogeneity of the ADHD phenotype, but also the huge
variability in the methodology across studies [37]. Again no specific finding
thus has sufficient positive or negative predictive value to be included in the
next generation of ADHD criteria in nosologic classifications [36].

As extensively revised by others, several neuropsychologic measures have
huge effects sizes in differentiating subjects who have ADHD from normal
control subjects. Effects sizes significantly decrease, however, when comparisons include other psychiatric control subjects (see the article by Sergeant and colleagues, elsewhere in this issue) [37]. In other words,
neuropsychologic measures tend to help clinicians for diagnostic purposes
where they need less—differentiating subjects who have ADHD from
normal control subjects who have no psychiatric symptoms.

As expected, no molecular genetic, neuropsychologic, neurophysiologic,
or neuroimaging marker thus has sufficient positive and negative predictive
value and diagnostic efficiency to deal with all heterogeneity inherent in
DSM or ICD criteria for ADHD.

Recently there has been a renewed interest in the concept of endophenotype
in psychiatry [38]. Deconstructing heterogeneous phenotypes such as ADHD
into smaller heritable intermediate endophenotypes may facilitate the search
for genetic markers. Theoretically this approach would facilitate the search

for more valid ADHD subtypes. In fact, there are even some proposals to include executive functioning deficits as an ADHD subtype [23]. Despite the increasing number of ADHD investigations in this field, no proposed ADHD endophenotype fulfilled sufficiently the criteria discussed to be incorporated into future modifications of the classification system at this moment.

Finally, a more ambitious approach to refining the heterogeneous ADHD phenotype has been proposed recently. Using modern statistical approaches and accumulating knowledge on a molecular genetics basis for ADHD, some investigators are pursuing a more causal pathway. They are departing from specific polymorphisms or haplotypes in candidate genes and trying to determine which specific aspects of the ADHD phenotype are associated with them [39,40]. Although innovative and promising, this approach needs also to document that it would be able to derive an even more heritable phenotype characterizing phenotypically a more homogeneous group of patients, presenting specific associated demographic and psychosocial factors with a more homogeneous course of symptoms and a specific pattern of response to treatment.

In sum, we are neither at a point that any molecular genetic, neuropsychologic, neurophysiologic, or neuroimaging marker is ready to be included in the classification system nor that any endophenotype might be included in the nosologic classification for ADHD to decrease the heterogeneity of the phenotype.

Do we need more data on construct validity for attention deficit hyperactivity disorder criteria as proposed to that in the DSM-IV?

Although there are enormous amounts of new data on ADHD each year—more than 500 articles in the PUBMED just in the first 6 months of 2007 using only the acronym ADHD for searching—there are several issues on the diagnostic criteria in both classification systems that deserve special attention. Some of them are (1) Is there validity for the age-of-onset of impairment criterion in the DSM-IV and age-of-onset of symptoms criterion in ICD-10? (2) Do we have enough data to support ADHD types as currently described in the DSM-IV? (3) Is there a need to better operationalize the criteria of frequency of symptoms? (4) Do all ADHD symptoms listed in the DSM/ICD have the same diagnostic efficiency? (5) How to solve the overlapping of some symptoms listed in the DSM/ICD and the presence of different issues assessed by the same criterion? (6) How to integrate different information sources in the diagnostic assessment? (7) Which is the rationale for excluding ADHD diagnosis in the presence of PDD?

Is there validity for the age-of-onset of impairment criterion in the DSM-IV and age-of-onset of symptoms criterion in ICD-10?

The DSM-IV requires that some of the core ADHD symptoms that cause significant impairment must be present before the age of 7 years [11]. In the

ICD-10, criteria for HD require that symptoms must begin before the age of 6 years, with no mention of age for impairment [12].

Although this age-of-onset/age-of-onset of impairment criterion for ADHD has been used for more than 2 decades, its implementation and retention was based on the clinical experience of the previous committees formed to create diagnostic criteria, not on empiric research. Several investigations clearly document that: (1) comparisons between the group having an age-on-onset after 7 years and the group with an age-of-onset before 7 years did not reveal significant differences in comorbid conditions or degree of impairment [41,42]; (2) no significant differences between late onset and full ADHD subjects were found in neuropsychologic impairment and family transmission [43,44]; and (3) subjects who had the full diagnosis did not have a better response to methylphenidate than did the late onset ADHD subjects in samples of children and adults [45].

Finally, Green and colleagues [46] showed that the recall of the exact age-of-onset of symptoms by parents has only moderate reliability after a 1-year period. This poses dilemmas for the diagnostic process that are even greater when assessing ADHD in adults [8]. This age-of-onset of impairment criterion thus might be expanded to children and adolescents in future classifications without mentioning any arbitrary age until there are investigations suggesting a clear specific cutoff point.

Do we have enough data to support attention deficit hyperactivity disorder types as currently described in the DSM-IV?

Findings from several investigations are consistent in suggesting a bidimensional construct for ADHD symptoms in non-referred samples [20,47]. There is thus evidence supporting the DSM-IV proposal of three ADHD types: combined, predominantly inattentive, and predominantly hyperactive/impulsive [11]. In addition, there are several studies suggesting different neuropsychologic profiles, neurobiologic substrates, patterns of comorbidity, gender distribution, and impairments according to these ADHD types [48–51].

Some recent studies, however, have challenged this DSM-IV proposal for ADHD types, suggesting that: (1) There is no developmental continuity for these ADHD types. Lahey and colleagues [52] documented that a significant proportion (50%) of children diagnosed as having ADHD, predominantly inattentive type, in preschool years met criteria for other ADHD types at least twice during a follow-up investigation (6 follow-up assessments). (2) There is a week association between DSM-IV ADHD types of the probands and relatives [53,54]. In other words, parents presenting one ADHD type might have children who have a completely different ADHD type. A family pattern of transmission was detectable only for ADHD inattentive type [54]. (3) There is no different pattern of response to methylphenidate according to ADHD type or dimension (inattentive versus hyperactive/impulsive) [55].

In addition, other strategies for decreasing ADHD phenotypic heterogeneity have also been proposed. Jensen and colleagues [4] suggested that dividing ADHD according to comorbidities (exophenotype) would result in improvements of classification systems. This strategy was not extensively assessed in further investigations, however. More recently the use of statistically-based classification methods—latent class analyses—has shown success in refining ADHD into homogenous and heritable subtypes [56,57].

Finally, there is a subgroup of patients presenting inattentive symptoms without hyperactivity that seem to show slow retrieval and information processing, low levels of alertness, and more problems with memory and orientation. These features of inconsistent alertness and orientation (sluggishness, drowsiness, and daydreaming) were considered a distinct factor, termed "sluggish cognitive tempo" (SCT). Such items were excluded from the final version of DSM-IV because of their poor predictive validity. Recently there has been renewed interest in assessing whether SCT symptoms might be included in the ADHD diagnosis, decreasing heterogeneity for ADHD inattentive type [58].

In sum, there is a clear need to reassess the current classification of ADHD types in light of the controversial data on its validity and the availability of new statistical techniques like latent class analyses.

Is there a need to better operationalize the criteria of frequency of symptoms?

In a qualitative assessment of families in the author's ADHD outpatient program, the author's asked parents what they understand "often" to mean. The DSM-IV requires that each of the 18 symptoms listed in criteria A must occur "often" to be positive. Not surprisingly, parents have an extremely diverse understanding of what "often" means. Although inserting an operational definition of what "often" means in any classification system may cause it to be more psychometrically precise [59], this approach makes the criteria less friendly for clinical purposes. These data, however, should raise attention to the fact that clinicians and interviewers need to discuss with families a common understanding when assessing frequency of symptoms.

Do all attention deficit hyperactivity disorder symptoms listed in the DSM/ICD have the same diagnostic efficiency? How to solve the overlapping of some symptoms listed in the DSM/ICD and the presence of different issues assessed by the same criterion?

The DSM-IV/ICD-10 attributes the same positive and negative predictive value for each of the 18 symptoms listed as ADHD criterion. In other words, clinicians have to count symptoms, checking to see if the threshold of six inattentive and hyperactive/impulsive symptoms was reached, attributing the same weight for each symptom (each count as one). Unfortunately this same weight for each symptom has never been tested in other investigations conducted after the work of the clinical trials for DSM-IV that were carried out before 1994. There are thus no data supporting, for instance, that the statement "is often easily distracted by extraneous stimuli" has the same diagnostic efficiency for ADHD diagnosis as does the statement "is often forgetful in daily activities." Moreover, all symptoms are equally required to occur often. Recent investigations on samples of adults have documented that different frequency levels for each symptom might have a better performance for ADHD diagnosis [60]. For instance, the symptom "have difficulty getting things in order when you have to do a task that requires organization" thus needs to be endorsed sometimes, whereas the symptom "when you have a task that requires a lot of thought, do you avoid or delay getting started?" needs to be endorsed often. All these assumptions need to be tested using modern statistical techniques like those from item response theory in non-referred samples [61,62].

There are even more problematic issues regarding the construct validity of the ADHD criteria in the DSM-IV, such as, for instance, the fact some items (symptoms) seem to be assessing the same concept—see, for example: "often leaves seat in classroom or in other situations in which remaining seated is expected" and "often runs about or climbs excessively in situations in which it is inappropriate." If this is the case, prevalence rates might be artificially inflated. Different neuropsychologic concepts are included in the same item, however: "often does not follow through instructions and fails to finish school work, chores, or duties in the workplace." Moreover, the DSM-IV criteria do not specify what happens when just one of the two symptoms presented in this criterion is endorsed.

It is fundamental that future classification systems might benefit from more research on all these issues to refine the list of symptoms from DSM-IV criterion A for ADHD.

How to integrate different information sources in the diagnostic assessment?

Considering that the information source is relevant for the variability of ADHD estimates as documented by Polanczyk and colleagues [14], there is an urgent need to solve the issue of "who should report on what." Symptoms must be pervasive in the subject's life as stated in the DSM-IV, but is information by parents on the school and the home environment sufficient for children and adolescents? Or do we need information from two different sources—parents for home and teachers for school? Although some overlap exists in the group of patients determined by these two approaches, there is evidence that they are not fully similar [63].

Which is the rationale for excluding attention deficit hyperactivity disorder diagnosis in the presence of pervasive development disorders?

The DSM-IV criteria exclude the diagnosis of ADHD in the presence of PDD [12]. There is no clear empiric background for this diagnostic decision however. Several recent investigations have documented that: (1) ADHD symptomatology can occur frequently in patients who have PDD [64], and autistic traits are also common in population-based children meeting diagnostic criteria for ADHD [65]; (2) there might be similar genetic susceptibility for the two disorders [66]; (3) children endorsing PDD criteria and high scores in a scale for ADHD had a significant worse outcome and a more broad psychopathology than those who had PDD and a low endorsement of ADHD symptoms [67]; (4) some measures of pragmatic language can differentiate children who have ADHD and PDD [68]; (5) impairment in executive functioning is more global in PDD than in ADHD [69]; and (6) ADHD symptoms might be successfully treated in children who have PDD, and the recognition of this dual diagnosis might be essential for conducting effective treatments [70].

Finally, there is no conceptual reason to exclude ADHD diagnosis in the presence of PDD if it is not excluded in the presence of mental retardation. At least revisiting this issue is thus mandatory for new classification systems.

Summary

There are several issues that clearly need to be addressed through more investigations to improve the validity of the ADHD diagnosis in future classifications systems. Three aspects deserve special attention: (1) improving ADHD diagnosis in adults; (2) making DSM/ICD classification for ADHD more similar; and (3) exclusion of the age-of-onset of impairment criteria.

It is important to bear in mind, however, that, despite the problems mentioned, ADHD is an extremely well investigated disorder with superior validity over most mental disorders and even over several medical conditions [71].

Finally, it is also important to realize that modifications in the classification system need to be empirically based and to encompass a more reliable description of patients. Moreover, any modification is not a mere academic exercise, because it has tremendous repercussions in the mental health systems worldwide.

References

[1] Zachar P, Kendler KS. Psychiatric disorders: a conceptual taxonomy. Am J Psychiatry 2007; 164:557–65.
[2] Caspi A, Moffitt TE. Gene-environment interactions in psychiatry: joining forces with neuroscience. Nat Rev Neurosci 2006;7:583–90.
[3] Robins E, Guze SB. Establishment of diagnostic validity in psychiatric illness: its application to schizophrenia. Am J Psychiatry 1970;126:983–7.
[4] Jensen PS, Martin D, Cantwell DP. Comorbidity in ADHD: implications for research, practice, and DSM-V. J Am Acad Child Adolesc Psychiatry 1997;36:1065–79.

[5] Kupfer DJ, First MB, Reiger DA. A research agenda for DSM-V. Washington, DC: American Psychiatric Press; 2002.

[6] Volkmar FR, Schwab-Stone M, First M. Classification in child and adolescent psychiatry: principles and issues. In: Lewis M, editor. Child and adolescent psychiatry. A comprehensive textbook. 3rd edition. Lippincott Williams & Wilkins. Philadelphia 2002. p. 499–505.

[7] Naglieri JA, Goldstein S. The role of intellectual processes in the DSM-V diagnosis of ADHD. J Atten Disord 2006;10:3–8.

[8] McGough J, McCracken J. Adult attention deficit hyperactivity disorder: moving beyond DSM-IV. Am J Psychiatry 2006;163:1673–5.

[9] American Psychiatric Association. Diagnostic and statistical manual of mental disorders. Washington, DC: American Psychiatric Association; 1980.

[10] American Psychiatric Association. Diagnostic and statistical manual of mental disorders. Washington, DC: American Psychiatric Association; 1986.

[11] American Psychiatric Association. Diagnostic and statistical manual of mental disorders. Washington, DC: American Psychiatric Association; 1994.

[12] World Health Organization. The ICD-10 classification of mental and behavioral disorders: diagnostic criteria for research. Geneva: WHO; 1993.

[13] Goodman R, Ford T, Richards H, et al. The development and well-being assessment: description and initial validation of an integrated assessment of child and adolescent psychopathology. J Child Psychol Psychiatry 2000;41:645–55.

[14] Polanczyk G, Lima MS, Horta BL, et al. The worldwide prevalence of attention-deficit/hyperactivity disorder: a systematic review and meta-regression analyses. Am J Psychiatry 2007;164:942–8.

[15] Santosh P, Taylor E, Swanson J, et al. Refining the diagnoses of inattention and overactivity syndromes: a reanalysis of the multimodal treatment study of attention deficit hyperactivity disorder (ADHD) based on ICD-10 criteria for hyperkinetic disorder. Clin Neurosci Res 2005;5:307–14.

[16] Tripp G, Luk SL, Schaughency EA, et al. DSM-IV and ICD-10: a comparison of the correlates of ADHD and hyperkinetic disorder. J Am Acad Child Adolesc Psychiatry 1999;38: 156–64.

[17] Levy F, Hay DA, McStephen M, et al. Attention-deficit hyperactivity disorder: a category or a continuum? Genetic analysis of a large-scale twin study. J Am Acad Child Adolesc Psychiatry 1997;36:737–44.

[18] Haslam N, Williams B, Prior M, et al. The latent structure of attention-deficit/hyperactivity disorder: a taxometric analysis. Aust N Z J Psychiatry 2006;40:639–47.

[19] Lahey BB, Applegate B, McBurnett K, et al. DSM-IV field trials for attention deficit hyperactivity disorder in children and adolescents. Am J Psychiatry 1994;151:1673–85.

[20] Faraone SV, Biederman J, Mick E. The age-dependent decline of attention deficit hyperactivity disorder: a meta-analysis of follow-up studies. Psychol Med 2006;36:159–65.

[21] Kooij JJ, Buitelaar JK, van den Oord EJ, et al. Internal and external validity of attention-deficit hyperactivity disorder in a population-based sample of adults. Psychol Med 2005; 35:817–27.

[22] Biederman J, Petty C, Fried R, et al. Impact of psychometrically defined deficits of executive functioning adults with attention-deficit/hyperactivity disorder. Am J Psychiatry 2006;163: 1673–5.

[23] Fayyad J, De Graaf R, Kessler R, et al. Cross-national prevalence and correlates of adult attention-deficit hyperactivity disorder. Br J Psychiatry 2007;190:402–9.

[24] Barkley RA. Symptoms and age of onset. The science of ADHD in adults: clinic-referred adults and children grown up. In: Barkley RA, Murphy KR, Fischer M, editors. New York: Guilford, in press.

[25] Graetz BW, Sawyer MG, Baghurst P. Gender differences among children with DSM-IV ADHD in Australia. J Am Acad Child Adolesc Psychiatry 2005;44:159–68.

[26] Biederman J, Faraone SV. The Massachusetts General Hospital studies of gender influences on attention-deficit/hyperactivity disorder in youth and relatives. Psychiatr Clin North Am 2004;27:225–32.
[27] Waschbusch DA, King S. Should sex-specific norms be used to assess attention-deficit/hyperactivity disorder or oppositional defiant disorder? J Consult Clin Psychol 2006;74: 179–85.
[28] Redberg RF. Coronary artery disease in women: understanding the diagnostic and management pitfalls. Medscape Womens Health 1998;3:1.
[29] Castellanos FX, Tannock R. Neuroscience of attention-deficit/hyperactivity disorder: the search for endophenotypes. Nat Rev Neurosci 2002;3:617–28.
[30] Swanson JM, Kinsbourne M, Nigg J, et al. Etiologic subtypes of attention-deficit/hyperactivity disorder: brain imaging, molecular genetic and environmental factors and the dopamine hypothesis. Neuropsychol Rev 2007;17:39–59.
[31] Faraone SV, Khan SA. Candidate gene studies of attention-deficit/hyperactivity disorder. J Clin Psychiatry 2006;67(Suppl 8):13–20.
[32] Valera EM, Faraone SV, Murray KE, et al. Meta-analysis of structural imaging findings in attention-deficit/hyperactivity disorder. Biol Psychiatry 2007;61:1361–9.
[33] Castellanos FX, Lee PP, Sharp W. Developmental trajectories of brain volume abnormalities in children and adolescents with attention-deficit/hyperactivity disorder. JAMA 2002; 288:1740–8.
[34] Halperin JM, Schulz CP. Revisiting the role of the prefrontal cortex in the pathophysiology of attention-deficit/hyperactivity disorder. Psychol Bull 2006;132:560–81.
[35] Serene JA, Ashtari M, Szeszko PR, et al. Neuroimaging studies of children with serious emotional disturbances: a selective review. Can J Psychiatry 2007;52:135–45.
[36] Castellanos FX. Proceed, with caution: SPECT cerebral blood flow studies of children and adolescents with attention deficit hyperactivity disorder. J Nucl Med 2002;43:1630–3.
[37] Willcutt EG, Doyle AE, Nigg JT, et al. Validity of the executive function theory of attention-deficit/hyperactivity disorder: a meta-analytic review. Biol Psychiatry 2005;57:1336–46.
[38] Gottesman II, Gould TD. The endophenotype concept in psychiatry: etymology and strategic intentions. Am J Psychiatry 2003;160:636–45.
[39] Lasky-Su J, Lange C, Biederman J, et al. Family-based association analysis of a statistically derived quantitative traits for ADHD reveal an association in DRD4 with inattentive symptoms in ADHD individuals. Am J Med Genet B Neuropsychiatr Genet 2007, in press.
[40] Lasky-Su J, Banaschewski T, Buitelaar J. Partial replication of a DRD4 association in ADHD individuals using a statistically derived quantitative trait for ADHD in a family-based association test. Biol Psychiatry; 2007 [Epub ahead of print]. PMID 17560555.
[41] Applegate B, Lahey BB, Hart EL, et al. Validity of the age-of-onset criterion for ADHD: a report from the DSM-IV field trials. J Am Acad Child Adolesc Psychiatry 1997;36:1211–21.
[42] Rohde LA, Biederman J, Zimmermann H, et al. Exploring ADHD age-of-onset criterion in Brazilian adolescents. Eur Child Adolesc Psychiatry 2000;9:212–8.
[43] Faraone SV, Biederman J, Doyle A, et al. Neuropsychological studies of late onset and subthreshold diagnoses of adult ADHD. Biol Psychiatry 2006;60:1081–7.
[44] Faraone SV, Biederman J, Spencer TJ, et al. Diagnosing adult ADHD: are late onset and subthreshold diagnoses valid? Am J Psychiatry 2006;163:1720–9.
[45] Reinhardt MC, Benetti L, Victor MM, et al. Is age-of-onset criterion relevant for the response to methylphenidate in attention-deficit/hyperactivity disorder? J Clin Psychiatry 2007;68:1109–16.
[46] Green S, Loeber R, Lahey BB. Stability of mothers' recall of the age of onset of their child's attention and hyperactivity problems. J Am Acad Child Adolesc Psychiatry 1991; 30:135–7.
[47] Rohde LA, Szobot C, Polanczyk G, et al. ADHD in a diverse culture: do research and clinical findings support the notion of a cultural construct for the disorder? Biol Psychiatry 2005; 57:1436–41.

[48] Gaub M, Carlson CL. Behavioral characteristics of DSM-IV ADHD subtypes in a school-based population. J Abnorm Child Psychol 1997;25:103–11.
[49] Baumgaertel A, Wolraich M, Dietrich M. Comparison of diagnostic criteria for ADHD in a German elementary school sample. J Am Acad Child Adolesc Psychiatry 1995;34: 629–38.
[50] Schmitz M, Cadore LP, Paczko MB, et al. Neuropsychological performance in DSM-IV ADHD types: an exploratory study with untreated adolescents. Can J Psychiatry 2002;47: 863–9.
[51] Hesslinger B, Thiel T, Tebartz van Elst L, et al. Attention-deficit disorder in adults with or without hyperactivity: where is the difference? A study in humans using short echo (1)H-magnetic resonance spectroscopy. Neurosci Lett 2001;304:117–9.
[52] Lahey BB, Pelham WE, Loney J, et al. Instability of the DSM-IV subtypes of ADHD from preschool through elementary school. Arch Gen Psychiatry 2005;62:896–902.
[53] Faraone SV, Biederman J, Mick E, et al. Family study of girls with attention deficit hyperactivity disorder. Am J Psychiatry 2000;157:1077–83.
[54] Stawicki JA, Nigg JT, von Eye A. Family psychiatric history evidence on the nosological relations of DSM-IV ADHD combined and inattentive subtypes: new data and meta-analysis. J Child Psychol Psychiatry 2006;47:935–45.
[55] Buitelaar JK, Danckaerts M, Gillberg C, et al. A prospective, multicenter, open-label assessment of atomoxetine in non-North American children and adolescents with ADHD. Eur Child Adolesc Psychiatry 2004;13:249–57.
[56] Rassmussen E, Todd RD, Neuman RJ, et al. Comparison of male adolescent report of ADHD symptoms across two cultures using latent class and principal component analysis. J Child Psychol Psychiatry 2002;43:797–805.
[57] Volk HE, Henderson C, Neuman RJ, et al. Validation of population-based ADHD subtypes and identification of three clinically impaired subtypes. Am J Med Genet B Neuropsychiatr Genet 2006;141:312–8.
[58] Todd RD, Rasmussen ER, Wood C. Should sluggish cognitive tempo symptoms be included in the diagnosis of attention-deficit/hyperactivity disorder? J Am Acad Child Adolesc Psychiatry 2004;43:588–97.
[59] ADHD molecular genetics network working group. Collaborative possibilities for molecular genetic studies of attention deficit hyperactivity disorder: report from an international conference. The ADHD Molecular Genetics Network. Am J Med Genet 2000;96: 251–7.
[60] Kessler RC, Adler L, Ames M, et al. The World Health Organization Adult ADHD Self-Report Scale (ASRS): a short screening scale for use in the general population. Psychol Med 2005;35:245–56.
[61] Merrell C, Tymms P. Rasch analysis of inattentive, hyperactive, and impulsive behavior in young children and the link with academic achievement. J Appl Meas 2005;6:1–18.
[62] Tennant A, Kucukdeveci AA, Sehim K, et al. Assessing normative cut points through differential item functioning analysis: an example from the adaptation of the Middlesex Elderly Assessment of Mental State (MEAMS) for use as a cognitive screening test in Turkey. Health Qual Life Outcomes 2006;4:18.
[63] Wolraich ML, Lambert EW, Bickman L, et al. Assessing the impact of parent and teacher agreement on diagnosing attention-deficit/hyperactivity disorder. J Dev Behav Pediatr 2004;25:41–7.
[64] Lee DO, Ousley OY. Attention-deficit hyperactivity disorder symptoms in a clinic sample of children and adolescents with pervasive developmental disorders. J Child Adolesc Psychopharmacol 2006;16:737–46.
[65] Reiersen AM, Constantino JN, Volk HE, et al. Autistic traits in a population-based ADHD twin sample. J Child Psychol Psychiatry 2007;48:464–72.
[66] Heiser P, Friedel S, Dempfle A, et al. Molecular genetic aspects of attention-deficit/hyperactivity disorder. Neurosci Biobehav Res 2004;28:625–41.

[67] Holtmann M, Bolte S, Poustka F. Attention deficit hyperactivity disorder symptoms in pervasive developmental disorders: association with autistic behavior domains and coexisting psychopathology. Psychopathology 2007;40:172–7.

[68] Geurts HM, Verte S, Oosterlaan J, et al. Can the children's communication checklist differentiate between children with autism, children with ADHD, and normal controls? J Child Psychol Psychiatry 2004;45(8):1437–53.

[69] Geurts HM, Verte S, Oosterlaan J, et al. How specific are executive functioning deficits in attention deficit hyperactivity disorder and autism? J Child Psychol Psychiatry 2004;45: 836–54.

[70] Hazell P. Drug therapy for attention-deficit/hyperactivity disorder-like symptoms in autistic disorder. J Paediatr Child Health 2007;43:19–24.

[71] Goldman LS, Gene M, Bezman RJ, et al. Diagnosis and treatment of attention-deficit/hyperactivity disorder in children and adolescents. Council on Scientific Affairs, American Medical Association. JAMA 1998;279(14):1100–7.

CHILD AND
ADOLESCENT
PSYCHIATRIC CLINICS
OF NORTH AMERICA

ELSEVIER
SAUNDERS

Child Adolesc Psychiatric Clin N Am
17 (2008) 421–437

Psychosocial Interventions in Attention Deficit Hyperactivity Disorder

Kevin M. Antshel, PhD[a],*, Russell Barkley, PhD[b]

[a]Department of Psychiatry & Behavioral Sciences, State University of New York Upstate
Medical University, 750 East Adams Street, Syracuse, NY 13210, USA
[b]Medical University of South Carolina, 171 Ashley Avenue, Charleston, SC 29425, USA

Attention deficit hyperactivity disorder (ADHD) is the most common reason for referral to child and adolescent psychiatry clinics and affects approximately 5% to 7% of youth worldwide [1]. ADHD is considered a chronic disorder and pharmacologic and psychosocial interventions often are used to manage the disorder. Stimulant medications are a front-line intervention for managing ADHD and are effective for approximately 80% of youth who have ADHD [2]. Although effective, stimulants are associated with side effects, such as decreased appetite and increased sleep-onset latencies. In addition, although having a positive impact on core ADHD symptoms (eg, inattention and impulsivity), there is less robust evidence that stimulants normalize peer relationships [3], lessen family dysfunction [4], or improve academic achievement [5]. Moreover, combining psychosocial treatments with ADHD medications can result in the need for lower doses of each form of treatment [6]. Parents are more enthusiastic and interested in treatments that include psychosocial components [7]. For these reasons, psychosocial interventions continue to play a prominent role in the management of youth who have ADHD.

Psychosocial interventions, such as behavioral modification, initially were used with children who had ADHD on an atheoretic basis; successful in the mental retardation population, psychosocial interventions, such as behavioral modification, were applied to ADHD, another behaviorally disordered population. Subsequent efforts to propose a rationale for behavioral treatments centered on the notion that faulty social contingencies of reinforcement could

Dr. Barkley is a consultant to and speaker for Eli Lilly Co., Shire, McNeil, Janssen-Ortho, and Novartis and receives royalties from Guilford Publications, Compact Clinicals, J & K Seminars, Continuing Education Online, and New England Educational Institute.

* Corresponding author.
E-mail address: antshelk@upstate.edu (K.M. Antshel).

generate or exacerbate the symptoms of the disorder and that correcting them through training of caregivers could lead to lasting changes in the behavioral problems associated with the disorder. Functional behavioral assessment still is predicated on this outdated view of the origins of ADHD symptoms. A more recent theory of ADHD, however, that it is a problem of response inhibition and self-regulation with secondary consequences these may create for poor self-motivation to persist at assigned tasks [8], provides a theoretically based rationale for using these interventions with ADHD. From Barkley's theoretic stance, these interventions are not done chiefly to increase skills or information, as if children who have ADHD are ignorant of them, but are done to enhance the deficient self-motivation and working memory of these children to help them to show what they already know. From this perspective, ADHD is a disorder of performance of skills, not knowledge. Thus, psychosocial interventions are used to cue the use of those skills at key points of performance in natural settings and to motivate their display through the use of artificial consequences that ordinarily do not exist at those points of performance in natural settings. Such theory-driven efforts into further psychosocial treatment development are to be encouraged in future research.

This review encompasses psychosocial treatments that have documented efficacy for managing ADHD. This literature is sizeable, however, and space prohibits an all-encompassing discussion and critique of each treatment. Rather, the focus is on describing those psychosocial interventions that merit consideration for managing youth who have ADHD in clinical practice. Special deference is given to the largest treatment outcome study of ADHD to date: the National Institute of Mental Health Multimodal Treatment Study of Children with ADHD (MTA). Finally, those interventions that have limited or no empiric support are highlighted, again, in an effort to help guide clinicians in knowing which interventions may not hold promise for managing ADHD. This review begins by highlighting the psychosocial treatments included in the MTA study, focusing on the empiric support for each intervention.

Parent training in behavioral management

Behavioral parent training (BPT) programs seem effective for children who have disruptive behaviors whether or not they have co-occurring attentional/hyperactive difficulties [9,10]. Although nonspecific to ADHD, parent training in behavioral management also seems efficacious for youth who have ADHD [11–17]. Nonetheless, most of the studies on BPT are of short duration and do not assess maintenance of treatment effects [18]. BPT generally results in improvements in child oppositional behavior rather than ADHD symptoms specifically, suggesting that the treatment is most useful where parent-child conflict exists [19]. Studies of preschool children who have ADHD, however, find significant improvements in symptoms of ADHD specifically as a function of BPT [15].

BPT techniques generally consist of training parents in general operant conditioning techniques, such as contingent application of reinforcement or punishment after appropriate/inappropriate behaviors. Reinforcement procedures typically rely on praise, privileges, or tokens, whereas punishment methods usually are loss of positive attention, privileges, or tokens or formal time out from reinforcement. Several similar, although not identical, parent training programs have been studied in children who have ADHD, including Cunningham and colleagues Community Parent Education Program [20] and those described in Webster-Stratton's [21] *The Incredible Years* and Barkley's [22] *Defiant Children*. Other programs used with oppositional or noncompliant children, some of whom undoubtedly also have ADHD, are those described in Eyberg and Robinson's [23] *Parent-Child Interaction Therapy* and Sanders and colleagues [24] *Triple P-Positive Parenting Program*, which recently were compared with each other and with control groups in a meta-analysis of the literature [25]. All of these programs are founded on a social learning model of disruptive child behavior (disrupted parenting and social coercion) and all demonstrate efficacy for disruptive children, including those who have ADHD [11].

BPT programs generally consist of weekly training sessions, in groups of parents or as individuals, each focusing on a discrete operant conditioning technique. These methods can be grouped into three basic types of procedures: (1) those that manipulate the setting events that may precede or surround a child's tasks or activities so as to increase positive or negative behavior (parental commands, task demands, teacher instructions, and so forth); (2) those that may restructure the tasks to be done (reduce work quotas, insert more interesting task materials, and so forth); (3) and those that manipulate the nature of the consequences for child behavior in that setting (attention, praise, token reinforcement, punishment, and so forth). Because of the authors' familiarity and experience with it, Barkley's [22] program serves as an example of a typical program used with parents of children who have ADHD; it consists of 10 steps: (1) reviewing information on ADHD; (2) reviewing the cause of oppositional defiant disorder; (3) developing and enhancing parental attention; (4) attending to child compliance and independent play; (5) establishing a home token economy; (6) implementing time out for noncompliance; (7) extending time out to additional noncompliant behaviors; (8) managing noncompliance in public places; (9) implementing a daily school behavior report card; and (10) managing future misconduct. A 1-month booster session also is included in Barkley's BPT. Data support the efficacy of this BPT [19,26]. In contrast to the typically positive results of research with clinic-referred families, Barkley and colleagues [27] found that if such a clinic-based parent training program is offered to parents who did not seek treatment but whose preschool children were identified at kindergarten enrollment as having significant levels of aggressive-hyperactive-impulsive behavior, most do not attend training or do not attend reliably and no treatment effect is evident. For teenagers who have ADHD and oppositional behavior, there is little research on BPT; that which exists shows significant pre- to post-treatment improvements, yet such changes are not different from an approach based more on problem-solving and communication training of parents and their teens [28]. It is the authors' opinion that BPT addresses primarily the parent-child conflicts and child oppositional behavior that often are associated with ADHD in children but is not likely to provide much benefit for ADHD symptoms specifically.

ADHD is a highly heritable condition [29,30] making it likely that one or both parents may have the same disorder. When present, maternal ADHD seems to limit the outcomes of BPT significantly [31]. Maternal depression, antisocial personality, and drug use, parenting stress, or marital distress likewise can limit the success of BPT but largely are not studied in families with children who have ADHD [11].

Teacher training in classroom behavior management

Teachers often receive explicit training in classroom behavioral management during their training and education. Thus, it is not surprising that more research has occurred on the application of behavior management methods in the classroom than with parent training. A meta-analysis on school interventions for ADHD was conducted that comprised 70 separate experiments of various within- and between-subjects designs and single-case designs [32]. An overall mean effect size for contingency management procedures was reported of 0.60 for between-subject designs, nearly 1.00 for within-subject designs, and approximately 1.40 for single-case experimental designs. Curriculum modifications, strategy training, and other cognitive-behavioral approaches are associated less reliably with classroom behavioral improvements [32].

Contingent application of reinforcers for reduced activity level or increased sustained attention can alter the levels of ADHD symptoms rapidly [32]. These contingency management programs generally incorporate token rewards, as praise may not be sufficient to increase or maintain normal levels of on-task behavior in hyperactive children [33,34]. Similar to BPT, few studies have assessed maintenance of these improvements after treatment withdrawal. In addition, none of these studies examined whether or not generalization of behavioral control occurred in other school settings where no treatment procedures were in effect. The role of punishment in the management of classroom behavior in ADHD children is less well studied. What data exist suggest that response cost is the most effective punishment technique [33,35]. Home-based contingencies for in-class behavior and performance (eg, daily report cards) also have some research support [36,37].

Summer treatment program

One of the most well-known and well-regarded multimodality intervention programs is the summer treatment program (STP) developed by

Pelham and colleagues [38] and conducted at Western Psychiatric Institute in Pittsburgh. This program relies on five major components of treatment: (1) parent training in child behavior management; (2) classroom implementation of behavior modification techniques; (3) academic and sports skills practice and tutoring; (4) social skills training (SST) (typically involving sports); and (5) stimulant medication.

The STP was developed largely by Pelham and colleagues and is conducted in a day-treatment environment with a summer school/camp-like format. Daily activities include a few hours of classroom instruction that incorporates behavior modification methods, such as token economies, response cost, and time out from reinforcement. In addition, 3 to 4 hours of sports and recreational activities are arranged each day during which behavioral management programs are operative. The program includes parent training, peer relationship training, and a follow-up protocol to enhance the likelihood that treatment gains are maintained after leaving the program. During their stay at the camp, some children may be tested on stimulant medication using a double-blind, placebo-controlled procedure in which the child is tested on several different doses of medication while teacher ratings and behavioral observations are collected across the different camp activities. Pelham and colleagues have used this setting and larger programmatic context to conduct more focused research investigations into the effectiveness of classroom behavior management procedures alone, stimulant medication alone, and their combination in managing ADHD symptoms and improving academic performance and social behavior.

The STP program was a part of the intensive multimodal treatment program for children who have ADHD studied in the MTA project. Other components of the program, such as SST, have not been evaluated as well for their efficacy with children who have ADHD. Results from parents' ratings before and after their children's participation indicate that 86% believe their ADHD children improved from their participation in the program. No data are published, however, on whether or not the gains made during the treatment program are maintained in subsequent normal school and home settings after children terminate their participation in this program.

These three interventions (BPT, teacher training, and STP) were the psychosocial treatments that were included in the MTA study.

National Institute of Mental Health Multimodal Treatment Study of Children with ADHD

Multimodal Treatment Study of Children with attention deficit hyperactivity disorder methodology

The MTA study was designed to provide more complete information regarding the long-term effectiveness of ADHD interventions, alone or in combination, on the multiple functional outcome areas on which ADHD has an impact [36,39]. Children ages 7 through 9.9 years of age randomly were assigned to one of four treatment groups: medication alone (MedMgt), behavior modification alone (Beh), a combination of medication and behavior modification (Comb), and community comparison (CC). The MTA included six United States sites and one collaborative site in Canada. Outcomes that were assessed in the MTA include ADHD symptoms, oppositional/aggressive symptoms, social skills, internalizing symptoms, parent-child relations, parental discipline, and academic achievement.

Children who had ADHD-Combined type in grades 1 through 4 were eligible to participate in the MTA. Diagnosis was made via the Diagnostic Interview Schedule for Children-Parent version (supplemented by teacher-reported symptoms if a case was near the diagnostic threshold). Youth who had comorbid internalizing or externalizing psychiatric disorders were included as long as these conditions did not require treatment incompatible with study treatments. Having an IQ less than 80 or a major medical illness was an exclusionary criterion for participation. The overall sample of 579 youth included girls (20%); those who had prior medication treatments (31%); those who had oppositional defiant disorder (ODD) or conduct disorder diagnoses (40% and 14%), respectively; those who had *Diagnostic and Statistical Manual of Mental Disorders, Revised Third Edition* (DSM-III-R Classified) anxiety disorder (34% who had simple phobia alone not included); and youth whose families were receiving welfare, public assistance, or SSI (19%). Of the total sample, these participants represent only 13% of those who expressed interest and contacted one of the sites [36,39].

Treatments were delivered over 14 months. Detailed assessments of functioning were conducted at baseline before randomization and at the 3-, 9-, and 14-month time points. Behavioral treatments (in Beh and Comb conditions) encompassed parent, child, and school domains. BPT was provided by experienced training consultants and based on models by Barkley [22] and Forehand and McMahon [40]. Behavioral intervention consisted of 27 group and 8 individual sessions. Child behavioral treatment consisted of an intensive STP (based on the Pelham STP model) [38] and school consultation services. The STP was an intensive 8-week, 9-hour per day program; study-training consultants supervised program staff and provided parent interventions during the summer. These same consultants provided school consultation services (10 to 16 sessions of teacher consultation and establishment of a daily report card), and the staff working with the children in the STP worked in the schools in the fall as paraprofessional aides (half time for 12 weeks). Families attended an average of 77.8% of parent training sessions, 36.2 of 40 possible STP days, 10.7 teacher consultation visits, and 47.6 of 60 possible days with a classroom aide. Delivery of behavioral treatments was diminished over the course of treatment; at the end of the 14-month study, therapists had contact with parents less than once per month.

Similar to the intensity with which the behavioral interventions were implemented, the medical treatments likewise were provided in a rigorous fashion. All medication treatment provided by the MTA included an initial 28-day, double-blind, placebo-controlled titration consisting of placebo plus four different doses of methylphenidate (5, 10, 15, and 20 mg) given randomly over the titration period. Three times per day dosing was used in the titration (and typically during treatment), the full dose given in the morning and at lunch and a half dose in the midafternoon. A "best dose" was chosen and the blind was broken; that dose became the initial dose for treatment. If the dose chosen was placebo, alternative medications were titrated openly until a satisfactory medication was chosen (or, in the case of a robust placebo response, the child was not medicated). Approximately 89% of youth assigned to MedMgt or Comb completed titration successfully; of these, 68.5% were assigned to initial doses of methylphenidate averaging 30.5 mg per day given 3 times per day; of the remaining group of youth who completed titration but were not started on methylphenidate, 26 received an unblinded titration of dextroamphetamine because of unsatisfactory methylphenidate response and 32 were given no medication because of a robust placebo response [36,39].

Those youth assigned to the CC group did not receive any MTA intervention yet sought treatment as usually provided in the community. Referrals to non-MTA providers were made as necessary for these families; all CC youth and families returned for assessments at the same time as youth in the other three conditions of the study. Approximately two-thirds of the children in the CC group received medication for ADHD [36,39].

Multimodal Treatment Study of Children with attention deficit hyperactivity disorder results—attention deficit hyperactivity disorder symptoms

All groups demonstrated symptom reduction over the 14-month time frame. Using group means, the MTA Collaborative Group concluded that the medication treatments (MedMgt and Comb) were superior to the Beh and CC groups. Based on significance tests of means, the Beh and CC conditions were equivalent statistically. Likewise, the MedMgt and Comb groups were comparable, indicating no advantage of Comb relative to intensive MedMgt [36,41]. Two thirds of the youth in the CC group were receiving medication. Thus, rather than a no-treatment control group, the CC group was a treatment-as-usual group, which involved predominately medications. At the 14-month follow-up, the average daily dose for Comb was 31.2 mg whereas the average daily dose for MedMgt was 37.7 mg [36]. (The average dose of the CC group that sought treatment in the community was 22.6 mg per day) [41]. Thus, it is possible that the intensive behavioral intervention allowed individuals to take lower doses of medication. Lower doses are advantageous because most stimulant side effects, including the mild growth suppression observed in the MTA, are dose dependent [42].

Although receiving less attention than the group means comparisons (described previously), alternative statistical tests have been applied to the

MTA data. When using an idiographic approach to individual outcomes, there is a clear advantage of combined treatment [43]. Swanson and colleagues [43] created a categoric measure of treatment outcome based on composite ADHD and ODD symptoms scores from teachers and parents using the revision of the Swanson, Nolan, and Pelham–Fourth Edition Rating Scale (SNAP-IV). Successful treatment was identified as scoring an average of 1 or below on a composite SNAP score at the end of treatment (representing symptoms falling in the "not at all" or "just a little" range of categories at treatment endpoint). Success rates were as follows: 68% for Comb, 56% for MedMgt, 34% for Beh, and 25% for CC. A similar, but less robust, pattern of results was observed at the 24-month follow-up. Specifically, the normalization rates were 48%, 37%, 32%, and 28%, for Comb, MedMgt, Beh, and CC [41]. Thus, although the group means comparisons do not suggest any difference between MedMgt and Comb group outcomes, the idiographic approach to individual outcomes suggests some advantage for Comb relative to MedMgt.

Multimodal Treatment Study of Children with attention deficit hyperactivity disorder results—other outcomes

Assessing outcomes other than symptoms is of critical importance as there are weak relationships between symptoms and functional impairments [44]. In addition to ADHD symptoms, oppositional/aggressive symptoms, internalizing symptoms, social skills, parent-child relations, and academic achievement also were assessed as dependent variables in the MTA study. Across all of these parameters, most of the MTA trends favor the Comb condition. For example, the MTA Cooperative Group ordered treatment conditions by the number of times each group placed first on the 19 outcome measures. Comb was rated as more efficacious (12) than MedMgt (4), Beh (2), and CC (1). (The four times that MegMgt was superior were for parent ratings of symptoms of inattention and hyperactivity and classroom observation of hyperactivity and impulsivity [36].) Parent satisfaction scores for the Comb and Beh were equivalent and significantly higher than parent satisfaction scores for the MedMgt condition [36]. The highest attrition rates were for the MedMgt condition.

Conners and colleagues [45] conducted post hoc analysis using a composite outcome measure. Using the composite measure, Comb outcomes were more positive than MedMgt, albeit with a low effect size of 0.28 (less than a quarter of a SD). MedMgt versus Beh alone (0.26) and an effect size of 0.35 for MedMgt versus CC also were reported by Conners and colleagues [45].

In the 24-month MTA outcome, oppositional symptoms, social skills, negative/ineffective parenting, and reading achievement were assessed. Relying on group means differences, the MTA intensive medication groups experienced a greater reduction in oppositional/aggressive symptoms. The oppositional/aggressive symptom mean for Comb versus MedMgt was somewhat lower (1.34 versus 1.42, respectively) with a P value approaching significance ($P = .081$) [41]. For the other three variables examined, Comb was better than MedMgt for social skills ($P = .05$) and negative/ineffective parenting ($P = .03$). No such differences were found for Beh versus CC.

Multimodal Treatment Study of Children with attention deficit hyperactivity disorder results—moderators and mediators of intervention success

Participant characteristics that could have an impact on outcome, positive or negative, are moderators. Knowledge of moderators helps in making decisions about who benefits from what treatment. Mediators are intervening variables that operate during treatment that could have an impact on outcome. Knowledge of mediators can help identify causal pathways from intervention to outcomes.

A priori selected moderators included gender, prior medication status, ODD or CD diagnoses, DSM-III-R anxiety disorder, and receipt of public assistance. Results suggest that MTA study outcomes did not vary as a function of gender, prior history of medication, or comorbid disruptive disorders. Youth who had comorbid anxiety disorders in all three MTA treatment groups outperformed the CC group. This is an interesting finding given that the MTA treatments did not target anxiety. For families receiving public assistance, parents in the MedMgt condition reported less closeness in parent-child interactions. Teachers also reported better social skills for the Comb group. This is another interesting finding, as no differences were seen between the treatment conditions in terms of positive parenting or family stress measures [46].

A MTA mediator analysis focused on treatment acceptance/attendance [39]. Operational definitions included accepting the treatment assignment and percentage of treatment sessions attended: 80% pharmacotherapy visits attended with prescriptions written/delivered during the sessions, and for Beh, 75% attendance at group parent training sessions and STP days and both the child and the paraprofessional present together in the classroom for 75% of the possible days of this aspect of the intervention. Participants then were defined as "as intended" or "below intended." Individual parent training session attendance and teacher/therapist consultation visits were not counted. In the as-intended subgroup, MedMgt was equivalent to Comb and both were better than CC and Beh. In the below intended subgroup, however, Comb was superior in terms of ADHD symptom reduction, with MedMgt was equivalent to Beh [39]. Thus, there was an effect of compliance with treatment outcome and the Comb condition seemed more robust to noncompliance.

Although there are a variety of ways to interpret the MTA data [47,48], the authors' general interpretation of the data is that for children who have uncomplicated ADHD (no psychiatric comorbidities, adequate social functioning, good academic performance, and so forth), the MTA data suggest that MedMgt may be the best treatment option. For those youth who have

ADHD complicated by oppositional symptoms, poor social functioning and negative/ineffective parenting, Comb seems the best treatment option.

Psychosocial therapies having limited or no evidence of effectiveness

Cognitive-behavioral therapy

Although once believed effective for youth who have ADHD [49], neither cognitive behavioral therapy (CBT) nor cognitive therapy has much research support in pediatric ADHD [32,50–53]. Meta-analyses of CBT typically have reported the effect sizes as less than one third a SD [52]. Because of its limited efficacy, CBT was not included in the MTA treatment protocols.

Social skills training

SST in youth who have ADHD similarly is limited in efficacy; results are discouraging [54–57]. For example, one of the only clinical trials of SST in ADHD reported negative results. Using a clinic-referred sample of 120 children who had ADHD, youth ages 8 to 12 were assigned randomly to one of three treatment conditions: a wait-list control group or one of two types of SST groups: diagnostically homogenous (only ADHD, Combined Type or ADHD, Predominently Inattentive Type youth) or diagnostically heterogeneous (both ADHD subtypes included in the group). No clinically significant benefits for most youth who had ADHD were reported. Moreover, some evidence of peer deviancy training was evident; some children who had ADHD-Inattentive type were rated by parents as worse after the treatment. All of these participants were in the diagnostically heterogeneous groups. There may be some risk for accelerating antisocial behavior, or deviancy training, involved in SST when delinquent youth are placed together in groups [58,59].

Children who have ADHD have peer difficulties [57]; nonetheless, the nature of the social interaction problems is heterogeneous [54]. Barkley's [8] theoretic model of ADHD posits that ADHD is not a knowledge deficit as much as a performance disorder. Thus, teaching youth who have ADHD additional skills is not as much the issue as is assisting them with performing the skills they have when it is useful to do so. Rather than in a clinic setting, this instruction likely should occur at the point of performance (the place and time in the natural setting), where such skills most likely prove useful to the long-term social acceptance of individuals.

Other therapies

Many questionable treatments have been attempted with children who have ADHD [7,60]. Among many others, vestibular stimulation [61], biofeedback and relaxation training [62], electroencephalographic biofeedback [63], and sensory integration exercises [64] are described as potentially effective treatments of ADHD in uncontrolled case reports, small series of case studies, or in some treatment versus no-treatment comparisons. All, however, lack well-controlled experimental replications of their efficacy. Traditional psychotherapy and play therapy also have not proved effective for ADHD [65].

Summary and future directions

ADHD is conceptualized now as a largely chronic disorder for most but not all children, similar in some respects to chronic medical disorders, such as diabetes or phenylketonuria. Although others have reported less promising results for psychosocial interventions in stimulant-responsive children [66,67], the MTA study documents that for ADHD symptoms and associated problems, a combined and intensive treatment protocol likely is most efficacious. Psychosocial interventions that seem most promising and, therefore, should be included in the combined treatment program include contingency management methods applied in classrooms and elsewhere (summer camps) and training of parents (BPT) in these same methods to be used in the home and elsewhere (community settings). Evidence for CBT, SST, and other psychosocial interventions is less encouraging. Electroencephalographic biofeedback, or sensory integration training likewise do not seem efficacious psychosocial interventions.

Psychosocial interventions as applied in the MTA may be difficult to replicate in everyday clinical practice. For example, STPs may not be readily available in all parts of the country (or world), and even in the United States this treatment can be more expensive than medical management with parent training and several school consultations or than managed care health plans are willing to reimburse for regarding this disorder. Despite these caveats, future research should continue to consider the role that psychosocial therapies will play in the treatment of ADHD across the lifespan. To that end, the authors recommend a particular emphasis on the following issues.

Theory-driven psychosocial treatment

Current psychosocial, largely cognitive-behavioral interventions were based on now outdated assumptions about ADHD and its associated disruptive behavior. Most treatments grew out of social learning theory—a theory that held that deviant or disruptive behavior should be believed developed or maintained as a result of exposure to faulty contingencies of reinforcement or social modeling. This view came to be supplemented with cognitive-behavioral theory that ascribed some importance to the cognitive (largely verbal) deficits associated with ADHD that should respond to direct cognitive training. The increased prosocial and decreased deviant behavior would be maintained as a consequence of the improved natural contingencies of reinforcement for those behaviors that would sustain them. Supplemental cognitive training in verbal self-regulation strategies would result in the internalization of such strategies that would further promote generalization and maintenance of treatment gains. Parents and that teachers would sustain their use of these procedures for the reinforcement they, too, received from the reductions in child disruptive behavior and increased positive behaviors shown by the children who have ADHD in their classrooms. This is not to say that local contingencies of reinforcement have no bearing on children's levels of ADHD and disruptive behavior in the classroom—clearly they can in individual cases. But such contingencies are not the primary origin of those behavioral problems and likely not the source of individual differences among children with those behavioral problems (population variation in ADHD traits) and will not, once changed, persist in sustaining any behavioral improvements once the formal interventions are withdrawn. Psychosocial treatments, especially behavioral ones, now are viewed as comparable to medication management in this sense, producing solid benefits as long as they are in place. They yield little evidence of maintenance or generalization, however, once withdrawn and are not considered the origin of the behavioral problems.

In the past 10 years, the usefulness of behavioral interventions has come to be based on a different view, which Barkley [8] calls, "designing prosthetic environments." Behavioral treatments, such as hearing aides, wheelchairs, ramps into public facilities, lower bathroom fixtures, glasses and large print books, and prosthetic limbs for amputees, are artificial means of altering environments designed to reduce the adverse impact of a biologic handicap on the performance of major life activities. No one would rationally claim that physical disabilities arise from the lack of wheelchairs and ramps. Similarly, no one would claim that using a wheelchair or associated ramps for a month or 2 would result in their being internalized or so alter the social environment that they would be sustained by changes in naturally occurring contingencies after the chairs and ramps are withdrawn. Likewise, no one should rationally claim that ADHD arises from faulty learning or that several months of contingency management would produce sustained benefits for ADHD once treatment is withdrawn. Behavioral methods are prostheses—means of rearranging environments by artificial means so as to yield improved participation in major life activities. A better theoretic understanding of ADHD is needed if novel psychosocial treatments are to be developed that offer greater hope for success than those currently available. A theory of ADHD is needed that explains why the use of artificial consequences scheduled more intensively in natural settings is even needed for management of ADHD when it is not required for typically developing children. Theories of ADHD as a motivational deficit, executive function disorder, disorder of self-regulation, and so forth are efforts to fill this theoretic void that have had only partial success. The authors encourage more work in this direction.

Adverse events in behavioral treatments

The authors study psychosocial and psychopharmacologic interventions for ADHD and repeatedly notice the routine absence of efforts to study the side effects or adverse events (AEs) associated with such interventions, especially given that such side effects and AEs not only are routine but also are a matter of utmost importance in drug research. Mental health professionals seem to believe that their therapies do no harm even if they are not beneficial. However, any intervention that truly is effective must produce AEs if only because of individual differences among people in their psychologic and physical makeup and the variance this must create in their reactions to interventions. AEs also are expected given the likely occasional ineptitude in the use of treatments by clinicians, parents, and teachers. There are other reasons, but these serve to make the point. Psychosocial treatments of any power to influence behavior will produce AEs in some subset of the treated population.

For instance, in a study by Barkley and colleagues [28] of various family therapy approaches to addressing parent-teen conflict in teens who have ADHD, the authors noted a significant increase in conflicts in a minority of the families (10%–20%) as a consequence of largely behavioral interventions. The probable reasons for this have to do with teaching parents to set limits on highly disruptive teenagers through contracting, time out, and other forms of behavioral containment and punishment that served to escalate rather than reduce conflict and teen temper outbursts within these families. Other studies have documented the adverse effect of group SST on a significant subset (20%–25%) of children who have ADHD that may result in increased aggressive behavior [57] by a process known as deviancy training [58]. The authors believe that these findings are not isolated instances but their rarity in articles is attributable to not evaluating routinely the potential AEs of psychosocial interventions. Does anyone doubt that time outs, response cost, overcorrection, or other coercive forms of punishment do not have some AEs in some subsets of these children? Postextinction bursts of heightened disruptive behavior are to be expected with the cessation of positive attention or other reinforcers for their previous occurrences. This common wisdom does not change the fact that this is a form of AE that potentially can occur even when using differential attention, probably perceived as the most benign and well-intentioned psychosocial recommendation. Had a medication produced such an effect, even temporarily, it dutifully would have been recorded as an AE in that treatment protocol as a matter of course. This same dutiful recording for AEs is needed in psychosocial treatment protocols as is consent to enter them by patients, families, and school staff to be truly informed.

Developmental causal pathways affecting various domains of impairment

As suggested previously, the different domains of major life activities affected in those who have ADHD probably do not have the same causal pathways or moderators and mediators across them all nor is ADHD necessarily always the most important source of influence on these impairments [44]. Thus, treating only the ADHD symptoms may not provide the most effective interventions for reducing certain domains of impairments. Even within the realm of ADHD symptoms, inattentive symptoms may lead to different impairments (ie, school and work) than hyperactive or impulsive ones (speeding citations, accidental injuries, and so forth). Research is exploring such pathways with regard to factors affecting various domains of impairment, such as academic achievement deficits versus parent-child interaction conflicts versus teen school behavioral problems [4,5,9,11,13,31]. The authors encourage these efforts to identify the multifactorially determined pathways associated with various impairments so as to guide treatment development to address those factors more explicitly.

Psychosocial treatments in adolescence

Although CBT is not demonstrated as efficacious in children who have ADHD, there are reasons to be optimistic that CBT may be more efficacious in adolescents who have ADHD. For example, CBT generally is more effective in adolescents relative to preadolescents [68]. Similarly, in the literature on adult ADHD, there is some evidence that CBT is efficacious for reducing functional impairments [69]. Future research should consider the extent to which CBT is effective for adolescents who have ADHD, either in combination with pharmacotherapy or in isolation.

Psychosocial treatments of ADHD frequently are a necessary and effective component of the total treatment package that must be assembled to address the clinical needs of most cases of ADHD.

References

[1] Association AP. DSM-IV-TR. Washington, DC: American Psychiatric Association; 2000.
[2] Faraone SV, Biederman J, Spencer TJ, et al. Comparing the efficacy of medications for ADHD using meta-analysis. MedGenMed 2006;8(4):4.
[3] Hoza B, Gerdes AC, Mrug S, et al. Peer-assessed outcomes in the multimodal treatment study of children with attention deficit hyperactivity disorder. J Clin Child Adolesc Psychol 2005;34(1):74–86.
[4] Johnston C, Mash EJ. Families of children with attention-deficit/hyperactivity disorder: review and recommendations for future research. Clin Child Fam Psychol Rev 2001;4(3): 183–207.
[5] Raggi VL, Chronis AM. Interventions to address the academic impairment of children and adolescents with ADHD. Clin Child Fam Psychol Rev 2006;9(2):85–111.
[6] Fabiano GA, Pelham WE Jr, Gnagy EM, et al. The single and combined effects of multiple intensities of behavior modification and methylphenidate for children with attention deficit hyperactivity disorder in a classroom setting. School Psych Rev 2007; 36:195–216.
[7] Pelham WE Jr, Fabiano GA, Gnagy EM, et al. The role of summer treatment programs in the context of comprehensive treatment for attention deficit hyperactivity disorder. In: Hibbs ED, Jensen PS, editors. Psychosocial treatments for child and adolescent disorders: empirically based strategies for clinical practice. 2nd edition. 2005. p. 377–409.
[8] Barkley RA. Behavioral inhibition, sustained attention, and executive functions: constructing a unifying theory of ADHD. Psychol Bull 1997;121(1):65–94.

[9] Hartman RR, Stage SA, Webster-Stratton C. A growth curve analysis of parent training outcomes: examining the influence of child risk factors (inattention, impulsivity, and hyperactivity problems), parental and family risk factors. J Child Psychol Psychiatry 2003;44(3): 388–98.

[10] Bor W, Sanders MR, Markie-Dadds C. The effects of the Triple P-Positive Parenting Program on preschool children with co-occurring disruptive behavior and attentional/hyperactive difficulties. J Abnorm Child Psychol 2002;30(6):571–87.

[11] Chronis AM, Chacko A, Fabiano GA, et al. Enhancements to the behavioral parent training paradigm for families of children with ADHD: review and future directions. Clin Child Fam Psychol Rev 2004;7(1):1–27.

[12] Chronis AM, Jones HA, Raggi VL. Evidence-based psychosocial treatments for children and adolescents with attention-deficit/hyperactivity disorder. Clin Psychol Rev 2006;26(4): 486–502.

[13] Chronis AM, Lahey BB, Pelham WE Jr, et al. Maternal depression and early positive parenting predict future conduct problems in young children with attention-deficit/hyperactivity disorder. Dev Psychol 2007;43(1):70–82.

[14] Anastopoulos AD, DuPaul GJ, Barkley RA. Stimulant medication and parent training therapies for attention deficit-hyperactivity disorder. J Learn Disabil 1991;24(4):210–8.

[15] Sonuga-Barke EJ, Daley D, Thompson M, et al. Parent-based therapies for preschool attention-deficit/hyperactivity disorder: a randomized, controlled trial with a community sample. J Am Acad Child Adolesc Psychiatry 2001;40(4):402–8.

[16] Sonuga-Barke EJ, Thompson M, Daley D, et al. Parent training for attention deficit/hyperactivity disorder: is it as effective when delivered as routine rather than as specialist care? Br J Clin Psychol 2004;43(Pt 4):449–57.

[17] Strayhorn JM, Weidman CS. Reduction of attention deficit and internalizing symptoms in preschoolers through parent-child interaction training. J Am Acad Child Adolesc Psychiatry 1989;28(6):888–96.

[18] Kazdin AE. Parent management training: evidence, outcomes, and issues. J Am Acad Child Adolesc Psychiatry 1997;36(10):1349–56.

[19] Anastopoulos AD, Shelton TL, DuPaul GJ, et al. Parent training for attention-deficit hyperactivity disorder: its impact on parent functioning. J Abnorm Child Psychol 1993;21(5): 581–96.

[20] Cunningham CE, Bremner R, Secord M. COPE: the community parent education program: a school-based family systems oriented workshop for parents of children with disruptive behavior disorders. Hamilton (Ont.): COPE Works; 1997.

[21] Webster-Stratton C. The incredible years. Toronto: Umbrella Press; 1992.

[22] Barkley RA. Defiant children: a clinician's manual for assessment and parent training. New York: Guilford Press; 1997.

[23] Eyberg SM, Robinson EA. Parent-child interaction training: effects on family functioning. J Clin Child Psychol 1982;11:130–7.

[24] Sanders MR, Markie-Dadds C, Tully LA, et al. The triple P-positive parenting program: a comparison of enhanced, standard, and self-directed behavioral family intervention for parents of children with early onset conduct problems. J Consult Clin Psychol 2000;68(4): 624–40.

[25] Thomas R, Zimmer-Gembeck MJ. Behavioral outcomes of parent-child interaction therapy and triple p-positive parenting program: a review and meta-analysis. J Abnorm Child Psychol 2007;35(3):475–95.

[26] Pisterman S, McGrath P, Firestone P, et al. Outcome of parent-mediated treatment of preschoolers with attention deficit disorder with hyperactivity. J Consult Clin Psychol 1989;57(5):628–35.

[27] Barkley RA, Shelton TL, Crosswait C, et al. Multi-method psycho-educational intervention for preschool children with disruptive behavior: preliminary results at post-treatment. J Child Psychol Psychiatry 2000;41(3):319–32.

[28] Barkley RA, Guevremont DC, Anastopoulos AD, et al. A comparison of three family therapy programs for treating family conflicts in adolescents with attention-deficit hyperactivity disorder. J Consult Clin Psychol 1992;60(3):450–62.

[29] Faraone SV, Doyle AE. The nature and heritability of attention-deficit/hyperactivity disorder. Child Adolesc Psychiatr Clin N Am 2001;10(2):299–316, viii-ix.

[30] Faraone SV, Perlis RH, Doyle AE, et al. Molecular genetics of attention-deficit/hyperactivity disorder. Biol Psychiatry 2005;57(11):1313–23.

[31] Sonuga-Barke EJ, Daley D, Thompson M. Does maternal ADHD reduce the effectiveness of parent training for preschool children's ADHD? J Am Acad Child Adolesc Psychiatry 2002; 41(6):696–702.

[32] DuPaul GJ, Eckert TL. The effects of school-based interventions for attention deficit hyperactivity disorder: a meta-analysis. Sch Psychol Dig 1997;26:5–27.

[33] Pfiffner LJ, Rosen LA, O'Leary SG. The efficacy of an all-positive approach to classroom management. J Appl Behav Anal 1985;18(3):257–61.

[34] Pfiffner LJ, DuPaul GJ, Barkley RA. Educational management. In: Barkley R, editor. Attention deficit hyperactivity disorder: a handbook for diagnosis and treatment, vol. 3. New York: Guilford Press; 2005. p. 547–89.

[35] Pfiffner LJ, O'Leary SG, Rosen LA, et al. A comparison of the effects of continuous and. intermittent response cost and reprimands in the classroom. J Clin Child Psychol 1985;14: 348–52.

[36] Group MC. A 14-month randomized clinical trial of treatment strategies for attention-deficit/hyperactivity disorder. The MTA Cooperative Group. Multimodal treatment study of children with ADHD. Arch Gen Psychiatry 1999;56(12):1073–86.

[37] Atkinson BM, Forehand R. Home-based reinforcement programs designed to modify classroom behavior: a review and methodological evaluation. Psychol Bull 1979;86: 1298–308.

[38] Pelham WE, Hoza B. Intensive treatment: a summer treatment program for children with ADHD. In: Jensen EHP, editor. Psychosocial treatments for child and adolescent disorders: empirically based strategies for clinical practice. New York: APA Press; 1996. p. 311–40.

[39] Group MC. Moderators and mediators of treatment response for children with attention-deficit/hyperactivity disorder: the Multimodal Treatment Study of children with Attention-deficit/hyperactivity disorder. Arch Gen Psychiatry 1999;56(12):1088–96.

[40] Forehand R, McMahon R. Helping the noncompliant child: a clinician's guide to parent training. New York: Guilford Press; 1981.

[41] Group MC. National Institute of Mental Health Multimodal Treatment Study of ADHD follow-up: 24-month outcomes of treatment strategies for attention-deficit/hyperactivity disorder. Pediatrics 2004;113(4):754–61.

[42] Group MC. National Institute of Mental Health Multimodal Treatment Study of ADHD follow-up: changes in effectiveness and growth after the end of treatment. Pediatrics 2004; 113(4):762–9.

[43] Swanson JM, Kraemer HC, Hinshaw SP, et al. Clinical relevance of the primary findings of the MTA: success rates based on severity of ADHD and ODD symptoms at the end of treatment. J Am Acad Child Adolesc Psychiatry 2001;40(2):168–79.

[44] Gordon M, Antshel K, Faraone S, et al. Symptoms versus impairment: the case for respecting DSM-IV's Criterion D. J Atten Disord 2006;9(3):465–75.

[45] Conners CK, Epstein JN, March JS, et al. Multimodal treatment of ADHD in the MTA: an alternative outcome analysis. J Am Acad Child Adolesc Psychiatry 2001;40(2):159–67.

[46] Wells KC, Epstein JN, Hinshaw SP, et al. Parenting and family stress treatment outcomes in attention deficit hyperactivity disorder (ADHD): an empirical analysis in the MTA study. J Abnorm Child Psychol 2000;28(6):543–53.

[47] Pelham WE Jr. The NIMH multimodal treatment study for attention-deficit hyperactivity disorder: just say yes to drugs alone? Can J Psychiatry 1999;44(10):981–90.

[48] Swanson JM, Arnold LE, Vitiello B, et al. Response to commentary on the multimodal treatment study of ADHD (MTA): mining the meaning of the MTA. J Abnorm Child Psychol 2002;30(4):327–32.

[49] Kendall PC, Braswell L. Cognitive-behavioral therapy for impulsive children. New York: Guilford Press; 1985.

[50] Abikoff H, Gittelman R. Hyperactive children treated with stimulants. Is cognitive training a useful adjunct? Arch Gen Psychiatry 1985;42(10):953–61.

[51] Dush DM, Hirt ML, Schroeder HE. Self-statement modification in the treatment of child behavior disorders: a meta-analysis. Psychol Bull 1989;106(1):97–106.

[52] Baer RA, Nietzel MT. Cognitive and behavioral treatment of impulsivity in children: a meta-analytic review of the outcome literature. J Clin Child Psychol 1991;20:400–12.

[53] Bloomquist ML, August GJ, Ostrander R. Effects of a school-based cognitive-behavioral intervention for ADHD children. J Abnorm Child Psychol 1991;19:591–605.

[54] Hinshaw SP. Interventions for social competence and social skill. In: Weiss G, editor. Child and adolescent psychiatric clinics of North America, vol. 1Philadelphia: W. B. Saunders; 1992. p. 539–52.

[55] Whalen CK, Henker B. Therapies for hyperactive children: comparisons, combinations, and compromises. J Consult Clin Psychol 1991;59:126–37.

[56] Sheridan SM, Dee CC, Moprgan JC, et al. A multi-method introduction for social skills deficits in children with ADHD and their parents. School Psych Rev 1996;25:401–16.

[57] Antshel KM, Remer R. Social skills training in children with attention deficit hyperactivity disorder: a randomized-controlled clinical trial. J Clin Child Adolesc Psychol 2003;32(1): 153–65.

[58] Dishion TJ, McCord J, Poulin F. When interventions harm. Peer groups and problem behavior. Am Psychol 1999;54(9):755–64.

[59] Mager W, Milich R, Harris MJ, et al. Intervention groups for adolescents with conduct problems: is aggregation harmful or helpful? J Abnorm Child Psychol 2005;33(3): 349–62.

[60] Ingersoll BD, Goldstein S. Attention deficit disorder and learning disabilities: realities, myths, and controversial treatments. New York: Doubleday; 1993.

[61] Arnold LE, Clark DL, Sachs LA, et al. Vestibular and visual rotational stimulation as treatment for attention deficit and hyperactivity. Am J Occup Ther 1985;39:84–91.

[62] Richter NC. The efficacy of relaxation training with children. J Abnorm Child Psychol 1984; 12:319–44.

[63] Linden M, Habib T, Radojevic V. A controlled study of the effects of EEG biofeedback on cognition and behavior of children with attention deficit disorder and learning disabilities. Biofeedback Self Regul 1996;21:35–50.

[64] Vargas S, Camilli G. A meta-analysis of research on sensory-integration treatment. Am J Occup Ther 1999;53:189–98.

[65] Pelham WE Jr, Wheeler T, Chronis A. Empirically supported psychosoical treatments for attention deficit hyperactivity disorder. J Clin Child Psychol 1998;27:190–205.

[66] Abikoff H, Hechtman L, Klein RG, et al. Social functioning in children with ADHD treated with long-term methylphenidate and multimodal psychosocial treatment. J Am Acad Child Adolesc Psychiatry 2004;43(7):820–9.

[67] Abikoff H, Hechtman L, Klein RG, et al. Symptomatic improvement in children with ADHD treated with long-term methylphenidate and multimodal psychosocial treatment. J Am Acad Child Adolesc Psychiatry 2004;43(7):802–11.

[68] Holmbeck GE, Greenley RN, Franks EA. Developmental issues and considerations in research and practice. In: Kazdin A, Weisz JR, editors. Evidence-based psychotherapies for children and adolescents. New York: Guilford Press; 2003. p. 21–40.

[69] Safren SA, Otto MW, Sprich S, et al. Cognitive-behavioral therapy for ADHD in medication-treated adults with continued symptoms. Behav Res Ther 2005;43(7):831–42.

CHILD AND
ADOLESCENT
PSYCHIATRIC CLINICS
OF NORTH AMERICA

ELSEVIER
SAUNDERS

Child Adolesc Psychiatric Clin N Am
17 (2008) 439–458

Psychopharmacological Interventions

Joseph Biederman, MD[a,b,*], Thomas J. Spencer, MD[a,b]

[a]Pediatric Psychopharmacology Research Unit, Massachusetts General Hospital,
32 Fruit Street, Yaw 6A, Boston, MA 02114, USA
[b]Department of Psychiatry, Harvard Medical School, 25 Shattuck Street Boston,
MA 02115, USA

Stimulant treatments

Stimulant drugs are the first class of compounds reported as effective in treating behavioral disturbances evident in children who have attention deficit hyperactivity disorder (ADHD). Stimulants are sympathomimetic drugs structurally similar to endogenous catecholamines. The most commonly used compounds in this class include methylphenidate (Ritalin), *d*-methylphenidate (Focalin), *d*-amphetamine (Dexedrine), and a mixed-amphetamine product (Adderall). These drugs have been shown to enhance dopaminergic and noradrenergic transmission [1,2]. Because the various stimulants have somewhat different mechanism of action, some patients may experience preferential response to one or another [3,4].

An extensive literature has clearly documented the short-term efficacy of methylphenidate treatment, mostly in latency-age Caucasian boys [5].

Dr. Thomas Spencer receives research support from, is a speaker for, or is on the Advisory Board of the following sources: Shire, Eli Lilly and Company, GlaxoSmithKline, Ortho-McNeil, Inc., Novartis, New River Pharmaceuticals, Cephalon, Pfizer, and the National Institute of Mental Health (NIMH). Dr. Joseph Biederman is currently receiving research support from the following sources: Bristol-Myers Squibb, Eli Lilly and Company, Janssen, L.P., Ortho-McNeil, Inc., Otsuka, Shire, NIMH, and the National Institute of Child Health and Human Development Dr. Joseph Biederman is currently a consultant/advisory board member for the following pharmaceutical companies: Janssen, L.P., Ortho-McNeil, Inc., Novartis, and Shire. Dr. Joseph Biederman is currently a speaker for the following speaker's bureaus: Janssen, Ortho-McNeil, Inc., Novartis, Shire, and UCB Pharma, Inc. In previous years, Dr. Joseph Biederman received research support, consultation fees, or speaker's fees for/from the following additional sources: Abbott, AstraZeneca, Celltech, Cephalon, Eli Lilly and Company, Esai, Forest, GlaxoSmithKline, Gliatech Inc., NARSAD, New River Behavioral HealthCare, the National Institute on Drug Abuse, Novartis, Noven, Neurosearch, Pfizer, Pharmacia, The Prechter Foundation, The Stanley Foundation, and Wyeth.
* Corresponding author.
  E-mail address: biederman@helix.mgh.harvard.edu (J. Biederman).

A much more limited literature exists for stimulants at other ages and for women and ethnic minorities. The literature clearly documents that treatment with stimulants improves not only abnormal behaviors of ADHD but also self-esteem, cognition, and social and family function, supporting the importance of treating patients who have ADHD beyond school or work hours to include evenings, weekends, and vacations. Controlled clinical trails have documented the efficacy of methylphenidate and amphetamine in adults who have ADHD [6,7].

Treatment with stimulants improves a wide variety of cognitive abilities [8–10], increases school-based productivity, and improves performance in academic testing (Howard Abikoff, PhD and colleagues, personal communication, 1996). However, despite these beneficial cognitive effects, one must be aware that patients who have ADHD can manifest additional learning disabilities that are not responsive to pharmacotherapy [11,12] but may respond to educational remediation.

In fact, most studies indicate that both behavior and cognitive performance improve with stimulant treatment in a dose-dependent fashion [9,13–19]. The literature on the association between clinical benefits in ADHD and plasma levels of stimulants has been equivocal and complicated by large inter- and intraindividual variability in plasma levels at constant oral doses [9]. Although initial and final doses for stimulants should be individualized, some guidelines can be found in Table 1.

Recently, some concern was shown about the long-term efficacy of methylphenidate based on the 36-month data from the Multimodal Treatment Study of Children with ADHD study [20]. Although the break of randomization after 14 months and the lack of precise information on type of medication, dose, and length of treatment between assessments make findings subject to several bias, clinicians should periodically assess the need for treatment.

The most commonly reported side effects associated with stimulant medication are appetite suppression and sleep disturbances [21]. The sleep disturbance commonly reported is delay of sleep onset and usually accompanies late afternoon or early evening administration of the stimulant medications. Although less commonly reported, mood disturbances ranging from increased tearfulness to a full-blown major depression-like syndrome can be associated with stimulant treatment [22]. Other infrequent side effects include headaches, abdominal discomfort, increased lethargy, and fatigue [23].

Adverse cardiovascular effects of stimulants have consistently documented mild increases in pulse and blood pressure of unclear clinical significance [24]. Recent concerns have been expressed about cardiovascular safety. The U.S. Food and Drug Administration (FDA) (www.fda.gov/cder/drug/advisory/adderall.htm) issued the following statement:

> Health Canada, the Canadian drug regulatory agency, has suspended the sale of Adderall XR in the Canadian market.... The Canadian action was based on U.S. post-marketing reports of sudden deaths in pediatric patients.... When one considers the rate of sudden death in pediatric

patients treated with Adderall products based on the approximately 30 million prescriptions written between 1999 and 2003 (the period of time in which these deaths occurred), it does not appear that the number of deaths reported is greater than the number of sudden deaths that would be expected to occur in this population without treatment. For this reason, the FDA has not decided to take any further regulatory action at this time. However, because it appeared that patients with underlying heart defects might be at increased risk for sudden death, the labeling for Adderall XR was changed in August 2004 to include a warning that these patients might be at particular risk, and that these patients should ordinarily not be treated with Adderall products.

Caution should be used in treating patients who have a family history of early cardiac death or arrhythmias or a personal history of structural abnormalities, chest pain, palpitations, or fainting episodes of unclear origin either before or during treatment with stimulants. In these cases, consultation with a cardiologist is recommended. Although less of a clinical concern in pediatric care, potential increases in blood pressure associated with stimulant drugs may be of greater clinical significance in the treatment of adults who have ADHD (for a broader discussion on cardiovascular risk of stimulants, see the article by Vitiello, elsewhere in this issue).

A stimulant-associated toxic psychosis has also been very rarely observed and usually in the context of either a rapid rise in the dosage or very high doses. The reported psychosis in children in response to stimulant medications resembles a toxic phenomenon (ie, visual hallucinosis) and is dissimilar from the exacerbation of the psychotic symptoms present in schizophrenia. The development of psychotic symptoms in a child exposed to stimulants requires careful evaluation to rule out the presence of a preexisting psychotic disorder.

Early reports indicate that children who had a personal or family history of tic disorders were at greater risk for developing a tic disorder when exposed to stimulants [25]. However, other work has increasingly challenged this view [26–29]. Until more is known, the risks and benefits should be weighed on an individual basis, with appropriate discussion with the child and family about the benefits and pitfalls of the use of stimulants in children who have ADHD and tics.

Similar uncertainties remain about the abuse potential of stimulants in children who have ADHD. Despite the concern that ADHD may increase the risk for abuse in adolescents and young adults (or his or her associates), no clear evidence shows that children who have ADHD treated with stimulants abuse prescribed medication when appropriately diagnosed and carefully monitored. Furthermore, additional reports provide statistical evidence documenting that using stimulants and other pharmacologic treatments for ADHD significantly decreased the risk for subsequent substance use disorders in youth who had ADHD [30,31]. The type of methylphenidate formulation might be relevant to the abuse liability of this medication.

Table 1
Medications for attention deficit hyperactivity disorder

	Dosage form	Starting dose	Final dose
Amphetamine preparations			
Short-acting			
Adderall	5.0, 7.5, 10.0, 12.5, 15.0, 20.0, 30.0 mg	3–5 y: 2.5 mg qd ≥6 y: 5 mg qd–bid	Lesser of 1.0 mg/kg per day or 40 mg
Dexedrine	5 mg	3–5 y: 2.5 mg qd	
Dextrostat	5, 10 mg	≥6 y: 5 mg qd–bid	
Long-acting			
Dexedrine Spansule	5, 10, 15 mg	≥6 y: 5–10 mg qd–bid	Lesser of 1.0 mg/kg per day or 40 mg
Adderall XR	5, 10, 15, 20, 25, 30 mg	≥6 y: 10 mg qd	Lesser of 1.0 mg/kg per day or 30 mg
Lisdexamfetamine	30, 50, 70 mg	30 mg qd	Lesser of 1.0 mg/kg per day or 70 mg
Methylphenidate preparations			
Short-acting			
Focalin	2.5, 5.0, 10.0mg	2.5 mg bid	Lesser of 1.0 mg/kg per day or 20 mg
Methylin Ritalin	5, 10, 20 mg	5 mg bid	Lesser of 2.0 mg/kg per day or 60 mg
Intermediate-acting			
Metadate ER	10, 20 mg	10 mg qam	Lesser of 2.0 mg/kg per day or 60 mg
Methylin ER	10, 20 mg		
Ritalin SR	20 mg		
Metadate CD	10, 20, 30, 40, 50, 60 mg	20 mg qam	Lesser of 2.0 mg/kg per day or 60 mg
Ritalin LA	10, 20, 30, 40 mg		
Long-acting			
Concerta	18, 27, 36, 54 mg	18 mg qam	Lesser of 2.0 mg/kg per day or 72 mg
Daytrana Patch	10, 15, 20, 30 mg patches	Begin with 10 mg patch qd, then titrate up by patch strength	Lesser of 1.0 mg/kg per day or 30 mg
Focalin XR	5, 10, 15, 20 mg	5 mg qam	Lesser of 1.0 mg/kg per day or 30 mg
Selective norepinephrine reuptake inhibitor			
Strattera	10, 18, 25, 40, 60, 80, 100 mg	Children and adolescents <70 kg: 0.5 mg/kg per day for 4 days; then 1 mg/kg per day for 4 days; then 1.2 mg/kg per day	Lesser of 1.4 mg/kg or 100 mg
Antidepressants			
Bupropion			
Wellbutrin	75, 100 mg tablet	Lesser of 3 mg/kg per day or 150 mg per day	Lesser of 6 mg/kg or 300 mg, with no single dose >150 mg
Wellbutrin SR	100, 150, 200 mg tablet		
Wellbutrin XL	150, 300 mg tablet		

(*continued on next page*)

Table 1 (*continued*)

	Dosage form	Starting dose	Final dose
Imipramine			
Tofranil	10, 25, 50, 75 mg tablet	1 mg/kg per day	Lesser of 4 mg/kg or 200 mg
Nortriptyline			
Pamelor, Aventyl	10, 25, 50, 75 mg capsule	0.5 mg/kg per day	Lesser of 2 mg/kg or 100 mg
α_2-Adrenergic agonists			
Clonidine			
Catapres	0.1, 0.2, 0.3 mg tablet	<45 kg: 0.05 mg qhs; titrate in 0.05 mg increments bid, tid, qid	27–40.5 kg: 0.2 mg
		>45 kg: 0.1 mg qhs; titrate in 0.1 mg increments bid, tid, qid	40.5–45 kg: 0.3 mg >45 kg: 0.4 mg
Guanfacine			
Tenex	1, 2 mg tablet	<45 kg: 0.5 mg qhs; titrate in 0.5 mg increments bid, tid, qid	27–40.5 kg: 2 mg
		>45 kg: 1 mg qhs; titrate in 1 mg increments bid, tid, qid	40.5– 45 kg: 3 mg >45 kg: 4 mg

Data from Pliszka S; AACAP Work Group on Quality Issues. Practice parameter for the assessment and treatment of children and adolescents with attention-deficit/hyperactivity disorder. J Am Acad Child Adolesc Psychiatry 2007;46:894–921; with permission.

In general, long-acting medications are less able to be abused. The pharmacodynamic properties of some long-acting methylphenidate (eg, OROS) seem to determine lower liability to abuse than those of immediate release formulations [32]. Finally, lisdexamphetamine is a prodrug, and therefore the rate-limiting enzymatic conversion to active drug provides a barrier to euphoric abuse.

Although the effect of long-term administration of stimulants on growth continues to be a concern, several studies have begun to question this issue. Recently, Faraone and colleagues [33] undertook a comprehensive analysis of existing growth studies with stimulant medication. For most patients, treatment with stimulant medication into adolescence leads to modest (at most) delays in growth. Weight deficits were greater than height deficits and the two were modestly associated. This effect is greatest for children who are taller and heavier and for children 6 to 12 compared with adolescents 12 to 18. The studies reviewed also suggest these deficits attenuate over time and do not differ between methylphenidate and amphetamine or between long- and short-acting formulations. Some studies suggest that

ADHD itself, and not its treatment, is associated with dysregulation of growth and that final adult height is not affected [34]. Thus, although treatment with stimulants can lead to some reductions in expected height and weight, these reductions are, on average, small, attenuate with time, and do not cause a greater proportion of children to become extremely short or thin. If confirmed, this finding would not support the common practice of drug holidays in children who have ADHD. However, providing drug holidays or alternative treatment to children who are believed to have stimulant-associated growth deficits seems prudent [21]. This recommendation should be carefully weighed against the risk for exacerbation of symptoms from drug discontinuation (for a broader discussion about effects of stimulants on height and weight, see the article by Vitiello, elsewhere in this issue).

A transient behavioral deterioration can occur on the abrupt discontinuation of stimulant medications in some children. The prevalence of this phenomenon and its cause are unclear. Rebound phenomena can also occur in some children between doses, creating an uneven, often disturbing clinical course. In those cases, alternative treatments should be considered.

New-generation stimulants

A new generation of highly sophisticated, well-developed, safe, and effective long-acting preparations of stimulant drugs has reached the market and revolutionized the treatment of ADHD. These compounds use novel delivery systems to overcome acute tolerance, termed *tachyphylaxis*.

Concerta uses an osmotic pump mechanism to create an ascending profile of methylphenidate in the blood to provide effective extended treatment approximating the three-times-daily dosing of methylphenidate immediate release (MPH IR). A laboratory classroom found that a single morning dose of Concerta was effective for 12 hours on social and task behaviors and academic performance [35]. This study was followed by a large multicenter trial that was used to show the safety and efficacy of Concerta in an outpatient setting [36]. A 1-year follow-up study of 407 children treated with Concerta found no marked effects on weight, height, blood pressure, pulse, or tic exacerbation [31,37,38].

Metadate CD is a capsule with a mixture of immediate and delayed release beads containing methylphenidate. In Metadate CD, 30% of the beads are immediate release and 70% delayed to provide effective methylphenidate treatment for 8 to 9 hours. The efficacy and safety of Metadate CD was shown in a large randomized multicenter trial [39]. Ritalin LA uses a bimodal release system that produces effective treatment for 8 hours [40]. Ritalin LA consists of a mixture of immediate and delayed release beads in a 50:50 ratio.

Adderall XR is a capsule with a 50:50 ratio of immediate- to delayed-release beads designed to release drug content in a time course similar to Adderall given twice daily (0 and 4 hours). An analog classroom study documented behavioral and academic improvement of 12 hours [41]. A multicenter, randomized, trial of Adderall XR documented improvement in morning and afternoon assessments [42]. A 1-year follow-up documented continued efficacy, safety, and good toleration [43].

Two controlled studies showed the specific d-threo-methylphenidate stereoisomer of methylphenidate (Focalin) to be efficacious [44,45]. A new extended-release dosage form of Focalin (Focalin XR) was developed to provide effective methylphenidate treatment for 12 hours. Focalin XR consists of a mixture of immediate- and delayed-release beads in a 50:50 ratio. Focalin XR was found to be effective in a large, randomized, outpatient trial [46].

A transdermal delivery system for methylphenidate was developed recently (the methylphenidate transdermal system [MTS]; Daytrana TM, Shire and Noven Pharmaceuticals). Methylphenidate is contained within a multipolymeric adhesive layer attached to a transparent backing. Patches are applied once daily and deliver a consistent amount of methylphenidate during the time the patch is worn. The drug does not go through first-pass metabolism in the liver, thereby allowing more methylphenidate to be bioavailable. Transdermal delivery of methylphenidate might represent a useful treatment option for patients who have difficultly swallowing or tolerating (eg, gastrointestinally) oral formulations or for patients who need flexible duration of medication effect. Previously, a randomized, double-blinded study of MTS [47] conducted in a summer treatment program showed significant improvement in measures of social behavior in recreational settings, classroom functioning, and parent ratings of evening behavior. However, patch wear-times of at least 12 hours resulted in insomnia for many participants. Ensuing trials [48] used MTS with a wear-time of 9 hours. A classroom analog study [49] showed more than 12 hours of effectiveness for a wear-time of 9 hours.

In addition, a large, randomized, study of MTS and OROS methylphenidate in children aged 6 to 12 years diagnosed with ADHD [50] showed that treatment with MTS was effective at reducing the symptoms of ADHD according to clinicians, teachers, and parents and was generally well tolerated. A large long-term follow-up study of MTS in children who had ADHD found consistent long-term efficacy and tolerability that was typical for methylphenidate. In addition, evaluation of dermal response indicated that most skin responses consisted of only mild erythema. Skin redness or itching at the application site is common and does not necessitate discontinuation. More severe rashes, as indicated by swelling, bumps, or blisters around the application site, may indicate a skin allergy to MTS and may necessitate discontinuation.

Lisdexamfetamine dimesylate (LDX; Vyvanse TM) is a novel prodrug in which d-amphetamine is covalently bound to the amino acid l-lysine. This chemical bond renders the amphetamine component therapeutically inactive. After oral administration, LDX is converted to the active d-amphetamine, after enzymatic hydrolysis in a rate-limited manner at or following absorption. The saturable rate-limited hydrolysis releases active amphetamine slowly, creating a predictable long-acting delivery of active drug (d-amphetamine). Furthermore, saturation of enzymatic hydrolysis at supratherapeutic doses suggests that LDX may be associated with diminished risk for abuse and toxicity at these doses. In a classroom analog study, LDX was shown to be effective and long lasting [51]. In a large randomized study, LDX was effective and well tolerated [52]. Improvements were observed throughout the day up to 6:00 PM. The tolerability profile was similar to currently marketed extended-release stimulants.

Nonstimulants

Although the stimulants are undoubtedly effective in the treatment of ADHD, it is estimated that at least 30% of affected individuals do not adequately respond or cannot tolerate stimulant treatment [8,53,54]. In addition, stimulants are short-acting drugs that require multiple administrations during the day, and therefore require compliance and must be taken during school or work hours. Although this problem may be offset by the development of an effective long-acting stimulant, this class of drugs often adversely impacts sleep, making evening use difficult when children and adults must concentrate to deal with daily demands and interact with family members and friends. In addition to these problems, the fact that stimulants are controlled substances continues to fuel concerns in children, families, and the treating community, further inhibiting their use. These fears are based on lingering concerns about the abuse potential of stimulant drugs by children, family members, or their associates; the possibility of diversion; and safety concerns about the use of controlled substances by patients who are impulsive and frequently have antisocial tendencies [55]. Similarly, the controlled nature of stimulant drugs poses important medicolegal concerns to the treating community that further increase the barriers to treatment.

Historically, the first nonstimulant treatments for ADHD that were extensively evaluated were the tricyclic antidepressants (TCAs). Of 33 studies (21 controlled, 12 open) evaluating TCAs in children, adolescents (N = 1139), and adults (N = 78), 91% reported positive effects on ADHD symptoms [5]. Imipramine and desipramine are the most studied TCAs, followed by a handful of studies on other TCAs. Although most TCA studies (73%) were brief, lasting a few weeks to several months, nine studies (27%) reported enduring effects for up to 2 years. Outcomes in both short- and long-term studies were equally positive. Although one study [56] reported a 50% dropout rate after 1 year, improvement was sustained for those who remained on imipramine. Other studies using aggressive doses of TCAs reported sustained improvement for up to 1 year with desipramine (>4 mg/kg) [57,58] and nortriptyline (2 mg/kg) [59]. Although response was equally positive in all dose ranges, it was more sustained in the studies using higher doses. A high interindividual variability in TCAs serum levels has been consistently reported for imipramine and desipramine, with little relationship between serum level to daily dose, response, or side effects. In contrast, nortriptyline seems to have a positive association between dose and serum level [59].

Of the 33 TCA studies (40%), 13 compared TCAs with stimulants. Five studies reported that stimulants were superior to TCAs [60–63], five showed that they were equal [64–67], and three reported that TCAs were superior to stimulants [68–70]. Analysis of response profiles indicate that TCAs more consistently improve behavioral symptoms as rated by clinicians, teachers, and parents than they impact on cognitive function as measured in neuro-psychological testing [56,69,71,72]. Studies of TCAs have uniformly reported a robust rate of ADHD symptom response in patients who had ADHD with comorbid depression or anxiety [59,73–75]. In addition, studies of TCAs have consistently reported a robust rate of response in subjects who had ADHD with comorbid tic disorders [76–81]. The potential benefits of TCAs in treating ADHD have been clouded by concerns about their safety stemming from reports of sudden unexplained death in four children who had ADHD treated with desipramine [82], although the causal link between this drug and the deaths remains uncertain.

Evaluations of short- and long-term effects of therapeutic doses of TCAs on the cardiovascular systems in children have found TCAs to be generally well tolerated with only minor EKG changes associated with TCA treatment in daily oral doses as high as 5 mg/kg. TCA-induced EKG abnormalities (conduction defects) have been consistently reported in children at doses higher than 3.5 mg/kg [83] (1 mg/kg for nortriptyline). Although of unclear hemodynamic significance, the development of conduction defects in children undergoing TCA treatment merits closer EKG and clinical monitoring, especially when high doses of these medicines are used. In the context of cardiac disease, conduction defects may have more serious clinical implications. When a patient's cardiovascular state is in doubt, a more comprehensive cardiac evaluation, including 24-hour EKG, and cardiac consultation are suggested before TCA treatment is initiated to help determine the risk-versus-benefit ratio of this intervention. Because of the potential lethality of TCA overdose, parents should be advised to carefully store the medication in a place inaccessible to the children or their siblings.

Bupropion hydrochloride is a novel structured antidepressant of the aminoketone class related to the phenylisopropylamines but pharmacologically distinct from known antidepressants. Although its specific site or mechanism of action remains unknown, bupropion seems to have an indirect mixed agonist effect on dopamine and norepinephrine neurotransmission. In a controlled multisite study (N = 72) [84–86] and in comparison with methylphenidate (N = 15) [87], bupropion was shown to be effective for ADHD in children. Side effects include irritability, anorexia, insomnia, and, rarely, edema, rashes, and nocturia. Exacerbation of tic disorders has also been reported with bupropion. Although bupropion has been associated a slightly increased risk (0.4%) for drug-induced seizures compared with other antidepressants, this risk has been linked to high doses, a previous history of seizures, and eating disorders. Bupropion was formulated into long-acting (SR, XR) preparations that can be administered twice daily.

Although a small number of studies suggested that monoamine oxidase inhibitors (MAOIs) may be effective in ADHD, the potential for hypertensive crisis associated with dietetic transgressions and drug interactions seriously limits their use. The MAOIs include the hydrazine (phenelzine) and nonhydrazine (tranylcypromine) compounds. Short-term adverse effects include orthostatic hypotension, weight gain, drowsiness, and dizziness. However, major limitations for MAOI use in children and adolescents are the severe dietetic restrictions of tyramine-containing foods (eg, most cheeses), pressor amines (eg, sympathomimetic substances), and severe drug interactions (eg, most cold medicines, amphetamines), which can induce a hypertensive crisis and a serotonergic syndrome. Although not available in the United States, a new family of reversible inhibitors of MAOI (also known as *RIMA*) has been developed and used in Europe and Canada that may be free of these difficulties.

Although a single, small, open study [88] suggested that fluoxetine may be beneficial in treating children who have ADHD, the usefulness of selective serotonin reuptake inhibitors (SSRIs) in treating core ADHD symptoms is not supported by clinical experience [89]. Similarly uncertain is the usefulness of mixed serotonergic/noradrenergic atypical antidepressant venlafaxine in the treatment of ADHD [90–93]. Currently, expert opinion does not support the usefulness of these serotonergic compounds in treating core ADHD symptoms [4,89]. Nevertheless, because of the high rates of comorbidity in ADHD, these compounds are frequently combined with effective anti-ADHD agents. Because many psychotropics are metabolized by the cytochrome P450 system [94], which can then be inhibited by SSRIs, caution should be exercised when combining agents, such as TCAs, with SSRIs.

Specific norepinephrine reuptake inhibitors (atomoxetine)

Atomoxetine (Strattera) is one of a new class of compounds being developed, known as specific norepinephrine reuptake inhibitors. An initial controlled clinical trial in adults documented proof of concept in the treatment of ADHD [95]. These initial encouraging results coupled with extensive safety data in adults encouraged efforts to develop this compound for treating pediatric ADHD. An open-label, dose-ranging study of this compound in pediatric ADHD documented strong clinical benefits with excellent tolerability, including a safe cardiovascular profile, and provided dosing guidelines for further controlled studies [96].

Further controlled trials led to FDA approval of atomoxetine for children and adults who have ADHD. In the first pediatric controlled studies, atomoxetine significantly reduced total scores on an investigator-rated *Diagnostic and Statistical Manual of Mental Disorders, Fourth Edition* (DSM-IV) ADHD rating scale and was well tolerated [97]. Mild appetite suppression and insomnia were reported. Additionally, mild increases in diastolic blood pressure and heart rate were noted with no changes in ECG intervals. In another large controlled study, atomoxetine was associated with a graded dose response; response was best at 1.2 or 1.8 mg/kg per day and superior to 0.5 mg/kg per day [98]. This study documented a dose-dependent enhancement of social and family function. Parents of children taking atomoxetine reported fewer emotional difficulties and behavioral problems and greater self-esteem in their children and less emotional worry and limitations in personal time for themselves. In a year-long open follow-up of atomoxetine, treatment continued to be effective and well tolerated. The acute mild increases in diastolic blood pressure and heart rate persisted with not worsening. Growth in height and weight were normal and no significant differences were seen between atomoxetine and placebo in laboratory parameters and ECG intervals [99,100]. Because atomoxetine is metabolized by the hepatic 2D6 enzymatic system, care should be taken with coadministration of medications that inhibit 2D6 (eg, fluoxetine, paroxetine). In addition, atomoxetine has been shown to have low abuse potential [101].

Since its approval, two cases of severe liver injury were reported among greater than 2 million patients who have taken atomoxetine. Both patients recovered with normal liver function after discontinuing the medication. Although rare and both cases recovered, severe drug-related liver injury may progress to acute liver failure resulting in death or the need for a liver transplant. Eli Lilly (www.lilly.com) announced that as of December 2004, a bolded warning was added to atomoxetine's product label indicating that the medication should be discontinued in patients who have jaundice (yellowing of the skin or whites of the eyes) or laboratory evidence of liver injury. Patients taking atomoxetine are cautioned to contact their doctor immediately if they develop pruritus, jaundice, dark urine, upper right-sided abdominal tenderness, or unexplained flu-like symptoms.

Modafinil

Modafinil is an antinarcoleptic agent that is structurally and pharmacologically different from other agents approved to treat ADHD. Although its mechanism of action is unknown, it may improve symptoms of ADHD by way of the same mechanism through which it improves wakefulness. Preclinically, modafinil selectively activates the cortex without causing widespread central nervous system stimulation [102]. Modafinil does not seem to activate areas of the brain that mediate reward and abuse and has a low potential for abuse [103].

Although initial studies showed significant improvement in ADHD symptoms, subsequent studies reported increased efficacy with higher doses

(340–425 mg/d) in children and adolescents [104]. A 9-week, randomized, double-blind, placebo-controlled, flexible-dosage trial evaluated the efficacy and tolerability of this new modafinil formulation in once-daily dosing [105]. The most commonly reported adverse events in the modafinil group were insomnia (29%), headache (20%), and decreased appetite (16%). Modafinil was not FDA-approved for treatment of ADHD because of concerns about a rare but potentially serious rash characteristic of Stevens-Johnson syndrome.

α-Adrenergic agents: clonidine and guanfacine

Clonidine is an imidazoline derivative with α-adrenergic agonist properties that has been used primarily to treat hypertension. At low doses, it seems to stimulate inhibitory, presynaptic autoreceptors in the central nervous system. The most common use of clonidine in pediatric psychiatry is for treating Tourette's syndrome and other tic disorders [106], ADHD, and ADHD-associated sleep disturbances [107,108]. Clonidine was also reported as useful for controlling aggression to self and others in patients with developmental disorders. Clonidine is a short-acting compound with a plasma half-life ranging from approximately 5.5 (in children) to 8.5 hours (in adults). Therapy is usually initiated at the lowest manufactured dose of a full or half tablet of 0.1 mg depending on the size of the child (approximately 1–2 μg/kg) and increased depending on clinical response and adverse effects. Initial dosage can be given more easily in the evening hours or before bedtime because of sedation. The most common short-term adverse effect of clonidine is sedation. It can also produce hypotension, dry mouth, depression, and confusion. Clonidine is not known to be associated with long-term adverse effects. In adults who have hypertension, abrupt withdrawal of clonidine has been associated with rebound hypertension, and it therefore requires slow tapering when discontinued. Clonidine should not be administered concomitantly with β-blockers because adverse interactions have been reported with this combination. In addition, evidence shows that the more selective α_2-adrenergic agonist guanfacine may have a spectrum of benefits similar to clonidine with less sedation and longer duration of action [109–111]. Usual daily dose ranges from 42 to 86 μg/kg given generally in divided doses twice or three times daily.

Despite its wide use in ADHD children, few studies (six studies, four which were controlled; N = 292 children) [79,112–116] support the efficacy of clonidine. A multisite study compared clonidine with methylphenidate in a sample of children who had ADHD and Tourette's syndrome [115]. They reported that clonidine worked as well as methylphenidate on teacher ratings of ADHD, but that clonidine was most helpful for treating impulsivity and hyperactivity and not as helpful for inattention. Moreover, sedation was a common side effect occurring in 28% of subjects. Equally limited is the literature on guanfacine. Three open studies (n = 36 total) and one controlled study (n = 34) of guanfacine were conducted in children and adolescents who had ADHD [109–111,117]. These studies reported beneficial effects on hyperactive behaviors and attentional abilities. In the controlled study of children who had tic disorders and ADHD, guanfacine improved attention according to teacher ratings and a continuous performance test [117]. In a study in adults who had ADHD (n = 17), guanfacine was shown to improve ADHD symptoms and performance on a cognitive test of response inhibition as measured with the Stroop [118]. Several cases of sudden death were reported in children treated with clonidine plus methylphenidate, raising concerns about the safety of this combination [119]. A study examining the combination in 33 children found no evidence of cardiac toxicity [115]. Although more work is needed to evaluate if an increased risk is associated with this combination, a cautious approach is advised, including increased surveillance and cardiovascular monitoring.

New-generation α-adrenergic agents

In attempt to increase convenience and decrease side effects such as sedation, Shire developed an extended-release formulation of guanfacine hydrochloride as monotherapy for treating ADHD in children and adolescents. This formulation received an approvable letter from the FDA but is not yet approved or marketed. As an extended release, it has a lower maximum serum concentration and a longer half-life. Two large 8- to 9-week randomized studies of guanfacine extended-release were conducted in children aged 6 to 17 years diagnosed with ADHD [120]. Doses of 1, 2, 3, and 4 mg were tested. Efficacy for ADHD was substantial and proportionate to weight-corrected dose. Adverse events were mild to moderate in severity, with most common events related to somnolence, sedation, or fatigue. Small to moderate changes in blood pressure and pulse rate were observed as expected for a medication with antihypertensive properties.

Integrating findings

Considering the huge amount of medications available for treating ADHD, a practical issue is how to choose drugs and formulations. Although individual choices should be made for each patient, a recent meta-analysis of the available literature suggested that effect sizes for stimulants are significantly greater than those for nonstimulants [121]. However, because of the diversity of methodological issues among studies, caution is warranted when comparing the effects of different medications across studies. The field definitively needs more confirmatory head-to-head studies.

Despite the benefits of long-acting preparations of stimulants for treating ADHD, immediate-release formulations still have their usefulness, mainly in initial treatment for many children because of cost and flexibility of dosing [122]. When starting an extended-release stimulant preparation, the choice of preparation will depend on the profile of action required over time. If a child does not experience response to a stimulant, an alternative stimulant might be the next logical option.

Although a stimulant will be the first choice in most patients, atomoxetine may be preferred in some cases, particularly when substance abuse or comorbid tics are a problem, if a strong family preference exists for a non-stimulant, if 24-hour action is strongly required, or if comorbid anxiety is present. In addition, in the presence of adverse events while using stimulants, the next step often will be atomoxetine.

Summary

ADHD is a heterogeneous disorder with strong neurobiologic basis that affects millions of individuals of all ages worldwide. Although the stimulants remain the mainstay of treatment for this disorder, a new generation of non-stimulant drugs is emerging that provides viable alternative for patients and families. When assessing patients who have ADHD, a careful differential diagnosis must be applied that considers psychiatric, social, cognitive, educational, and medical/neurologic factors that may contribute to the clinical presentation. Realistic expectations of interventions, careful definition of target symptoms, and careful assessment of the potential risks and benefits of each type of intervention for these patients are major ingredients for success.

References

[1] Bymaster FP, Katner JS, Nelson DL, et al. Atomoxetine increases extracellular levels of norepinephrine and dopamine in prefrontal cortex of rat: a potential mechanism for efficacy in attention deficit/hyperactivity disorder. Neuropsychopharmacology 2002;27:699–711.

[2] Volkow ND, Wang G, Fowler JS, et al. Therapeutic doses of oral methylphenidate significantly increase extracellular dopamine in the human brain. J Neurosci 2001;21:RC121.

[3] Greenhill L, Halperin J, Abikoff H. Stimulant medications. J Am Acad Child Adolesc Psychiatry 1998;38:503–12.

[4] Pliszka S, AACAP work group on quality issues. Practice parameter for the assessment and treatment of children and adolescents with attention-deficit/hyperactivity disorder. J Am Acad Child Adolesc Psychiatry 2007;46:894–921.

[5] Spencer T, Biederman J, Wilens T. Pharmacotherapy of ADHD: a life span perspective. In: Oldham J, Riba M, editors. American psychiatric press review of psychiatry. Washington: APA Press; 1997. p. 87–128.

[6] Spencer T, Wilens T, Biederman J, et al. A double-blind, crossover comparison of methylphenidate and placebo in adults with childhood-onset attention-deficit hyperactivity disorder. Arch Gen Psychiatry 1995;52:434–43.

[7] Wilens TE, Biederman J, Spencer TJ, et al. Controlled trial of high doses of pemoline for adults with attention- deficit/hyperactivity disorder. J Clin Psychopharmacol 1999;19:257–64.

[8] Barkley RA. A review of stimulant drug research with hyperactive children. J Child Psychol Psychiatry 1977;18:137–65.

[9] Gittleman-Klein R. Pharmacotherapy of childhood hyperactivity: an update. In: Meltzer HY, editor. Psychopharmacology: the third generation of progress. New York: Raven Press; 1987. p. 1215–24.

[10] Rapport MD, Stoner G, DuPaul GJ, et al. Attention deficit disorder and methylphenidate: a multilevel analysis of dose-response effects on children's impulsivity across settings. J Am Acad Child Adolesc Psychiatry 1988;27:60–9.

[11] Bergman A, Winters L, Cornblatt B. Methylphenidate: effects on sustained attention. In: Greenhill L, Osman B, editors. Ritalin: theory and patient management. New York: Mary Ann Liebert, Inc.; 1991. p. 223–31.

[12] Faraone SV, Biederman J, Lehman BK, et al. Intellectual performance and school failure in children with attention deficit hyperactivity disorder and in their siblings. J Abnorm Psychol 1993;102:616–23.

[13] Douglas V, Barr R, Amin K, et al. Dosage effects and individual responsivity to methylphenidate in attention deficit disorder. J Child Psychol Psychiatry 1988;29:453–75.

[14] Kupietz SS, Winsberg BG, Richardson E, et al. Effects of methylphenidate dosage in hyperactive reading-disabled children: I. Behavior and cognitive performance effects. J Am Acad Child Adolesc Psychiatry 1988;27:70–7.

[15] Pelham WE, Bender ME, Caddell J, et al. Methylphenidate and children with attention deficit disorder. Arch Gen Psychiatry 1985;42:948–52.

[16] Rapport MD, DuPaul GJ, Kelly KL. Attention deficit hyperactivity disorder and methylphenidate: the relationship between gross body weight and drug response in children. Psychopharmacol Bull 1989;25:285–90.

[17] Rapport MD, Jones JT, DuPaul GJ, et al. Attention deficit disorder and methylphenidate: group and single-subject analyses of dose effects on attention in clinic and classroom settings. J Clin Child Psychol 1987;16:329–38.

[18] Rapport MD, Quinn SO, DuPaul GJ, et al. Attention deficit disorder with hyperactivity and methylphenidate: the effects of dose and mastery level on children's learning performance. J Abnorm Child Psychol 1989;17:669–89.

[19] Tannock R, Schachar RJ, Carr RP, et al. Dose-response effects of methylphenidate on academic performance and overt behavior in hyperactive children. Pediatrics 1989;84:648–57.

[20] Jensen PS, Arnold LE, Swanson JM, et al. 3-year follow-up of the NIMH MTA study. J Am Acad Child Adolesc Psychiatry 2007;46:989–1002.

[21] Martins S, Tramontina S, Polanczyk G, et al. Weekend holidays with Methylphenidate use in ADHD children: a randomized clinical trial. J Child Adolesc Psychopharmacol 2004;14: 195–206.

[22] Wilens TE, Biederman J. The stimulants. Psychiatr Clin North Am 1992;15(1):191–222.

[23] Barkley RA, Murray MB, Edelbrock C, et al. Side effects of methylphenidate in children with attention-deficit hyperactivity disorder: a systemic, placebo-controlled evaluation. Pediatrics 1990;86:184–92.

[24] Brown RT, Wynne ME, Slimmer LW. Attention deficit disorder and the effect of methylphenidate on attention, behavioral, and cardiovascular functioning. J Clin Psychiatry 1984; 45:473–6.

[25] Lowe TL, Cohen DJ, Detlor J. Stimulant medications precipitate Tourette's syndrome. JAMA 1982;247:1168–9.

[26] Comings DE, Comings BG. Tourette's syndrome and attention deficit disorder. In: Cohen DJ, Bruun RD, Leckman JF, editors. Tourette's syndrome and tic disorders: clinical understanding and treatment. New York: John Wiley and Sons; 1988. p. 119–36.

[27] Gadow K, Sverd J, Sprafkin J, et al. Efficacy of methylphenidate for attention-deficit hyperactivity disorder in children with tic disorder. Arch Gen Psychiatry 1995;52:444–55, [published erratum appears in Arch Gen Psychiatry 1995 Oct;52(10):836].

[28] Gadow KD, Nolan EE, Sverd J. Methylphenidate in hyperactive boys with comorbid tic disorder: II. Short-term behavioral effects in school settings. J Am Acad Child Adolesc Psychiatry 1992;31:462–71.

[29] Spencer T, Biederman J, Coffey B, et al. The 4-year course of tic disorders in boys with attention-deficit/hyperactivity disorder. Arch Gen Psychiatry 1999;56:842–7.

[30] Biederman J, Wilens T, Mick E, et al. Pharmacotherapy of attention-deficit/hyperactivity disorder reduces risk for substance use disorder. Pediatrics 1999;104:e20.

[31] Wilens T, McBurnett K, Stein M, et al. ADHD treatment with once-daily OROS methylphenidate: final results from a long-term open-label study. J Am Acad Child Adolesc Psychiatry 2005;44(10):1015–23.

[32] Spencer TJ, Biederman J, Ciccone PE, et al. PET study examining pharmacokinetics, detection and likeability, and dopamine transporter receptor occupancy of short- and long-acting oral methylphenidate. Am J Psychiatry 2006;163:387–95.

[33] Faraone SV, Biederman J, Morley CP, et al. The effect of stimulants on height and weight: a review of the literature. J Am Acad Child Adolesc Psychiatry, in press.

[34] Spencer T, Biederman J, Wilens T. Growth deficits in children with attention deficit hyperactivity disorder. Pediatrics 1998;102:501–6.

[35] Pelham WE, Gnagy EM, Burrows-Maclean L, et al. Once-a-day Concerta methylphenidate versus three-times-daily methylphenidate in laboratory and natural settings. Pediatrics 2001;107:E105.

[36] Wolraich M, Greenhill LL, Pelham W, et al. Randomized controlled trial of OROS methylphenidate qd in children with attention deficit/hyperactivity disorder. Pediatrics 2001;108:883–92.

[37] Palumbo D, Spencer T, Lynch J, et al. Emergence of tics in children with ADHD: impact of once-daily OROS methylphenidate therapy. J Child Adolesc Psychopharmacol 2004;14(2): 185–94.

[38] Spencer TJ, Faraone SV, Biederman J, et al. Does prolonged therapy with a long-acting stimulant suppress growth in children with ADHD? J Am Acad Child Adolesc Psychiatry 2006;45(5):527–37.

[39] Greenhill LL, Findling RL, Swanson JM. A double-blind, placebo-controlled study of modified-release methylphenidate in children with attention-deficit/hyperactivity disorder. Pediatrics 2002;109:E39.

[40] Biederman J, Quinn D, Weiss M, et al. Efficacy and safety of Ritalin LA, a new, once daily, extended-release dosage form of methylphenidate, in children with attention deficit hyperactivity disorder. Paediatr Drugs 2003;5(12):833–41.

[41] McCracken JT, Biederman J, Greenhill LL, et al. Analog classroom assessment of a once-daily mixed amphetamine formulation, SLI381 (Adderall XR), in children with ADHD. J Am Acad Child Adolesc Psychiatry 2003;42(6):673–83.

[42] Biederman J, Lopez FA, Boellner SW, et al. A randomized, double-blind, placebo-controlled, parallel-group study of SLI381 in children with attention deficit hyperactivity disorder. Pediatrics 2002;110:258–66.

[43] McGough JJ, Biederman J, Wigal SB, et al. Long-term tolerability and effectiveness of once-daily mixed amphetamine salts (Adderall XR) in children with ADHD. J Am Acad Child Adolesc Psychiatry 2005;44(6):530–8.

[44] Wigal S, Swanson JM, Feifel D, et al. A double-blind, placebo-controlled trial of dexmethylphenidate hydrochloride and d,l-threo-methylphenidate hydrochloride in children with attention-deficit/hyperactivity disorder. J Am Acad Child Adolesc Psychiatry 2004;43(11):1406–14.

[45] Arnold LE, Lindsay RL, Conners CK, et al. A double-blind, placebo-controlled withdrawal trial of dexmethylphenidate hydrochloride in children with attention deficit hyperactivity disorder. J Child Adolesc Psychopharmacol 2004;14(4):542–54.

[46] Greenhill LL, Muniz R, Ball RR, et al. Efficacy and safety of dexmethylphenidate extended-release capsules in children with attention-deficit/hyperactivity disorder. J Am Acad Child Adolesc Psychiatry 2006;45(7):817–23.

[47] Pelham WE, Manos MJ, Ezzell CE, et al. A dose-ranging study of a methylphenidate transdermal system in children with ADHD. J Am Acad Child Adolesc Psychiatry 2005; 44:522–9.

[48] Pelham WE, Burrows-Maclean L, Gnagy EM, et al. Transdermal methylphenidate, behavioral, and combined treatment for children with ADHD. Exp Clin Psychopharmacol 2005;13:111–26.

[49] McGough JJ, Wigal SB, Abikoff H, et al. A randomized, double-blind, placebo-controlled, laboratory classroom assessment of methylphenidate transdermal system in children with ADHD. J Atten Disord 2006;9:476–85.

[50] Findling RL, Bukstein OG, Melmed RD, et al. A Randomized, Double-Blind, Placebo-Controlled, Parallel-Group Study of Methylphenidate Transdermal System in Pediatric Patients With Attention-Deficit/Hyperactivity Disorder. J Clin Psychiatry. 2008; in press.

[51] Biederman J, Boellner SW, Childress A, et al. Lisdexamfetamine dimesylate and mixed amphetamine salts extended-release in children with ADHD: a double-blind, placebo-controlled, crossover analog classroom study. Biol Psychiatry 2007;62(9):970–6.

[52] Biederman J, Krishnan S, Zhang Y, et al. Efficacy and safety of Lisdexamfetamine (LDX; NRP104) in children with attention-deficit/hyperactivity disorder: a phase 3, randomized, multicenter, double-blind, parallel-group study. Clin Ther 2007;29:450–63.

[53] Gittleman R, et al. Childhood disorders. In: Klein D, Quitkin F, Rifkin A, editors. Drug treatment of adult and child psychiatric disorders. Baltimore: Williams and Wilkins; 1980. p. 576–756.

[54] Spencer TJ, Biederman J, Wilens T, et al. Pharmacotherapy of attention deficit hyperactivity disorder across the lifecycle: a literature review. J Am Acad Child Adolesc Psychiatry 1996;35:409–32.

[55] Goldman L, Genel M, Bezman R, et al. Diagnosis and treatment of attention-deficit/hyperactivity disorder in children and adolescents. JAMA 1998;279:1100–7.

[56] Quinn PO, Rapoport JL. One-year follow-up of hyperactive boys treated with imipramine or methylphenidate. Am J Psychiatry 1975;132:241–5.

[57] Biederman J, Gastfriend DR, Jellinek MS. Desipramine in the treatment of children with attention deficit disorder. J Clin Psychopharmacol 1986;6:359–63.

[58] Gastfriend DR, Biederman J, Jellinek MS. Desipramine in the treatment of attention deficit disorder in adolescents. Psychopharmacol Bull 1985;21:144–5.

[59] Wilens TE, Biederman J, Geist DE, et al. Nortriptyline in the treatment of attention deficit hyperactivity disorder: a chart review of 58 cases. J Am Acad Child Adolesc Psychiatry 1993;32:343–9.

[60] Garfinkel BD, Wender PH, Sloman L, et al. Tricyclic antidepressant and methylphenidate treatment of attention deficit disorder in children. J Am Acad Child Adolesc Psychiatry 1983;22:343–8.

[61] Gittleman-Klein R. Pilot clinical trial of imipramine in hyperkinetic children. In: Conners CK, editor. Clinical use of stimulant drugs in children. The Hague, Netherlands: Excerpta Medica; 1974. p. 192–201.

[62] Greenberg L, Yellin A, Spring C, et al. Clinical effects of imipramine and methylphenidate in hyperactive children. Int J Ment Health 1975;4:144–56.

[63] Rapoport JL, Quinn P, Bradbard G, et al. Imipramine and methylphenidate treatment of hyperactive boys: a double-blind comparison. Arch Gen Psychiatry 1974;30:789–93.

[64] Gross M. Imipramine in the treatment of minimal brain dysfunction in children. Psychosomatics 1973;14:283–5.

[65] Huessy H, Wright A. The use of imipramine in children's behavior disorders. Acta Paedopsychiatr 1970;37:194–9.

[66] Kupietz SS, Balka EB. Alterations in the vigilance performance of children receiving amitriptyline and methylphenidate pharmacotherapy. Psychopharmacology 1976;50:29–33.

[67] Yepes LE, Balka EB, Winsberg BG, et al. Amitriptyline and methylphenidate treatment of behaviorally disordered children. J Child Psychol Psychiatry 1977;18:39–52.

[68] Watter N, Dreyfuss FE. Modifications of hyperkinetic behavior by nortriptyline. Va Med Mon 1973;100:123–6.

[69] Werry J. Imipramine and methylphenidate in hyperactive children. J Child Psychol Psychiatry 1980;21:27–35.

[70] Winsberg BG, Bialer I, Kupietz S, et al. Effects of imipramine and dextroamphetamine on behavior of neuropsychiatrically impaired children. Am J Psychiatry 1972;128: 1425–31.

[71] Gualtieri CT, Evans RW. Motor performance in hyperactive children treated with imipramine. Percept Mot Skills 1988;66:763–9.

[72] Rapport M, Carlson G, Kelly K, et al. Methylphenidate and desipramine in hospitalized children: I. Separate and combined effects on cognitive function. J Am Acad Child Adolesc Psychiatry 1993;32:333–42.

[73] Biederman J, Baldessarini RJ, Wright V, et al. A double-blind placebo controlled study of desipramine in the treatment of attention deficit disorder: III. Lack of impact of comorbidity and family history factors on clinical response. J Am Acad Child Adolesc Psychiatry 1993;32:199–204.

[74] Cox W. An indication for the use of imipramine in attention deficit disorder. Am J Psychiatry 1982;139:1059–60.

[75] Wilens TE, Biederman JB, Mick E, et al. A systematic assessment of tricyclic antidepressants in the treatment of adult attention-deficit hyperactivity disorder. J Nerv Ment Dis 1995;183:48–50.

[76] Dillon DC, Salzman IJ, Schulsinger DA. The use of imipramine in Tourette's syndrome and attention deficit disorder: case report. J Clin Psychiatry 1985;46:348–9.

[77] Hoge SK, Biederman J. A case of Tourette's syndrome with symptoms of attention deficit disorder treated with desipramine. J Clin Psychiatry 1986;47:478–9.

[78] Riddle MA, Hardin MT, Cho SC, et al. Desipramine treatment of boys with attention-deficit hyperactivity disorder and tics: preliminary clinical experience. J Am Acad Child Adolesc Psychiatry 1988;27:811–4.

[79] Singer S, Brown J, Quaskey S, et al. The treatment of attention-deficit hyperactivity disorder in Tourette's syndromes: a double-blind placebo-controlled study with clonidine and desipramine. Pediatrics 1994;95:74–81.

[80] Spencer T, Biederman J, Kerman K, et al. Desipramine in the treatment of children with tic disorder or Tourette's syndrome and attention deficit hyperactivity disorder. J Am Acad Child Adolesc Psychiatry 1993;32:354–60.

[81] Spencer T, Biederman J, Wilens T, et al. Nortriptyline in the treatment of children with attention deficit hyperactivity disorder and tic disorder or Tourette's syndrome. J Am Acad Child Adolesc Psychiatry 1993;32:205–10.

[82] Abramowicz M. Sudden death in children treated with a tricyclic antidepressant. In: The medical letter on drugs and therapeutics. New Rochelle, NY: The Medical Letter; 1990. p. 53.

[83] Biederman J, Baldessarini RJ, Wright V, et al. A double-blind placebo controlled study of desipramine in the treatment of ADD: I. Efficacy. J Am Acad Child Adolesc Psychiatry 1989;28:777–84.

[84] Casat CD, Pleasants DZ, Schroeder DH, et al. Bupropion in children with attention deficit disorder. Psychopharmacol Bull 1989;25:198–201.

[85] Casat CD, Pleasants DZ, Van Wyck Fleet J. A double-blind trial of bupropion in children with attention deficit disorder. Psychopharmacol Bull 1987;23:120–2.

[86] Conners K, Casat C, Gualtieri T, et al. Bupropion hydrochloride in attention deficit disorder with hyperactivity. J Am Acad Child Adolesc Psychiatry 1996;35:1314–21.

[87] Barrickman L, Perry P, Allen A, et al. Bupropion versus methylphenidate in the treatment of attention-deficit hyperactivity disorder. J Am Acad Child Adolesc Psychiatry 1995;34: 649–57.

[88] Barrickman L, Noyes R, Kuperman S, et al. Treatment of ADHD with fluoxetine: a preliminary trial. J Am Acad Child Adolesc Psychiatry 1991;30:762–7.

[89] NIMH. Alternative pharmacology of ADHD, 1996.

[90] Adler L, Resnick S, Kunz M, et al. Open-label trial of venlafaxine in attention deficit disorder. Orlando: New Clinical Drug Evaluation Unit Program; 1995.

[91] Findling R, Schwartz M, Flannery D, et al. Venlafaxine in adults with ADHD: an open trial. J Clin Psychiatry 1996;57:184–9.

[92] Hornig-Rohan M, Amsterdam J. Venlafaxine vs. stimulant therapy in patients with dual diagnoses of ADHD and depression. Orlando (FL): New Clinical Drug Evaluation Unit Program; 1995, -pp. Poster #92.

[93] Reimherr F, Hedges D, Strong R, et al. An open-trial of Venlaxine in adult patients with attention deficit hyperactivity disorder. Orlando (FL): New Clinical Drug Evaluation Unit Program; 1995.

[94] Nemeroff C, DeVane L, Pollock B. Newer antidepressants and the cytochrome P450 system. Am J Psychiatry 1996;153:311–20.

[95] Spencer T, Biederman J, Wilens T, et al. Effectiveness and tolerability of tomoxetine in adults with attention deficit hyperactivity disorder. Am J Psychiatry 1998;155:693–5.

[96] Spencer T, Biederman J, Heiligenstein J, et al. An open-label, dose-ranging study of atomoxetine in children with attention deficit hyperactivity disorder. J Child Adolesc Psychopharmacol 2001;11:251–65.

[97] Spencer T, Heiligenstein J, Biederman J, et al. Results from 2 proof-of-concept, placebo-controlled studies of atomoxetine in children with attention-deficit/hyperactivity disorder. J Clin Psychiatry 2002;63:1140–7.

[98] Michelson D, Faries D, Wernicke J, et al. Atomoxetine in the treatment of children and adolescents with attention-deficit/hyperactivity disorder: a randomized, placebo-controlled, dose-response study. Pediatrics 2001;108:E83.

[99] Kratochvil CJ, Bohac D, Harrington M, et al. An open-label trial of tomoxetine in pediatric attention deficit hyperactivity disorder. J Child Adolesc Psychopharmacol 2001;11:167–70.

[100] Spencer T, Newcorn J, Kratochvil C, et al. Effects of atomoxetine on growth after 2-year treatment in pediatric patients with ADHD. Pediatrics 2005;116:e74–80.

[101] Heil SH, Holmes HW, Bickel WK, et al. Comparison of the subjective, physiological, and psychomotor effects of atomoxetine and methylphenidate in light drug users. Drug Alcohol Depend 2002;67:149–56.

[102] Engber TM, Koury EJ, Dennis SA, et al. Differential patterns of regional c-Fos induction in the rat brain by amphetamine and the novel wakefulness-promoting agent modafinil. Neurosci Lett 1998;241:95–8.

[103] Myrick H, Malcolm R, Taylor B, et al. Modafinil: preclinical, clinical, and post-marketing surveillance–a review of abuse liability issues. Ann Clin Psychiatry 2004;16:101–9.

[104] Swanson JM, Greenhill LL, Lopez FA, et al. Modafinil film-coated tablets in children and adolescents with attention-deficit/hyperactivity disorder: results of a randomized, double-blind, placebo-controlled, fixed-dose study followed by abrupt discontinuation. J Clin Psychiatry 2006;67(1):137–47.

[105] Biederman J, Swanson JM, Wigal SB, et al. Efficacy and safety of modafinil film-coated tablets in children and adolescents with attention-deficit/hyperactivity disorder: results of a randomized, double-blind, placebo-controlled, flexible-dose study. Pediatrics 2005; 116(6):e777–84.

[106] Leckman JF, Hardin MT, Riddle MA, et al. Clonidine treatment of Gilles de la Tourette's syndrome. Arch Gen Psychiatry 1991;48:324–8.

[107] Hunt RD, Capper L, O'Connell P. Clonidine in child and adolescent psychiatry. J Child Adolesc Psychopharmacol 1990;1:87–102.

[108] Prince J, Wilens T, Biederman J, et al. Clonidine for ADHD related sleep disturbances: a systematic chart review of 62 cases. J Am Acad Child Adolesc Psychiatry 1996;35: 599–605.

[109] Chappell P, Riddle M, Scahill L, et al. Guanfacine treatment of comorbid attention-deficit hyperactivity disorder and Tourette's syndrome. J Am Acad Child Adolesc Psychiatry 1995;34:1140–6.

[110] Horrigan JP, Barnhill LJ. Guanfacine for treatment of attention-deficit hyperactivity disorder in boys. J Child Adolesc Psychopharmacol 1995;5:215–23.

[111] Hunt R, Arnsten A, Asbell M. An open trial of guanfacine in the treatment of attention-deficit hyperactivity disorder. J Am Acad Child Adolesc Psychiatry 1995;34:50–4.

[112] Gunning B. A controlled trial of clonidine in hyperkinetic children. Thesis: Department of Child and Adolescent Psychiatry. Academic Hospital Rotterdam- Sophia Children's Hospital Rotterdam. The Netherlands. Rotterdam, The Netherlands, Department of Child and Adolescent Psychiatry. Academic Hospital Rotterdam- Sophia Children's Hospital Rotterdam, 1992.

[113] Hunt RD. Treatment effects of oral and transdermal clonidine in relation to methylphenidate: an open pilot study in ADD-H. Psychopharmacol Bull 1987;23:111–4.

[114] Hunt RD, Minderaa RB, Cohen DJ. Clonidine benefits children with attention deficit disorder and hyperactivity: report of a double-blind placebo-crossover therapeutic trial. J Am Acad Child Psychiatry 1985;24:617–29.

[115] Tourette's Syndrome Study Group. Treatment of ADHD in children with tics: a randomized controlled trial. Neurology 2002;58:527–36.

[116] Steingard R, Biederman J, Spencer T, et al. Comparison of clonidine response in the treatment of attention deficit hyperactivity disorder with and without comorbid tic disorders. J Am Acad Child Adolesc Psychiatry 1993;32:350–3.

[117] Scahill L, Chappell PB, Kim YS, et al. A placebo-controlled study of guanfacine in the treatment of children with tic disorders and attention deficit hyperactivity disorder. Am J Psychiatry 2001;158:1067–74.

[118] Taylor FB, Russo J. Comparing guanfacine and dextroamphetamine for the treatment of adult attention-deficit/hyperactivity disorder. J Clin Psychopharmacol 2001;21(2):223–8.

[119] Wilens TE, Spencer TJ. Combining methylphenidate and clonidine: a clinically sound medication option. J Am Acad Child Adolesc Psychiatry 1999;38:614–22.

[120] Biederman J, Melmed RD, Patel A, et al. A randomized, double-blind, placebo-controlled study of guanfacine extended release in children and adolescents with attention-deficit/hyperactivity disorder. Pediatrics 2008;121(1):e73–84.

[121] Faraone SV, Biederman J, Spencer TJ, et al. Comparing the efficacy of medications for ADHD using meta-analysis. MedGenMed 2006;8:4.

[122] Banaschewski T, Coghill D, Santosh P, et al. Long-acting medications for the hyperkinetic disorders. A systematic review and European treatment guideline. Eur Child Adolesc Psychiatry 2006;15:476–95.

ELSEVIER
SAUNDERS

Child Adolesc Psychiatric Clin N Am
17 (2008) 459–474

CHILD AND
ADOLESCENT
PSYCHIATRIC CLINICS
OF NORTH AMERICA

Understanding the Risk of Using Medications for Attention Deficit Hyperactivity Disorder with Respect to Physical Growth and Cardiovascular Function

Benedetto Vitiello, MD

Child and Adolescent Treatment and Preventive Intervention Research Branch,
Division of Services and Intervention Research, National Institute of Mental Health,
Room 7147, 6001 Executive Boulevard, Bethesda, MD 20892-9633, USA

The treatment of attention deficit hyperactivity disorder (ADHD) with stimulant medications dates back to the late 1930s and has been common practice for decades. Hundreds of research reports have documented the therapeutic and adverse effects of methylphenidate and amphetamines have been well characterized, and stimulants in children. Frequent and less frequent adverse effects of methylphenidate and amphetamines are characterized and a dose-effect relationship demonstrated for some of them in school-aged children and preschoolers [1,2]. Decrease in appetite, stomachache, nausea, headache, insomnia, and nervousness are frequent on starting treatment but lead to treatment discontinuation in less than 5% of school-aged children, although higher rates were observed in preschoolers (approximately 9%) and in children who had pervasive developmental disorders (approximately 18%) [1–4]. The still lively debate about certain aspects of the safety of these medications attests to the difficulty of establishing safety issues conclusively and the need to evaluate risk in the context of the evolving clinical practice.

The use of medications for the treatment of ADHD has expanded considerably over the past decade, becoming common in adolescents and adults in addition to prepubertal children [5,6]. New formulations of

The opinions and assertions contained in this report are the private views of the author and are not to be construed as official or as reflecting the views of the Department of Health and Human Services, the National Institutes of Health, or the National Institute of Mental Health.

E-mail address: bvitiell@mail.nih.gov

1056-4993/08/$ - see front matter. Published by Elsevier Inc.
doi:10.1016/j.chc.2007.11.010

stimulants have been developed to allow extended pharmacologic activity with single dosing, and a novel, nonstimulant compound, atomoxetine, was introduced in 2003. These factors have contributed to bringing new attention to short- and long-term risks for pharmacologic treatment of ADHD [7,8].

Two distinct, persisting concerns about medications approved for the treatment of ADHD relate to their impact on physical growth, with possible implications for development and adult height, and to their cardiovascular effects, with possible implications for serious cardiotoxicity. The purpose of this review is to discuss these issues critically in light of current clinical practice and the need for further research.

Stimulants and physical growth

That long-term stimulant treatment of children can decrease growth velocity has been recognized for more than 30 years [9]. Several studies conducted in the 1970s and 1980s investigated the extent, persistence, and possible mechanisms of stimulant-induced growth suppression [10–16]. It was observed that the effect on weight typically emerges in the first few months of treatment, followed by attenuation, whereas the effect on height takes at least 1 year to become detectable. From these studies, the loss of expected growth in height was estimated at approximately 1 cm per year for children treated continuously (with daily doses above 20 mg of methylphenidate for 3 years or longer). Growth rebound was reported after drug discontinuation, and interruptions of stimulant treatment (drug holidays) attenuated this effect on growth [10,12]. Furthermore, no difference in final height was found between young adults treated with methylphenidate (average daily dose of 45 mg for 6 months to 5 years) and untreated peers [13]. Almost all these children, however, had discontinued stimulant treatment before age 13, leaving open the question of whether or not continuous treatment throughout puberty may have an impact on final growth.

Consequent to this considerable body of work, recommendations for periodic monitoring of weight and height were included in treatment guidelines and drug product labeling instructions, but the effect of stimulants on growth generally had been considered minor, transient, and of negligible practical importance [17,18]. More recently, with the continuous expansion on the use of stimulant medications and the increasingly longer duration of treatment of ADHD, which now is recognized as a persistent, lifelong condition rather than a spontaneously resolving developmental phenomenon, more attention is paid to possible long-term treatment effects, including effects on physical growth. It also is postulated that growth delay may be intrinsic in the ADHD condition rather than drug induced [19], but other studies have not found evidence that unmedicated ADHD are smaller than expected [20,21].

Several recently reported long-term treatment studies have provided an opportunity to evaluate the effects of stimulants on growth in greater detail.

A dozen studies addressing this issue have been published since 2000 (Table 1) [20–33]. These studies vary considerably in sample size, design, and methodology. Although most relied on prospective, longitudinal assessments of naturalistically treated children, others were retrospective chart reviews. Some used a normal control comparison, others an unmedicated ADHD sample. Most referred to population norms using z scores (ie, deviation from the population mean measured in SD units), but some relied on percentile changes (ie, movement from one population growth trajectory to another). A systematic review of studies addressing growth during stimulant treatment was published in 2005 and identified 29 studies, 11 of which reported an attenuation of growth with chronic treatment that was estimated at approximately 1 cm per year for the first 1 to 3 years of treatment [34]. The pattern that emerges from these studies is of early weight loss in the first 3 to 4 months of treatment, more marked among the heaviest children, followed by a resumption of weight growth; slowing in height growth becomes evident after approximately 1 year of continuous treatment and persists, although attenuated, over the years.

Among these studies, the Multimodal Treatment Study of ADHD (MTA) took advantage of a large sample size of children (N = 579), homogeneous for age (7–9 years), and randomly assigned to nonpharmacologic intervention, community treatment (average methylphenidate dose 23 mg per day), combined psychosocial and medication treatment (31 mg per day), or intensive medication treatment (38 mg per day) for 14 months [27,35,36]. Treatment consisted of immediate-release methylphenidate, given 3 times a day and continued 7 days a week with no drug holidays. In these treatment groups, mean growth was 6.19 cm, 5.58 cm, 4.85 cm, and 4.25 cm, respectively, for height, with a mean estimated loss of growth of 1.23 cm per year for the group medicated most intensively. For weight, growth was 4.53 kg, 3.13 kg, 2.52 kg, and 1.64 kg, respectively, with a mean estimated loss of growth of 2.48 kg per year for the group medicated most intensively [27]. These data strongly suggest that the effect of stimulants on growth is dose dependent, as also reported by other investigators [31].

One limitation of the MTA was that several children had received stimulant treatment before entering the study. Because the effect of medication on growth is strongest in the first few months of treatment and may be followed by rebound on discontinuation, prestudy treatment can bias the estimates of treatment effect during the study. Thus, stimulant effect on growth is assessed best in treatment-naïve subjects not exposed to stimulants [34]. The MTA sample has been followed naturalistically after the end of the 14-month controlled trial. Analyses of the data from the children who were medicated consistently, never medicated, or newly medicated confirmed a growth suppression effect, which was evident especially during the first 2 years of treatment and still detectable after 3 years, when the newly medicated group had grown on average 2.0 cm and 2.7 kg less than the unmedicated group [21].

Table 1
Recently reported studies of growth during stimulant treatment

Study	N	Age (years)	Drug	Dose[a]	Duration	Design	Findings
Kramer, et al, 2000 [22]	97	4–12	MPH	10–40 mg	36 months	Retrospective	Adult height and weight not affected
Sund and Zeiner, 2002 [23]	91	3–10	MPH AMP	24 mg 12 mg	12 months	Observational	Smaller weight growth on AMP
Lisska and Rivkees, 2003 [24]	84	–	MPH	22 mg	24 months	Observational	Decrease in height z scores
Poulton and Cowell, 2003 [25]	51	3–11	MPH AMP	27 mg 14 mg	6–42 months	Observational	1 cm/y and 1.2 kg less than expected
Biederman, et al, 2003 [26]	124	6–17	Multiple	Unspecified	Unspecified	Observational	No treatment effect on growth
MTA Cooperative, 2004 [27]	579	7–10	MPH[b]	0–39 mg[c]	14 months	Randomized	1.23 cm/y and 2.48 kg/y less growth
Faraone, et al, 2005 [28]	569	6–12	AMP-XR	10–30 mg	6–30 months	Observational	Decrease in height (−0.31) and weight (−0.63) z scores
Spencer, et al, 2006 [29]	178	6–13	OROS MPH	1.2 mg/kg 43.7 mg	21 months	Observational	0.23 cm less than expected 1.23 kg less than expected; no change in mean z scores
Pliszka, et al, 2006 [30]	113 66	8.5 (mean) 9.0 (mean)	MPH AMP	34.8 mg 22.7 mg	32 months 29 months	Retrospective	No change in mean z scores
Charach, et al, 2006 [31]	79	6–12	MPH or AMP	Unspecified	60 months	Observational	Dose-dependent decrease in height and weight z scores
Zachor, et al, 2006 [32]	81	8.5 (mean)	MPH or AMP	Unspecified	36 months	Retrospective	Decrease in z scores for weight but not for height

Study	N	Age	Medication	Dose	Duration	Design	Findings
Swanson, et al, 2006 [20]	95	3–5	MPH	14.2 mg	12 months	Observational	1.4 cm/y less than expected; 1.3 kg/y less than expected; 0.30 decrease in height z; 0.53 decrease in weight z
Swanson, et al, 2007 [21][d]	320	7–10	MPH	Unspecified	36 months	Observational	Dose-related decrease in height and weight z scores; consistently medicated children were 2.3 cm shorter and 1.5 kg lighter than normal controls
Farietta-Murray, 2007 [33]	50	4–10	MPH AMP	Unspecified	24 months	Retrospective	Decrease in weight percentile only

Studies included were of at least 50 children and of at least 12-month duration.

Abbreviations: AMP, amphetamine; MPH, methylphenidate.

[a] Highest mean daily dose.

[b] A few children received dextroamphetamine or other medications.

[c] The mean daily MPH doses were 0 mg in the behavioral therapy group, 23 mg in the community control, 31 mg in the combined medication management/behavior therapy group, and 38 mg in the medication management group.

[d] Based on the MTA study sample and reporting on the 36-month naturalistic follow-up.

Although the preponderance of the evidence indicates that there is a statistically significant suppression of growth with stimulants, whether or not this effect is clinically significant is a subject of debate. A difference in height of 2 cm over a 3-year period may be considered by some of borderline practical significance, but this consideration is based on group mean differences: some children can present with larger differences, which, in the context of individual children's situations, may be important. Case reports describe particular clinical situations where growth suppression was of concern. For example, a 10-year-old boy presented with an almost complete growth arrest after being treated with methylphenidate for 15 months concurrently with corticosteroids for asthma; bone age indicated a delay of 10 months with a 7-cm loss of projected adult height [37]. No generalizations are possible from such case descriptions, except that the growth of individual patients should be monitored carefully during stimulant treatment, especially if other medications known for affecting growth are prescribed concomitantly.

An indirect concern is whether or not the effect on height is paralleled by delayed growth in organs of the body besides the skeletal system. At this time, there are no data to support this concern. Although no effect on the onset of puberty is reported, this issue has not been addressed fully.

A critical question is whether this loss of growth velocity merely is a transient delay or if final height can be affected. Prior studies indicate that rebound occurs during drug holidays (with some reports suggesting that it occurs even when treatment is continued), and that, in any case, adult height is not affected [10,12,13,38]. Not all the studies, however, have found evidence of growth rebound or confirmed the benefit of drug holidays [24,25,29]. Current evidence indicates that stimulant treatment does not, on average, influence final height, but further data from children medicated continuously for more than 3 years and during puberty seem to be needed before settling this issue. Few studies have examined bone age in the context of stimulant treatment [37]. An investigation of the dental development of children who had received methylphenidate daily, at the average 30 mg for more than 4 years, did not find evidence of delay in dental maturation [39].

Relevant to understanding the effect of stimulants on growth is the elucidation of the underlying mechanism of action. Stimulants are known for decreasing appetite in children and adults. For instance, in a randomized controlled clinical trial involving 282 children, ages 6 to 12 years, the incidence of decreased food intake after 2 weeks of treatment was greater in the osmotic-controlled release formulation (OROS) of methylphenidate (22.5%) or in immediate-release methylphenidate (18.8%) group as compared with placebo (12.0%) [40]. During the 14-month treatment in the MTA, approximately 10% of 198 treated with methylphenidate required a dose decrease because of anorexia, making this the most common reason for dose reduction in this study [36]. Similar findings emerged from a retrospective review of children treated naturalistically [32]. Children under age 6 seem even more sensitive to the anorexic effects of stimulants. In the Preschoolers with ADHD Treatment Study, approximately 40% of the children showed decrease in appetite, a rate that remained basically unchanged during the 10-months' duration of treatment, in spite of the low doses used [2,41]. It is possible, therefore, that the effect on height is caused by the reduced caloric intake during stimulant treatment [34]. The effect on weight seems limited, however, to the first few months after starting treatment.

It is hypothesized that the persistant, stimulant-induced, increase in hypothalamic dopamine may affect pituitary function, thus slowing growth [42]. Such an explanation is consistent with dopamine antagonists increasing weight and seeming to accelerate height growth [43]. Studies in the late 1970s and early 1980s examined the possible effect of stimulants on diurnal and nocturnal plasma levels of growth hormone and prolactin. Acute administration of methylphenidate increased growth hormone and decreased prolactin, but no consistent changes in the plasma levels of these hormones were detected during chronic treatment [14–16]. More recently, a transient decrease in insulin-dependent growth factor after 4 months of treatment, which, however, was not evident at months 8 and 14 assessment, was reported in a few children [44]. Despite these hypotheses, the basic mechanism through which stimulants affect growth remains unknown and deserves further investigation.

Atomoxetine and physical growth

Atomoxetine is a nonstimulant, selective noradrenergic reuptake inhibitor approved for the treatment of ADHD since 2003. Gastrointestinal adverse effects, such as appetite decrease, vomiting, gastric upset, and abdominal pain, frequently emerge early in treatment but seldom lead to drug discontinuation [45]. Acute treatment is on average accompanied by a slight decrease in weight of approximately 1 kg over a period of 2 to 3 months. Several open-label studies of atomoxetine administered for 2 years or longer have been conducted and two meta-analyses reported recently.

One meta-analysis included data from 13 studies of 6- to 7-year-old children who were treated with atomoxetine (up to a mean dosage of 1.47/kg per day). At the end at the 24-month treatment, weight was on average 2.5 kg and height on average 2.7 cm less than expected based on baseline percentile [46]. The other meta-analysis pooled data from children and adolescents ages 6 to 16 [47]. After 24 months of treatment, there was a decrease of 2.7 percentile points for weight (corresponding to a mean 0.87 kg less than expected) and a decrease of 2.2 percentile points for height (0.44 cm less than expected). These differences between observed and estimated growth in these studies were statistically significant. The slowing in growth velocity was most evident after 18 months of treatment and tended to attenuate afterwards.

The clinical significance of this effect is considered negligible at the group mean level [46,47] but may be important at the individual patient level with extended treatment beyond 2 years. The mechanism of the effect is speculated to be through a decrease in caloric intake. Caloric supplementation is suggested as a possible remedy, but its efficacy has not been tested. Because the therapeutic effect of atomoxetine requires continuous dosing, drug holidays are not an option during the academic year but may be considered for selected patients during summer vacations.

Stimulants and cardiovascular function

Stimulants are sympathomimetic agents that increase noradrenergic and dopaminergic transmission. An effect on heart rate and blood pressure can be considered an intrinsic feature of their pharmacologic activity [48]. Hypertension and tachycardia are common in case of overdosing with these compounds [49]. Several placebo-controlled studies have documented a slight, but statistically significant, increase in blood pressure and heart rate in children and adults during short-term administration of methylphenidate or amphetamine preparations [50–54]. The magnitude of the increase over placebo is approximately 2 to 6 bpm for heart rate, 2 to 4 mm Hg for systolic blood pressure, and 1 to 3 mm Hg for diastolic blood pressure. This conclusion is supported by 24-hour ambulatory recordings of blood pressure and heart rate of children medicated with stimulants, which found increases in diastolic blood pressure (75.5 mm Hg on medication versus 72.3 off medication) and heart rate (85.5 versus 79.9 bpm) [55].

Some studies, however, in spite of large sample sizes, did not find any differences in blood pressure or heart rate as compared with placebo [56,57]. In a large, open-label study involving almost 3000 children, ages 6 to 12 years, who were treated with extended release mixed amphetamine salts (up to 40 mg per day for up to 15 weeks), increase in systolic and diastolic blood pressure of less 1 mm Hg and increase in heart rate of approximately 1 bpm were detected, which were statistically significant mainly because of the large sample size but were considered without clinical relevance [58]. In this study, sustained blood pressure measurements above the 95th percentile were found in 2.5% and heart rate above 110 bpm in 3.6% of children. Although it is difficult to interpret causality in the absence of a control, as these changes might have happened regardless of treatment, these findings suggest that there are individual subjects who have clinically significant changes.

Open-label studies of children during long-term treatment indicate that these modest changes in heart rate and blood pressure tend to persist, a sign that full tolerance does not develop during chronic treatment [56,58]. Besides an increase in rhythm, no consistent ECG changes are attributed to stimulant medications. In particular, no clinically significant prolongation of the QT interval has been detected, although some studies found a statistically significant increase [53,57–59].

From a clinical point of view, two questions seem especially relevant. First, does even a slight elevation in blood pressure and heart rate increase the risk for cardiovascular pathology in the long run? The risk for cardio-vascular disease increases monotonically with increasing values of blood pressure without any specified cutoff point for no risk. Currently, there is no evidence that adults who were medicated as children are at increased risk for hypertension or cardiovascular events. This issue has not been inves-tigated fully, however, especially as stimulant treatment can start early in childhood and last for years into adulthood.

The second question relates to the debate about a possible link between stimulant treatment and sudden cardiovascular death [60,61]. In young peo-ple (first 3 decades of life), the incidence of sudden death from cardiac causes, defined as death that is instantaneous or occurs within 24 hours of an acute collapse [62], is estimated to range from 1.3 to 8.5 per 100,000 per-son-years, and a specific cardiac cause is identified in two thirds of the cases [63]. In older adults, sudden death typically occurs in the context of coro-nary atherosclerosis and is the result of ventricular fibrillation. Given the widespread use of stimulants for the treatment of ADHD in children and the increasing use in adults, it is not surprising that several cases of sudden death were reported to the Adverse Event Reporting System (AERS) of the Food and Drug Administration.

From January 1992 to February 2005, 20 cases of sudden death during treatment with amphetamine products were reported: 14 in children (under age 19) and 6 in adults; 6 of the 14 children had structural cardiovascular abnormalities or other predisposing factors for sudden death. During the same period, 18 cases of sudden death during treatment with methylpheni-date were reported: 14 in children (6 had structural cardiovascular abnor-malities) and 4 in adults [64]. The apparently similar incidence for amphetamine as for methylphenidate, despite the more common use of the latter, is intriguing, but may be due to reporting biases.

The estimated rates of sudden death based on these reports is below the background rates in the general population, but only a fraction of actual ad-verse events typically are reported to the AERS, so that accurate estimates of true incidence are not possible. Conclusions about presence or absence of a causal link cannot be drawn, therefore, from these data. Future analyses of systematically collected data from large numbers of patients in commu-nity settings treated naturalistically might be informative. Given the increas-ing use of stimulants for the treatment of ADHD in adults, it is important to investigate further possible adverse cardiovascular effects in this age group, with special attention to patients who have risks factors for heart disease, such as hypertension, atherosclerosis, smoking, or concomitant use of other drugs.

Even though a causal effect is not proved, it is plausible that stimulants, because of their sympathomimetic activity, may increase the risk for sudden cardiac death at usual therapeutic doses, especially in individuals who have predisposing factors. Therefore, the current product labeling for methylphe-nidate and amphetamine preparations informs that sudden deaths are reported during treatment with these stimulant medications at usual doses in children and adolescents who have structural cardiac abnormalities or other serious heart problems and warns that these medications generally should not be used in individuals who have known serious structural cardiac abnormalities, cardiomyopathy, or serious heart rhythm abnormalities [65].

The current practice guidelines recommend a careful medical evaluation of children before starting stimulant treatment, including physical examination and collection of personal history of structural heart or rhythm abnormalities or of cardiovascular events, such as syncope, dizziness, palpitations, or chest pain at rest or during physical exercise, and of family history of sudden cardiac or unexplained death before age 30 [61,66]. Pulse, blood pressure, and adverse events during treatment should be monitored periodically during treatment. ECG or echocardiographic examinations currently are not required for individuals who do not have known personal or family risk factors but should be conducted in selected cases.

Not uncommonly, stimulants are prescribed concomitantly with other medications. In particular, α_2-adrenergic agents, such as clonidine or guanfacine, are prescribed off-label together with stimulants to children who have ADHD [67]. After the report of four cases of sudden death in children taking methylphenidate and clonidine in the mid-1990s, concerns were raised about the safety of this combination [68]. No causal link could be established, however, and no additional evidence of possible cardiotoxicity has emerged thus far.

Atomoxetine and cardiovascular function

Atomoxetine is a selective norepinephrine reuptake inhibitor and an effect on the cardiovascular system can be expected given its pharmacologic properties. A review of five placebo-controlled clinical trials involving 612 children, adolescents, or adults treated with therapeutic doses of atomoxetine up to 10 weeks confirmed an increase 5 to 9 bpm in mean heart rate with suggestions of a dose-effect relationship [69]. Moreover, 3.6% of the children and adolescents on atomoxetine versus 0.5% of those on placebo ($P = .02$) had an increase of at least 25 bpm to a value of 110 bpm or greater. Palpitations were more common in adults but not children or adolescents on atomoxetine. Systolic blood pressure was increased in adults but not in children and adolescents, whereas an increase in diastolic blood pressure was seen in children and adolescents but not in adults. In children and adolescents, the mean change in diastolic blood pressure was 2.1 mm Hg on atomoxetine versus −0.5 on placebo ($P = .002$). These changes occurred in the first few weeks of treatment and stabilized afterwards, with no further increases during long-term treatment of 1 year and longer [69]. No evidence that atomoxetine prolongs that QT interval were found [46,69].

Forty cases of overdose on atomoxetine (up to 480 mg) in children and adolescents were reviewed: tachycardia (mean 131 $\pm$ SD 14 bpm) and hypertension up to 136/95 mm Hg occurred, but no other arrhythmias were detected [70]. Between November 2002 and February 2005, seven cases of sudden death during atomoxetine treatment were reported to the AERS, including three in children (ages 2.5–12 years) and four in adults. No evidence of causality can be derived from these cases, as there are multiple confounders and alternative explanations for these deaths other than atomoxetine [64].

Based on this information, physical examination (with heart rate and blood pressure measurements) and history taking should be part of the routine assessments before starting atomoxetine, followed by periodic checking of heart rate and blood pressure during treatment.

α_2-Agonists and cardiovascular function

Clonidine and guanfacine are marketed as antihypertensive drugs and do not have an official indication for the treatment of ADHD. They are, however, prescribed off-label alone or in combination with stimulants to children who have ADHD, especially in the presence of tic disorders or when other treatments prove insufficient [71]. Clonidine and guanfacine have prominent cardiovascular effects. They decrease blood pressure and can cause orthostatic hypotension, with dizziness, palpitations, and rapid heartbeat, when standing. Bradycardia also is a possible side effect. For these reasons, blood pressure and heart rate must be measured before and during treatment. ECG monitoring usually is not required, unless there is personal or family history of arrhythmias, cardiac malformations, or sudden unexpected death. With chronic treatment, tolerance to the hypotensive effects develops so that if the drug is discontinued abruptly, rebound hypertension can occur. Gradual tapering (decreasing the daily dose by 0.05 mg every 3 to 4 days) therefore is recommended.

Tricyclics and cardiovascular function

Although their use in children has decreased, tricyclic antidepressants still may be prescribed off-label for the treatment of ADHD in particular cases when stimulants or atomoxetine do not prove effective [71]. Tricyclics delay cardiac conduction and their use requires special attention to possible cardiotoxicity. Before starting treatment, children should receive a complete physical examination with ECG recording. Treatment should be considered only if the following limits are not exceeded on an ECG: 200 milliseconds for the PR interval, 120 milliseconds for the QRS interval, and 450 milliseconds for the corrected QT interval; and the heart rate should be regular and not higher than 100 bmp. If there is personal history of arrhythmias, dizziness, fainting, palpitation, or heart abnormalities, a more thorough evaluation by a cardiologist is appropriate. Family history of sudden, unexpected death or life-threatening arrhythmias may be reason for avoiding use of tricyclics. There are reports of sudden death in children receiving therapeutic doses of tricy-clics, even though a causal association is not demonstrated [72].

During treatment, ECG evaluation should be repeated after reaching a plasma steady state (usually after 4 days on a stable dose) and again if the dose is increased above 3 mg/kg per day. Plasma levels should be checked to make sure the subject is not a slow metabolizer. Plasma levels of imipramine and desipramine combined usually are approximately 80 to 225 ng/mL and should not exceed 300 ng/mL.

Summary

In past few years, there has been a flurry of studies investigating growth in children treated with stimulants because of ADHD. Overall, the findings confirm that stimulants cause a slowing in growth velocity for weight and height, which can persist, although attenuated, for at least to 4 years, during continuous treatment. A slight decrease in weight and height velocity also is observed during treatment with atomoxetine. The clinical and practical sig-nificance of this effect on growth is debatable, and further investigations are needed to clarify the exact mechanism of the effect and the impact on final height. From a clinical perspective, weight and height should be assessed at least semiannually in children receiving pharmacologic treatment, and the appropriateness of the treatment, or its intensity, reconsidered if there is substantial deviation from the individual child growth trajectory.

Stimulants and atomoxetine have cardiovascular effects with increase in heart rate and blood pressure. These changes usually are not clinically sig-nificant in the short term, but their possible significance for the long-term deserves further investigation. Although a causal link between therapeutic stimulant use and sudden cardiac death is not established, there are concerns that treatment may increase the risk for sudden death in patients who have structural cardiac abnormalities, so that careful pretreatment assessment and clinical screening currently is recommended.

Most important, safety considerations must be evaluated in the context of the therapeutic benefit from these medications, which is proved. Overall, when pharmacologic treatment of ADHD is prescribed correctly and mon-itored carefully, the balance between anticipated benefits and risks for harm is favorable.

References

[1] Greenhill LL, Swanson JM, Vitiello B, et al. Impairment and deportment responses to dif-ferent methylphenidate doses in children with ADHD: the MTA titration trial. J Am Acad Child Adolesc Psychiatry 2001;40:180–7.
[2] Wigal T, Greenhill LL, Chuang S, et al. Safety and tolerability of methylphenidate in pre-school children with ADHD. J Am Acad Child Adolesc Psychiatry 2006;45:1294–303.

[3] Efron D, Jarman F, Barker M. Side effects of methylphenidate and dexamphetamine in children with attention deficit hyperactivity disorder: a double-blind, crossover trial. Pediatrics 1997;100:662–6.

[4] Research Units on Pediatric Psychopharmacology (RUPP) Autism network. A randomized controlled crossover trial of methylphenidate in pervasive developmental disorders with hyperactivity. Arch Gen Psychiatry 2005;62:1266–74.

[5] Zuvekas SH, Vitiello B, Norquist NS. Recent trends in stimulant medication use among U.S. children. Am J Psychiatry 2006;163:579–85.

[6] Scheffler RM, Hinshaw SP, Modrek S, et al. The global market for ADHD medications. Health Aff 2007;26:450–7.

[7] Ross RG. Psychotic and manic-like symptoms during stimulant treatment of attention deficit hyperactivity disorder. Am J Psychiatry 2006;163:1149–52.

[8] Wilens TE, Faraone SV, Biederman J, et al. Does stimulant therapy of attention-deficit/hyperactivity disorder beget later substance abuse? A meta-analytic review of the literature. Pediatrics 2003;111:179–85.

[9] Safer DJ, Allen RP, Barr E. Depression of growth in hyperactive children with stimulant drugs. N Engl J Med 1972;287:217–20.

[10] Safer DJ, Allen RP, Barr E. Growth rebound after termination of stimulant drugs. J Pediatr 1975;86:113–6.

[11] Mattes JA, Gittelman R. Growth of hyperactive children on maintenance regimen of methylphenidate. Arch Gen Psychiatry 1983;40:317–21.

[12] Klein RG, Landa B, Mattes JA, et al. Methylphenidate and growth in hyperactive children. A controlled withdrawal study. Arch Gen Psychiatry 1988;45:1127–30.

[13] Klein RG, Mannuzza S. Hyperactive boys almost grown up. III. Methylphenidate effects on ultimate height. Arch Gen Psychiatry 1988;45:1131–4.

[14] Gualtieri CT, Hicks RE, Patrick K, et al. Growth hormone and prolactin secretion in adults and hyperactive children: relation to methylphenidate serum levels. Psychoneuroendocrinology 1981;6:331–9.

[15] Greenhill LL, Puig-Antich J, Novacenko H, et al. Prolactin, growth hormone and growth responses in boys with attention deficit disorder and hyperactivity treated with methylphenidate. J Am Acad Child Psychiatry 1984;23:58–67.

[16] Greenhill LL, Puig-Antich J, Chambers W, et al. Growth hormone, prolactin, and growth responses in hyperkinetic males treated with d-amphetamine. J Am Acad Child Psychiatry 1981;20:84–103.

[17] American Academy of Pediatrics. Clinical practice guideline: treatment of the school-aged child with attention-deficit/hyperactivity disorder. Pediatrics 2001;108:1033–44.

[18] Greenhill LL, Pliszka S, Dulcan MK, et al. Practice parameter for the use of stimulant medications in the treatment of children, adolescents, and adults. J Am Acad Child Adolesc Psychiatry 2002;41:26S–49S.

[19] Spencer T, Biederman J, Harding M, et al. Growth deficits in ADHD children revisited: evidence for disorder-associated growth delays? J Am Acad Child Adolesc Psychiatry 1996;35:1460–9.

[20] Swanson J, Greenhill L, Wigal T, et al. Stimulant-related reductions of growth rates in the PATS. J Am Acad Child Adolesc Psychiatry 2006;45:1304–13.

[21] Swanson JM, Elliott GR, Greenhill LL, et al. Effects of stimulant medication on growth rates across 3 years in the MTA follow-up. J Am Acad Child Adolesc Psychiatry 2007;46:1014–26.

[22] Kramer JR, Loney J, Ponto LB, et al. Predictors of adult height and weight in boys treated with methylphenidate for childhood behavior problems. J Am Acad Child Adolesc Psychiatry 2000;39:517–24.

[23] Sund AN, Zeiner P. Does extended medication with amphetamine or methylphenidate reduce growth in hyperactive children? Nord J Psychiatry 2002;56:53–7.

[24] Lisska MC, Rivkees SA. Daily methylphenidate use slows the growth of children: a community based study. J Pediatr Endocrinol Metab 2005;16:711–8.

[25] Poulton A, Cowell CT. Slowing of growth in height and weight on stimulants: a characteristic pattern. J Paediatr Child Health 2003;39:180–5.

[26] Biederman J, Faraone SV, Monuteaux MC, et al. Growth deficits and attention-deficit/ hyperactivity disorder revisited: impact of gender, development, and treatment. Pediatrics 2003;111:1010–6.

[27] MTA Cooperative Group. National institute of mental health multimodal treatment study of ADHD follow-up: changes in effectiveness and growth after the end of treatment. Pediatrics 2004;113:762–9.

[28] Faraone SV, Biederman J, Monuteaux M, et al. Long-term effects of extended-release mixed amphetamine salts treatment of attention-deficit/hyperactivity disorder on growth. J Child Adolesc Psychopharmacol 2005;15:191–202.

[29] Spencer TJ, Faraone SV, Biederman J, et al. Does prolonged therapy with a long-acting stimulant suppress growth in children with ADHD? J Am Acad Child Adolesc Psychiatry 2006; 45:527–37.

[30] Pliszka SR, Matthews TL, Braslow KJ, et al. Comparative effects of methylphenidate and mixed salts amphetamine on height and weight in children with attention-deficit/hyperactivity disorder. J Am Acad Child Adolesc Psychiatry 2006;45:520–6.

[31] Charach A, Figueroa M, Chen S, et al. Stimulant treatment over 5 years: effect on growth. J Am Acad Child Adolesc Psychiatry 2006;45:415–21.

[32] Zachor DA, Roberts AW, Hodgens JB, et al. Effects of long-term psychostimulant medication on growth of children wth ADHD. Res Dev Disabil 2006;27:162–74.

[33] Farietta-Murray T, Castellanos D, Katsikas S. Effects of stimulants on Hispanic boys' height and weight. J Am Acad Child Adolesc Psychiatry 2007;46:150–1.

[34] Poulton A. Growth on stimulant medication; clarifying the confusion: a review. Arch Dis Child 2005;90:801–6.

[35] MTA Cooperative Group. A 14-Month randomized clinical trial of treatment strategies for attention-deficit/hyperactivity disorder (ADHD). Arch Gen Psychiatry 1999;56:1073–86.

[36] Vitiello B, Severe JB, Greenhill LL, et al. Methylphenidate dosage for children with ADHD over time under controlled conditions: lessons from the MTA. J Am Acad Child Adolesc Psychiatry 2001;40:188–96.

[37] Holtkamp K, Peters-Wallraf B, Wueller S, et al. Methyphenidate-related growth impairment. J Child Adolesc Psychopharmacol 2002;12:55–61.

[38] Satterfield JH, Cantwell DP, Schell A, et al. Growth of hyperactive children with methylphenidate. Arch Gen Psychiatry 1979;36:212–7.

[39] Batterson KD, Southard KA, Dawson DV, et al. The effect of chronic methylphenidate administration on tooth maturation in a sample of Caucasian children. Pediatr Dent 2005;27: 292–7.

[40] Wolraich ML, Greenhill LL, Pelham W, et al. Randomized, controlled trial of OROS methylphenidate once a day in children with attention-deficit/hyperactivity disorder. Pediatrics 2001;108:883–92.

[41] Vitiello B, Abikoff HB, Chuang SZ, et al. Effectiveness of methylphenidate in the 10-month continuation phase of the Preschoolers with ADHD Treatment Study (PATS). J Child Adolesc Psychopharmacol 2007;17:593–603.

[42] Bosse R, Fumagalli F, Jaber M, et al. Anterior pituitary hypoplasia and dwarfism in mice lacking the dopamine transporter. Neuron 1997;19:127–38.

[43] Dunbar F, Kusumakar V, Daneman D, et al. Growth and sexual maturation during long-term treatment with risperidone. Am J Psychiatry 2004;161:918–20.

[44] Bereket A, Turan S, Karaman MG, et al. Height, weight, IGF-1, IGFBP-3 and thyroid functions in prepubertal children with attention deficit hyperactivity disorder: effect of methylphenidate. Horm Res 2005;63:159–64.

[45] Cheng JY, Chen RY, Ko JS, et al. Efficacy and safety of atomoxetine for attention-deficit hyperactivity disorder in children and adolescents—meta-analysis and meta-regression analysis. Psychopharmacol 2007;194:197–209.

[46] Kratochvil CJ, Wilens TE, Greenhill LL, et al. Effects of long-term atomoxetine treatment for young children with attention-deficit/hyperactivity disorder. J Am Acad Child Adolesc Psychiatry 2006;45:919–27.

[47] Spencer TJ, Newcorn JH, Kratochvil CJ, et al. Effects of atomoxetine on growth after 2-year treatment among pediatric patients with attention-deficit/hyperactivity disorder. Pediatrics 2005;116:e74–80.

[48] Volkow ND, Wang GJ, Fowler J, et al. Cardiovascular effects of methylpenidate in humans are associated with increases of dopamine in brain and of epinephrine in plasma. Psychopharmacol 2003;166:264–70.

[49] Klein-Schwartz W. Abuse and toxicity of methylphenidate. Curr Opin Pediatr 2002;14: 219–23.

[50] Findling RL, Short EJ, Manos MJ. Short-term cardiovascular effects of methylphenidate and Adderall. J Am Acad Child Adolesc Psychiatry 2001;40:525–9.

[51] Wilens T, Biederman J, Lerner M. Effects of once-daily osmotic-release methylphenidate on blood pressure and hear rate in children with attention-deficit/hyperactivity disorder. J Clin Psychopharmacol 2004;24:36–41.

[52] Wilens T, Spencer T, Biederman J. Short- and long-term cardiovascular effects of mixed amphetamine salts extended-release in adolescents with ADHD. CNS Spectr 2005;10: 22–30.

[53] Biederman J, Mick E, Surman C, et al. A randomized, placebo-controlled trial of OROS methylphenidate in adults with attention-deficit/hyperactivity disorder. Biol Psychiatry 2006;59:829–35.

[54] Wilens TE, Hammerness PG, Biederman J, et al. Blood pressure changes associated with medication treatment of adults with attention-deficit/hyperactivity disorder. J Clin Psychiatry 2005;66:253–9.

[55] Samuels JA, Franco K, Wan F, et al. Effect of stimulants on 24-h ambulatory blood pressure in children with ADHD: a double-blind, randomized, cross over trial. Pediatr Nephrol 2006; 21:92–5.

[56] Findling RL, Biederman J, Wilens TE, et al. Short- and long-term cardiovascular effects of mixed amphetamine salts extended release in children. J Pediatr 2005;57:147–54.

[57] Spencer T, Biederman J, Wilens T, et al. A large, double-blind, randomized clincial trial of methylphenidate in the treatment of adults with ADHD. Biol Psychiatry 2005;57:456–63.

[58] Donner R, Michaels MA, Ambrosini PJ. Cardiovascular effects of mixed amphetamine salts extended release in the treatment of school-aged children with attention-deficit/hyperactivity disorder. Biol Psychiatry 2007;61:706–12.

[59] Weisler RH, Biederman J, Spencer TJ, et al. Long-term cardiovascular effects of mixed amphetamine salts extended release in adults with ADHD. CNS Spectr 2005;10(S20): 35–43.

[60] Nissen SE. ADHD drugs and cardiovascular risk. N Engl J Med 2006;354:1445–8.

[61] Wilens TE, Prince JB, Spencer TJ, et al. Stimulants and sudden death: what is a physician to do? Pediatrics 2006;118:1215–9.

[62] Roberts WC. Sudden cardiac death: definitions and causes. Am J Cardiology 1986;57:1410–13.

[63] Liberthson RR. Sudden death from cardiac causes in children and young adults. N Engl J Med 1996;334:1039–44.

[64] Villalba L, Racoosin J. Postmarketing safety review of sudden death during treatment with drugs used to treat ADHD. Food and Drug Administration 2006. Available at: http://www.fda.gov/ohrms/dockets/ac/06/briefing/2006-4210b_07_01_safetyreview.pdf. Accessed September 5, 2007.

[65] Mc Neil Pharmaceuticals. Product label for concerta. 2007. Available at: http://www.fda.gov/cder/foi/label/2007/021121s014lbl.pdf. Accessed September 5, 2007.

[66] Gutgesell H, Atkins D, Barst R, et al. AHA scientific statement: cardiovascular monitoring of children and adolescents receiving psychotropic drugs. J Am Acad Child Adolesc Psychiatry 1999;38:1047–50.

[67] Wilens T, Spencer TJ. Combining methylphenidate and clonidine: a clinically sound medication option. J Am Acad Child Adolesc Psychiatry 1999;38:614–6.

[68] Swanson J, Flockhart D, Udrea D, et al. Clonidine in the treatment of ADHD: questions about safety and efficacy. J Child Adolesc Psychopharmacol 1995;5:301–4.

[69] Wernicke JF, Faries D, Girod D, et al. Cardiovascular effects of atomoxetine in children, adolescents, and adults. Drug Saf 2003;26:729–40.

[70] Spiller HA, Lintner CP, Winter ML. Atomoxetine ingestions in children: a report from poison centers. Ann Pharmacother 2005;39:1045–8.

[71] Pliszka SR, Crimson ML, Hughes CW, et al. The Texas children's medication algorithm project: revision of the algorithm for pharmacotherapy of attention-deficit/hyperactivity disorder. J Am Acad Child Adolesc Psychiatry 2006;45:642–57.

[72] Biederman J, Thisted RA, Greenhill LL, et al. Estimation of the association between desipramine and the risk for sudden death in 5 to 14 year old children. J Clin Psychiatry 1995;56: 87–93.

ELSEVIER
SAUNDERS

Child Adolesc Psychiatric Clin N Am
17 (2008) 475–490

CHILD AND
ADOLESCENT
PSYCHIATRIC CLINICS
OF NORTH AMERICA

The Pharmacogenomic Era: Promise for Personalizing Attention Deficit Hyperactivity Disorder Therapy

Mark A. Stein, PhD[a],*, James J. McGough, MD[b,c]

[a]Department of Psychiatry, Institute for Juvenile Research, University of Illinois at Chicago, (MC 747), 1747 W. Roosevelt Road, Chicago, IL 60608, USA
[b]Division of Child and Adolescent Psychiatry, UCLA Semel Institute for Neuroscience and Human Behavior, 760 Westwood Plaza, C8-183 Semel Institute, Los Angeles, CA 90095, USA
[c]UCLA Child and Adolescent Psychopharmacology Program and ADHD Clinic, 300 UCLA Medical Plaza, Suite 1414, Los Angeles, CA 90095, USA

Attention deficit hyperactivity disorder (ADHD) is a common and treatable behavioral syndrome that typically emerges during childhood or adolescence and often persists into adulthood. The number of stimulant and nonstimulant medication options is increasing for ADHD, with numerous new compounds in development [1]. In acute treatment studies, stimulant medications generally show large effect sizes on ADHD symptom reduction relative to placebo, with slightly smaller effect sizes in adult studies [2]. Surprisingly, only few children and adolescents who have ADHD remain on medication consistently [3], despite persistence of symptoms and impairments. Even among individuals who experience a response, marked variability is seen in optimal dosage, duration of effect, and tolerability. Moreover, despite acute symptom reduction from ADHD medications, little evidence of long-term response and improvement in functioning exists among children who underwent treatment [4,5]. Furthermore, few reliable predictors of medication response exist. Without these data, treatment is often

Dr. Stein received support for this manuscript from the National Institute of Mental Health Grant No. MH70564.

Dr. Stein has received research support from McNeil, Novartis, Eli Lilly and Company, Shire, Cortex Pharmaceuticals, and Pfizer and serves as a consultant for Novartis. Dr. McGough has received research support from and serves as a consultant to Eli Lilly and Company, Janssen, Novartis, and Shire.

* Corresponding author. 1747 West Roosevelt Road, Room 155, Chicago, IL 60008.

E-mail address: mstein@uic.edu (M.A. Stein).

determined empirically in clinical practice through a gradual titration of different dosages and trial-and-error approach to different medications.

ADHD is a highly heritable disorder [6]. The search for candidate genes associated with ADHD has been largely driven by the understanding that medications for the disorder have drug targets in the catecholamine system [7]. Conversely, variability in individual drug response is probably related to genetic factors. Spurred by completion of the human genome project [8], considerable interest has been shown in translating molecular genetics research into meaningful clinical applications. Emerging findings in ADHD pharmacogenetics and pharmacogenomics underlie attempts to apply molecular genetics findings to optimize individual patient therapies. Two prior reviews summarized findings in ADHD pharmacogenetics [9,10]. This article reviews definitions, summarizes and updates research advances, makes recommendations for future investigations, and discusses the potential clinical implications of pharmacogenetics and pharmacogenomics in managing ADHD.

Pharmacogenetics and pharmacogenomics

Pharmacogenetics is the study of genetic variability in medication response [11]. Pharmacogenetics encompasses how genetic variation influences both pharmacokinetics, particularly drug metabolism, and pharmacodynamics, in terms of symptom response and side effect profiles. Pharmacogenetics had its beginnings in the 1950s when clinicians noted increased patterns of adverse reactions within certain families and ethnic groups. In contrast to pharmacogenetics, *pharmacogenomics* is a more recent term, which broadly encompasses efforts to use the human genome to better understand and develop pharmacologic treatments [12]. Pharmacogenomics refers more specifically to the study of variations in genes and gene products and their relationship to medication response [13]. Based on advances in molecular biology, such as the advent of economical, high-throughput gene sequencing and genotyping, and the mapping of the human genome, pharmacogenetic and pharmacogenomic studies have the potential to inform individualized treatment decisions in medicine and subsequently improve long-term patient outcomes [14]. The promise of ADHD pharmacogenetics is far-reaching and includes the potential to develop individualized medication regimens that improve symptom response, decrease risk for side effects, improve long-term tolerability, and thus contribute to long-term treatment compliance and improved general effectiveness.

Obvious candidates for pharmacogenomic investigations include polymorphic drug-metabolizing enzymes, drug transporters, and targets that affect disease and drug-related pathways [15]. The dramatic and rapid effects of stimulant medications in managing ADHD symptoms suggest several strong candidates for pharmacogenetic analysis. Numerous candidate gene studies have examined the relationships between polymorphisms in the dopaminergic system and ADHD susceptibility, although only a small percentage of the variance in ADHD susceptibility can be attributed to any one gene [7]. Genome-wide linkage and association studies, including haplotype mapping, also have potential relevance to ADHD pharmacogenomics [16]. With increased identification of single nucleotide polymorphisms (SNPs), SNP tagging of common haplotypes can be economically used to identify regions of interest that better represent common genetic variation in association studies with drug response [17].

Candidate genes associated with increased risk for ADHD based on pooled odds ratios across three or more studies are the dopamine receptors (*DRD4* and *DRD5*), dopamine transporter (*DAT1*), dopa-β-hydroxylase (*DBH*), serotonin receptor (*HTR1B*), serotonin transporter (*5-HTT*), and synaptosomal-associated protein (*SNAP-25*) [7]. Other genes of potential interest in pharmacogenetic studies of ADHD include catechol-O-methyltransferase (*COMT*), and the adrenergic α_2-receptor (*ADRA2A*). In each of these genes, deep resequencing and association analysis has not been reported.

Pharmacogenetic research studies

Although knowledge about the presumed mechanisms of action of ADHD medications initially informed searches for polymorphisms related to increased risk for the disorder, these same polymorphisms are logical candidates to predict medication outcomes [9]. Several preliminary studies suggest that candidate genes involved in catecholamine pathways (ie, genes related to dopamine or norepinephrine) influence individual responses to ADHD treatments (Table 1). However, results from several of these reports are contradictory and the nature, magnitude, and direction of purported genetic effects remain unclear. Moreover, most studies examined predictors of response to methylphenidate, whereas little attention was given to other agents. Nonetheless, this seminal research suggests that genetic variability contributes to treatment response variability in individual patients and provides a foundation for definitive investigations in larger trials.

Dopamine transporter

Several reasons support the choice of *DAT1* as a candidate gene for ADHD treatment response. An association between ADHD and the 10-repeat (480-base-pair) allele of a variable number tandem repeat (VNTR) in the 3'-untranslated region of *DAT1* was initially described in 1995 [18] and replicated in multiple, but not all, follow-up reports [7]. Methylphenidate, and to some extent amphetamine, specifically targets and blocks the dopamine transporter [19–21]. Numerous neuroimaging studies reveal that ADHD patients express increased dopamine transporter densities in striatal regions [22], and that individuals with the 10-repeat allele exhibit approximately 50% greater densities than other genotypes [23]. This suggests that ADHD medications which block the dopamine transporter densities might

Table 1
Pharmacogenetic studies of methylphenidate in attention deficit hyperactivity disorder

Gene	Study	Sample size	Study location	Design	Outcome
Dopamine transporter (DAT1)	Winsberg and Comings [23]	30	New York	Prospective, open-label	Decreased response with homozygous 10-repeat
	Roman, et al [24]	50	Brazil	Prospective, open-label	Decreased response with homozygous 10-repeat
	Kirley, et al [26]	119	Ireland	Retrospective report	Increased response with number of 10-repeat
	Hamarman, et al [37]	45	New York	Prospective, open-label	No effect
	Cheon, et al [25]	11	Korea	Prospective, open-label with SPECT imaging	Decreased response with homozygous 10-repeat
	Stein, et al [27]	47	Washington, DC	Prospective, double-blind, placebo-controlled, dose-response	Different dose-response curves by DAT1 genotype, decreased response with homozygous nine-repeat
	Joober, et al [28]	159	Montreal	Prospective, double-blind, placebo-controlled	Worsening with homozygous nine-repeat on parent ratings
	Van der Meulen, et al [30]	82	Netherlands	Retrospective report	No effect
	Langley, et al [31]	236	Wales	Retrospective report	No effect
	McGough, et al [33]	81 (preschoolers)	United States (six sites)	Prospective, double-blind, placebo-controlled	No effect on primary outcome composite measure
	Mick, et al [34]	66 (adults)	Boston	Prospective study of methylphenidate arm	No effect
	Zeni, et al [32]	111	Brazil	Prospective, open-label	No effect

Gene/protein	Study	N	Location	Study design	Result
Dopamine receptor (DRD2)	Winsberg and Comings [23]	30	New York	Prospective, open-label	No effect
Dopamine receptor (DRD4)	Winsberg and Comings [23]	30	New York	Prospective, open-label	No effect
	Hamarman, et al [37]	45	New York	Prospective, open-label	Higher doses for normalization needed for seven-repeat
	McGough, et al [33]	81	United States (six sites)	Prospective, double-blind, placebo-controlled	No effect on symptoms; increased picking, irritability, social withdrawal
	Cheon, et al [38]	83	Korea	Prospective, open-label	Decreased response with seven-repeat allele
Synaptosomal-associated protein (SNAP-25)	Zeni, et al [32]	111	Brazil	Prospective, open-label	No effect
	McGough, et al [33]	81	United States (six sites)	Prospective, double-blind, placebo-controlled	Increased irritability and abnormal movements
Norepinephrine transporter protein 1 (NET)	Yang, et al [44]	45	China	Prospective, open-label	Decreased response for homozygous A-allele
Adrenergic α2A receptor (ADRA2A)	Polanczyk, et al [45]	106	Brazil	Prospective, open-label	Improved response on Inattention symptoms with G-allele
Serotonin receptors (HTR1B, HTR2A)	Zeni, et al [32]	111	Brazil	Prospective, open-label	No effect
Serotonin transporter (5-HTT)	Zeni, et al [32]	111	Brazil	Prospective, open-label	No effect

Abbreviations: ADHD, attention deficit hyperactivity disorder; SPECT, single-photon emission computed tomography.

serve to attenuate the effects of underlying brain pathophysiology. Similarly, functional polymorphisms in *DAT1* might influence response to ADHD medications.

The first pharmacogenetic study of ADHD examined the ability of catecholamine-related genes to predict response to methylphenidate [24]. This report found a significant difference in response rate among 30 stimulant-naïve, African-American youths based on *DAT1* genotype. Specifically, 86% of nonresponders were homozygous for the 10-repeat allele compared with 31% of responders (N = 16; 31%) (χ^2 $_{(1)}$ = 6.9; P = .008). Two subsequent studies reported a similar relationship between *DAT1* genotypes and symptom response. The first examined symptom reductions in 50 European-Brazilian men who had ADHD after open titration with methylphenidate up to 0.7 mg/kg per day [24]. Response was defined as a 50% or greater reduction in baseline ADHD ratings, and individuals who did not meet this threshold were more likely to be homozygous for the 10-repeat allele (Fisher's exact test; one-tailed P = .04). A second study that assessed dopamine transporter binding in addition to ADHD symptom reduction in 11 Korean individuals found that only 27% of subjects homozygous for the 10-repeat allele met response criteria compared with 100% of subjects who did not have this genotype (χ^2 $_{(1)}$ = 5.2; P = .06) [25].

In contrast, one retrospective and three prospective, placebo-controlled studies reported improved response to methylphenidate in youths who had ADHD who were homozygous or heterozygous for the 10-repeat polymorphism. One analysis based on parental retrospective report in 119 Irish children found that individuals who had one or two copies of the 10-repeat allele were more likely to have experienced improvement, and a linear relationship existed between the number of 10-repeats and degree of improvement [26]. Similarly, the presence of one or two 10-repeat alleles was associated with higher rates of symptom reduction and reduced impairment in 47 children and adolescents treated with 18 mg, 36 mg, and 54 mg of osmotic release oral system methylphenidate [27]. Individuals homozygous for the less-common 9-repeat allele showed a nonlinear dose–response curve, experienced more stimulant-related side effects, and remained more impaired during treatment.

Similar findings were reported for the 9/9 genotype group in a double-blind, placebo-controlled trial of 159 children who had ADHD conducted in Montreal [28]. Although children who had either the 9/10 or 10/10 genotypes showed a significant positive response to 10 mg of methylphenidate, the 9/9 genotype group displayed a negative response on parent symptom ratings only (effect size = −0.43). The effect of *DAT1* genotype on response was not found on teacher ratings.

In one of the few studies not conducted with methylphenidate, Lott and colleagues [29] reported that college student volunteers with the 9/9 genotype were less able to "feel" amphetamine effects relative to other genotype groups. However, this sample consisted of college student volunteers who did not have ADHD. These recent studies suggest a differential effect of stimulants on individuals homozygous for the 9-repeat genotypes relative to those containing the 10-repeat.

However, several uncontrolled studies found no association between *DAT1* and methylphenidate response, including a sample of 82 Dutch children treated prospectively with less than 0.6 mg/kg per day [30] and a retrospective analysis of 186 youth who had ADHD (dose not specified) in the United Kingdom [31]. In addition, an attempt to replicate previous findings in Brazilian youth [25] examined response rates during open-label treatment in 111 subjects and detected no association between *DAT1* genotype and outcomes [32].

In a study of 81 preschoolers who had ADHD treated with methylphenidate, no genotype effects of *DAT1* were seen on a composite measure based on parent and teacher symptom ratings [33], However, on parent ratings of ADHD symptoms, a negative effect size (-0.58) was seen for the homozygous nine-repeat genotype. The difference between parent and teacher ratings and pharmacogenetic effects of *DAT1* is similar to that reported by Joober and colleagues [28].

Recently, the first pharmacogenetic study of adults who had ADHD reported no relationship between *DAT1* genotype and response in 66 subjects titrated to a maximum methylphenidate dose of 1.3 mg/kg per day [34]. However, the sample included only three individuals who had the 9/9 genotype, and therefore had limited statistical power to detect an effect for this genotype group.

Dopamine receptor

The dopamine receptor DRD4 is a presumed target of postsynaptic catecholaminergic activity and a likely candidate for predicting variability in medication response. The association of the seven-repeat (48-base-pair) VNTR polymorphism in the coding region of DRD4 with ADHD is one of the most replicated findings in psychiatric genetics, yielding odds ratios ranging from 1.4 to 1.9 [7]. In vitro studies further indicate that the seven-repeat allelic variant is functionally less responsive to dopamine [35,36]. Consistent with this idea, one study showed that of 45 patients, those who had at least one copy of the seven-repeat allele required higher doses of methylphenidate for optimal symptom reduction [37]. Conversely, in a separate report on 83 Korean children, subjects who were homozygous for the four-repeat polymorphism were much more likely to exhibit positive responses on parent and teacher behavioral ratings than those who had other genotypes [38]. Other studies found no relationship between DRD4 genotype and ADHD symptom change [24,30,32,33].

The Preschool ADHD Treatment Study (PATS) was notable in that it not only focused on symptom reduction but also examined the potential role of genotype in predicting side effects [33]. PATS participants homozygous for the four-repeat allele were three times more likely to develop abnormal picking behaviors with methylphenidate treatment, whereas those who had one or two copies of the seven-repeat allele were more than four times as likely to exhibit social withdrawal with increasing dose. A second study found no association between genotype and side effects, particularly appetite loss and sleep difficulties [31].

One of the few studies to examine pharmacogenetic predictors of response to ADHD treatments other than methylphenidate found that children who had at least one copy of the DRD4 four-repeat allele showed a trend toward improved response on atomoxetine [39]. Response to methylphenidate, in contrast, was unrelated to DRD4 genotype. Furthermore, improvement on the hyperactivity subscale of the ADHD Rating Scale was maximized with the absence of any seven-repeat variant.

Synaptosomal-associated protein

A relatively unstudied gene with potential effects on ADHD medication response is SNAP-25, a neuron-specific protein implicated in exocytotic catecholamine release. Several studies of SNAP-25 have shown small but significant increased ADHD risk associated with two SNPs (T1069C and T1065G) separated by four base pairs at the 3' end of the gene [7]. In the coloboma mouse, chromosome deletion of SNAP-25 produces hyperactive symptoms that are relieved by amphetamine but not methylphenidate [40]. This finding is consistent with presumed differences in the mechanisms of action for these compounds, in which amphetamine but not methylphenidate compensates for reduced exocytotic catecholamine release through reversing the catecholamine diffusion gradient across the transporter.

Among preschool children who had ADHD treated with methylphenidate, those homozygous for the T allele at 1065 showed moderately increased improvements, whereas those who were homozygous for T at 1069 exhibited poorer medication response [32]. Children who were homozygous for the less-common G allele at 1065 were two to three times more likely to develop sleep difficulties and irritability than those who had at least one copy of the T allele. Additionally, those who were homozygous for the less-common C allele at 1069 were two to four times more likely to develop tics and other abnormal movements.

Norepinephrine transporter protein 1 and adrenergic α2A receptor

In addition to their effects on the dopamine system, stimulants also block reuptake at norepinephrine transporters and indirectly act to increase norepinephrine concentrations at adrenergic alpha receptors. Genes for the norepinephrine transporter (NET) and ADRA2A are therefore also likely candidates to assess genetic contributions to variability in ADHD treatment response. Although not confirmed in meta-analysis, polymorphisms at two SNPs in NET have been associated with ADHD [41]. An association between ADRA2A and ADHD was also shown [42]. NET blockade is also the presumed mechanism of activity for the nonstimulant ADHD medication atomoxetine [43].

One study evaluated the relationship between the G1278A polymorphism at NET and methylphenidate in 45 Han Chinese youth who had ADHD and found that individuals homozygous for the less-common A/A genotype had decreased symptom reductions compared with the G/A or AA groups [44]. The authors noted that, because the G1278A allele has no known functional activity, the allele might be in linkage disequilibrium with another allele responsible for outcome differences.

Potential effects for polymorphisms at the noradrenergic receptor ADRA2A were assessed in 104 children and adolescents after 1 and 3 months of methylphenidate treatment [45]. After post hoc secondary analyses, the investigators reported an interaction between the C1291G polymorphism and improvement over time that explained 30% of the variance in the inattentive score of the Swanson, Nolan, and Pelham (SNAP-IV) Rating Scale. Subjects who had at least one copy of the less-common G allele showed improved responses in the inattentive domain ($F_{1,104} = 8.5$; $P < .004$). No effect on overall SNAP-IV ratings or hyperactive–impulsive scores was seen, nor any direct effect of genotype on response.

Metabolic pathways and pharmacokinetics

ADHD pharmacogenetic studies have principally examined the potential effects of genetic variability on drug targets (ie, transporters and receptors) [9,10]. Little attention has been devoted to the potential effects of genetic variability on drug metabolism and pharmacokinetics, although these lines of inquiry frequently provide the basis for pharmacogenetic investigations [14]. This fact may be because although methylphenidate is specific in terms of its site of action, its metabolic pathways are poorly understood. d,l-Methylphenidate is believed to undergo esterification in the bloodstream through enzymatic activity of carboxylesterase to d,l-ritalinic acid and l-ethylphenidate. One recent report showed inhibition of this metabolic pathway with alcohol ingestion and also identified one subject as a methylphenidate poor–metabolizer associated with a polymorphism at the carboxylesterase-1 gene [46]. Further study and replication are required to see if this finding underlies the pharmacokinetic variability of methylphenidate generally seen in clinical practice.

Unlike the metabolic products of methylphenidate that are renally excreted, amphetamine undergoes metabolism through hepatic cytochrome P450 (CYP) isozymes. In mammals, amphetamine is metabolized along two major pathways that are differentially used by various species [47]. In the first pathway, hydroxylation of amphetamine by way of cytochrome P450 2D6 (CYP2D6) yields p-hydroxy amphetamine. Many psychotropic medications are metabolized by CYP2D6, although it is believed to play a minor role for amphetamine [48]. However, up to 20% of Caucasians and varying percentages of other racial groups are poor metabolizers because of polymorphisms at CYP2D6, which can have implications for individual patients [49]. In the second pathway amphetamine is presumably deaminated via CYP3A4 and excreted as inactive benzoic acid. The CYP3A4 amphetamine pathway is dominant in humans.

In a study of an extended-release preparation of mixed amphetamine salts, mean drug plasma concentrations after acute dosing were 25% higher in African American children [50,51]. Previous studies have noted ethnic differences in CYP3A4-mediated drug metabolism, with Caucasian subjects showing the highest levels of activity [52]. One allelic variant is heterozygous in 64% of African Americans and has been shown to have decreased metabolic activity [52]. Although racial differences in amphetamine pharmacokinetics have not been otherwise examined and a definitive association between amphetamine metabolism and polymorphisms at CYP3A4 has not been shown, these findings represent a unique lead for further examination of the potential role of genetic variability in explaining the pharmacokinetic variability of amphetamines used to treat ADHD.

Atomoxetine, a currently approved nonstimulant medication for ADHD, is metabolized by the CYP2D6 isozyme system. Drug development trials for atomoxetine were notable in that subjects' CYP2D6 status influenced dosing titration algorithms and subsequently derived approved dosing limits. One recent meta-analysis pooled outcome data from several atomoxetine clinical trials [53]. Subjects who were poor metabolizers displayed greater symptom improvement than extensive metabolizers, most likely because of higher plasma drug concentration levels, and were more likely to remain in therapy. Higher rates of appetite decrease and insomnia were reported more frequently in poor metabolizers, who also exhibited greater increases in medication-related pulse and blood pressure changes.

Genomewide investigations

Candidate gene studies presume some knowledge of the biologic system under investigation and require specific hypotheses on putative effects of particular polymorphisms. In contrast, genomewide investigations require no a priori hypotheses related to specific genes but scan the entire genome in an attempt to identify areas harboring genes that contribute some effect on outcome. Several genomewide scans have identified regions linked with ADHD risk [7,54], including fine mapping by one group to DAT1 [55]. Genomewide approaches also have potential use in pharmacogenetic investigations. One study used quantitative trait analysis in a genomewide scan to assess for linkage with methylphenidate response [56]. A linkage peak of moderate significance was identified on chromosome 7, with additional peaks on chromosomes 3, 5, and 9. Further study, including genomewide association with high-density SNP chips, is necessary to identify the specific genes that influence medication response.

Research challenges

Preliminary evidence suggests that genetic variability plays some role in predicting treatment response, but that results differ depending on whether parents or teachers are informants. Current studies are also constrained by the type of outcome measures used. Many studies rely on simple dichotomous outcomes, such as responder versus nonresponder, which have limited power to detect effects compared with analyses of quantitative measures. Correlations between multiple outcome measures in the same subjects are also known to be fairly weak, raising the question as to which outcome measure best defines positive response [57]. Future pharmacogenetic studies would benefit from consensus on the optimal measures to assess outcome. These measures remain uncertain, particularly regarding symptom reduction, the relative contributions of direct genetic effects and effects resulting from medication dose and formulation, and individual patient variables, including diet and gut motility.

Another contributor to differences in study findings is that pharmacogenetic effects may vary among ethnic groups. This finding implies the variants being studied may only be in linkage disequilibrium with other variants.

Most published ADHD pharmacogenetic studies examine response to methylphenidate. Although this is an obvious choice given the known pathophysiology of DAT1, its association with ADHD, and its serving as a specific target for stimulant action, results from preliminary reports have been inconsistent and contradictory. Some of these discrepant findings might be caused by methodological issues, because more consistent findings seem to be emerging from placebo-controlled, prospective studies. In addition to small sample sizes, other limitations of most existing trials include openlabel or retrospective assessment and medication doses that are not specified or considerably lower than used in community practice for optimal benefit [9]. Because the effects of methylphenidate on ADHD symptoms often follow a linear dose–response curve [27], these lower doses may bias against finding significant treatment effects when a less-robust dose is used.

A critical methodological issue that remains unaddressed is the proper approach to defining genotypes for analysis. To minimize the potential for spurious findings and increased type I errors, investigators must limit analysis to minimal genotype combinations. For some genes, the risk polymorphisms for ADHD are the less-common variants (eg, the seven-repeat allele of DRD4), whereas for others, such as DAT1, the more-common variant is associated with the disorder. For DAT1, the 10/10 and 10/9 genotypes are most common. Earlier studies of DAT1 combined these two common genotypes [23–25], which assumed a dominant effect of either the 9- or 10-repeat allele, but failed to test for a recessive effect of the 9/9 genotype. Alternative grouping of genotypes based on the presence of one or more 9-repeat allele has led to different results. Future candidate gene studies would benefit from consensus on optimal strategies to define genotype groupings. Without previous evidence of dominance of one allele, genotypes should not be lumped together. Statistical power is a combination of sample and effect sizes. Dominance (or lack thereof) may differ between association with origin of disorder and response to treatment.

At a recent meeting of the ADHD Molecular Genetics Network in Brussels, Belgium, the Pharmacogenetics Working Group proposed several principals to promote research in future ADHD pharmacogenetic studies, including

1. Pharmacogenetic studies of ADHD should be methodologically rigorous in terms of the pharmacologic intervention, which means the trial should meet criteria for being published on its own. Typically, this means that there should be random assignment to treatment and a placebo or other control group;
2. Response should be measured several ways and at different time points. Secondary functional outcomes and adverse events and symptom ratings should be evaluated;
3. Different doses or optimal dose should be evaluated, recognizing that dose-ranging and forced-titration designs are more likely to elicit pharmacogenetic effects than flexible-dosing designs;
4. Multiple genes should be examined;
5. Genotyping quality control must be performed, ideally including cross-laboratory and cross-method reliability checks;
6. Samples large enough to look at gene-by-environment interactions should be obtained;
7. Trials sponsored by pharmaceutical companies should routinely collect DNA for pharmacogenetic and subgroup analysis.

Clinical applications

Stimulant medications are acknowledged as first-line treatments for ADHD [58], although the evidence supporting sustained benefit from pharmacotherapy remains less clear [59]. One 5-year prospective study showed that more than half of the participants failed to continue medication into the second treatment year, and many of those who continued therapy reported clinically significant side effects [3]. The authors concluded that side effects and perceived tolerability were major factors in the decisions to discontinue treatment. Open-label follow-up studies of subjects in clinical trials taking either methylphenidate or amphetamine showed that fewer than 60% of previously stabilized patients remained on medication after 12 months of treatment, although those who remained in therapy showed sustained improvements from baseline [60,61]. Therefore, despite the overall effectiveness of stimulant medications in the short-term relief of ADHD symptoms, clearly considerable impediments exist to remaining on long-term treatment.

Although most published ADHD pharmacogenetic studies emphasize genetic predictors of symptom improvement, a more practical clinical application might lie in predicting side effect risk and medication tolerability. Side effects are major impediments to long-term treatment adherence. In PATS, development of irritability and increased emotionality were two major reasons subjects discontinued medication therapy [62]. Pharmacogenetic analyses from that trial showed genetic predictors of irritability, social withdrawal, and abnormal movements [33]. Conceivably, an awareness of increased side effect risk could guide clinicians toward treatment choices that are more likely to be tolerated over time, with less patient exposure to medications that are unlikely to provide benefit.

The most promising clinical application of ADHD pharmacogenetics and pharmacogenomics may lie in the development of novel ADHD treatments. The identification of genes that increase susceptibility for ADHD or predict ADHD treatment response might promote the discovery of new drug targets for future pharmaceutical development. It should also be possible, as the cost of genotyping individual patients decreases, to enroll in clinical trials subsets of patients who are more likely to exhibit positive responses and less likely to experience untoward effects. The hope is that this type of research will allow clinicians to tailor individual treatment choices based on genotype.

Summary

ADHD pharmacogenetic and pharmacogenomic research efforts in children, adolescents, and adults are expanding worldwide. Several promising findings related to diminished response and specific side effects have been reported. Future efforts will also examine a wider range of stimulant and non-stimulant medications on a range of outcome measures and time periods. The hope is that ADHD treatment outcomes will eventually be improved by a more personalized approach to determining treatments, which could result in better understanding of treatment failures and the development of more targeted ADHD treatments. Although research on positive and negative predictive value is necessary before preliminary findings are applied to contemporary practice, these studies are currently ongoing. If successful, personalized ADHD therapy will move quickly from the "promise" to the "practical" phase.

Acknowledgments

The authors would like to thank Edwin H. Cook, Jr, MD, for his thoughtful review and helpful comments.

References

[1] Prince J. Pharmacotherapy of attention-deficit hyperactivity in children and adolescents: update on new stimulant preparations, atomoxetine, and novel treatments. Child Adolesc Psychiatr Clin N Am 2006;15:15–30.

[2] Faraone SV, Biederman J, Spencer TJ, et al. Comparing the efficacy of medications for ADHD using meta-analysis. MedGenMed 2006;8:4.

[3] Charach A, Ickowicz A, Schachar R. Stimulant treatment over five years; adherence, effectiveness, and adverse events. J Am Acad Child Adolesc Psychiatry 2004;43:559–67.

[4] Schachar RJ, Tannock R. Childhood hyperactivity and psychostimulants: a review of extended treatment studies. J Child Adolesc Psychopharmacol 1993;3:81–97.

[5] MTA Cooperative Group. National Institute of Mental Health Multimodal Treatment Study of ADHD follow-up: 24-month outcomes of treatment strategies for attention-deficit/hyperactivity disorder. Pediatrics 2004;113:754–61.

[6] Faraone SV, Doyle AE. The nature and heritability of attention-deficit/hyperactivity disorder. Child Adolesc Psychiatr Clin N Am 2001;10:299–316.

[7] Faraone SV, Perlis R, Doyle AE, et al. Molecular genetics of attention-deficit/hyperactivity disorder. Biol Psychiatry 2005;57:1313–23.

[8] Lander ES, Linton LM, Birren B, et al. Initial sequencing and analysis of the human genome. Nature 2001;409:860–1.

[9] McGough JJ. Attention-deficit/hyperactivity disorder pharmacogenomics. Biol Psychiatry 2005;57:1367–73.

[10] Polanczyk G, Zeni C, Genro J, et al. Attention-deficit/hyperactivity disorder: advancing on pharmacogenomics. Pharmacogenomics 2005;6:225–34.

[11] Weber WW. Pharmacogenetics. New York: Oxford Press; 1997.

[12] Aitchison KJ, Gill M, et al. Pharmacogenetics in the postgenomic era. In: Plomin R, Devries J, Craig I, editors. Behavioral genetics in the postgenomic era. Washington, DC: American Psychological Association; 2003. p. 335–61.

[13] Meyer UA. Pharmacogenetics and adverse drug reactions. Lancet 2000;356:1667–71.

[14] Staddon S, Aranz MJ, Mancama D, et al. Clinical applications of pharmacogenetics in psychiatry. Psychopharmacology 2002;162:18–23.

[15] Masellis M, Basile V, Muglia P, et al. Psychiatric pharmacogenetics: personalizing psychostimulant therapy in attention-deficit/hyperactivity disorder. Behav Brain Res 2002;130:85–90.

[16] Sklar P. Principles of haplotype mapping and potential applications to attention-deficit hyperactivity disorder. Biol Psychiatry 2005;57:1357–66.

[17] Goldstein DB. Pharmacogenetics in the laboratory and the clinic. N Engl J Med 2003;348:553–6.

[18] Cook EH, Stein MA, Krasowski MD, et al. Association of attention-deficit disorder and the dopamine transporter gene. Am J Hum Genet 1995;56:993–8.

[19] Melega WP, Williams AC, Schmitz DA, et al. Pharmacokinetic and pharmacodynamic analysis of the actions of d-amphetamine and d-methamphetamine on the dopamine terminal. J Pharmacol Exp Ther 1995;274:90–6.

[20] Volkow ND, Wang G, Fowler JS, et al. Evidence that methylphenidate enhances the saliency of a mathematical task by increasing dopamine in the human brain. Am J Psychiatry 2004; 161:1173–80.

[21] Spencer TJ, Biederman J, Madras BK, et al. In vivo neuroreceptor imaging in attention-deficit/hyperactivity disorder: a focus on the dopamine transporter. Biol Psychiatry 2005; 57:1293–300.

[22] VanNess SH, Owens MJ, Kilts CD. The variable number of tandem repeats element in DAT1 regulates in vitro dopamine transporter density. BMC Genet 2005;6:55.

[23] Winsberg BG, Comings DE. Association of the dopamine transporter gene (DAT1) with poor methylphenidate response. J Am Acad Child Adoelsc Psychiatry 1999;38:1474–7.

[24] Roman T, Szobot C, Martine S, et al. Dopamine transporter gene and response to methylphenidate in attention-deficit/hyperactivity disorder. Pharmacogenetics 2002;12:497–9.

[25] Cheon KA, Ryu YH, Kim JW, et al. The homozygosity for the 10-repeat allele at dopamine transporter gene and dopamine transporter density in Korean children with attention deficit hyperactivity disorder: relating to treatment response to methylphenidate. Eur Neuropsychopharmacol 2005;15:95–101.

[26] Kirley A, Lowe N, Hawi A, et al. Association of the 480 bp DAT1 allele with methylphenidate response in a sample of Irish children with ADHD. Am J Med Genet 2003;121B:50–4.

[27] Stein MA, Waldman ID, Sarampote CS, et al. Dopamine transporter genotype and methylphenidate dose response in children with ADHD. Neuropsychopharmacology 2005;30: 1374–82.

[28] Joober R, Grizenko N, Sengupta S, et al. Dopamine transporter 3′-UTR VNTR genotype and ADHD: a pharmaco-behavioral genetic study with methylphenidate. Neuropsychopharmacology 2006;32:1370–6.

[29] Lott D, Kim S, Cook E, et al. Dopamine transporter genotype and amphetamine response. Neuropsychopharmacology 2003;30:602–9.

[30] Van der Meulen EM, Bakker SC, Pauls DL, et al. High sibling correlation on methylphenidate response but no association with DAT1-10R and DRD4-7 alleles in Dutch sibpairs with ADHD. J Child Psychol Psychiatry 2005;46:1074–80.

[31] Langley K, Turic D, Peirce TR, et al. No support for association between the dopamine transporter (DAT1) gene and ADHD. Am J Med Genet B Neuropsychiatr Genet 2005;139B:7–10.

[32] Zeni CP, Guimarães AP, Polanczyk GV, et al. No significant association between response to methylphenidate and genes of the dopaminergic serotonergic systems in a sample of Brazilian children with attention-deficit/hyperactivity disorder. Am J Med Genet B Neuropsychiatr Genet 2007;144:391–4.

[33] McGough JJ, McCracken JT, Swanson J, et al. Pharmacogenetics of methylphenidate response in preschoolers with ADHD. J Am Acad Child Adolesc Psychiatry 2006;45: 1314–22.

[34] Mick E, Biederman J, Spencer T, et al. Absence of association with DAT1 polymorphism and response to methylphenidate in a sample of adults with ADHD. Am J Med Genet 2006;141:890–4.

[35] Asghari V, Sanyal S, Buchwaldt S, et al. Modulation of intracellular cyclic AMP levels by different human dopamine D4 receptor variants. J Neurochem 1995;65:1157–65.

[36] Van Tol HH, Wu CM, Guan HC, et al. Multiple dopamine D4 receptor variants in the human population. Nature 1992;358:149–52.

[37] Hamarman S, Fossella J, Ulger C, et al. Dopamine receptor 4 (DRD4) 7-repeat allele predicts methylphenidate dose response in children with attention deficit hyperactivity disorder. J Child Adolesc Psychopharmacol 2004;14:564–74.

[38] Cheon K, Kim B, Cho S. Association of 4-repeat allele of the dopamine D4 receptor gene III polymorphism and response to methylphenidate treatment in Korean ADHD children. Neuropsychopharamcology 2007;32:1377–83.

[39] Sallee F, Newcorn JA, Allen AJ, et al. Pharmacogenetics of atomoxetine: relevance of DRD4. Scientific Proceedings of the 51st Annual Meeting of the American Academy of Child and Adolescent Psychiatry, Washington, DC, October 23, 2004.

[40] Wilson MC. Coloboma mouse mutant as an animal model of hyperkinesis and attention deficit hyperactivity disorder. Neurosic Biobehav Rev 2000;24:51–7.

[41] Bobb AJU, Addington AM, Sidransky E, et al. Support for association between ADHD and two candidate genes: NET1NET and DRD1. Am J Med Genet B Neuropsychiatr Genet 2005;134:67–72.

[42] Roman T, Schmitz M, Polanczyk GV, et al. Is the α-2A adrenergic receptor gene (ADRA2A) associated with attention-deficit/hyperactivity disorder? Am J Med Genet B Neuropsychiatr Genet 2003;120:116–20.

[43] Michelson D, Faries D, Wernicke J, et al. Atomoxetine in the treatment of children and adolescent with attention-deficit/hyperactivity disorder: a randomized, placebo-controlled, dose-response study. Pediatrics 2001;108:E83.

[44] Yang L, Wang Y-F, Li J, et al. Association of norepinephrine transporter gene (NET) with methylphenidate response. J Am Acad Child Adolesc Psychiatry 2004;43:1154–8.

[45] Polanczyk G, Zeni C, Genro JP, et al. Association of the adrenergic α2A receptor gene with methylphenidate improvement of inattentive symptoms in children and adolescents with attention-deficit/hyperactivity disorder. Arch Gen Psychiatry 2007;64:218–24.

[46] Patrick KS, Straughn AB, Minhinnett RR, et al. Influence of ethanol and gender on methylphenidate pharmacokinetics and pharmacodynamics. Clin Pharmacol Ther 2007;81:346–53.

[47] Dring LG, Smith RL, Williams RT. The metabolic fate of amphetamine in man and other species. Biochem J 1970;116:425–35.

[48] Markowitz JS, Patrick KS. Pharmacokinetic and pharmacodynamic drug interactions in the treatment of attention-deficit hyperactivity disorder. Clin Pharmacokinet 2001;40:753–72.

[49] Meyer UA, Zanger UM. Molecular mechanism of genetic polymorphisms of drug metabolism. Annu Rev Pharmacol Toxicol 1997;37:269–96.

[50] McGough JJ, Biederman J, Greenhill LL, et al. Pharmacokinetics of SLI381 (Adderall XR), and extended-release formulation of Adderall. J Am Acad Child Adolesc Psychiatry 2003;42:684–91.

[51] Xie H-G, Kim RB, Wood AJJ, et al. Molecular basis of ethnic differences in drug disposition and response. Annu Rev Pharmacol Toxicol 2001;41:815–50.

[52] Wandel C, Witte JS, Hall JM, et al. CYP3A activity in African American and European American men; population differences and functional effect of the CYP3A4*1B5′-promoter region polymorphisms. Clin Pharmacol Ther 2000;68:82–91.

[53] Michelson D, Read HA, Ruff D, et al. CY2D6 and clinical response to atomoxetine in children and adolescents with ADHD. J Am Acad Child Adolesc Psychiatry 2007;46:242–51.

[54] Waldman ID, Gizer IR. The genetics of attention deficit hyperactivity disorder. Clin Psychol Rev 2006;26:396–432.

[55] Friedel S, Saar K, Demple A, et al. Association and linkage of allelic variants of the dopamine transporter gene in ADHD. Mol Psychiatry 2007;12:923–33.

[56] Van der Meulen EM, Bakker SC, Pauls DL, et al. A genome-wide Quantitative Trait Locus analysis on methylphenidate response rate in Dutch sibpairs with attention-deficit/hyperactivity disorder. Scientific Proceedings of the 16th World Congress of the International Association for Child and Adolescent Psychiatry and Allied Professions, Berlin, Germany, August 22, 2004.

[57] Pelham WE, Millich R. Individual differences in response to Ritalin in class work and social behavior. In: Greenhill LL, Osman B, editors. Ritalin: theory and patient management. New York: Mary Ann Liebert; 1991. p. 203–21.

[58] Plizska SR, Crismon ML, Hughes CW, et al. The Texas Children's Medication Algorithm Project; revision of the algorithm for pharmacotherapy of attention-deficit/hyperactivity disorder. J Am Acad Child Adolesc Psychiatry 2006;45:642–57.

[59] Spencer T, Biederman J, Wilens T, et al. Pharmacotherapy of attention deficit hyperactivity disorder across the lifespan. J Am Acad Child Adolesc Psychiatry 1996;35:409–28.

[60] McGough JJ, Biederman J, Wigal S, et al. Long-term tolerability and effectiveness of once-daily mixed amphetamine salts (Adderall XR) in children with ADHD. J Am Acad Child Adolesc Psychiatry 2005;44:530–8.

[61] Wilens T, Pelham W, Stein M, et al. ADHD treatment with once-daily OROS methylphenidate: interim 12-month results from a long-term open-label study. J Am Acad Child Adolesc Psychiatry 2003;42:424–33.

[62] Wigal T, Greenhill L, Chuang S, et al. Safety and tolerability of methylphenidate in preschool children with ADHD. J Am Acad Child Adolesc Psychiatry 2006;45:1294–303.

ELSEVIER
SAUNDERS

Child Adolesc Psychiatric Clin N Am
17 (2008) 491–496

CHILD AND
ADOLESCENT
PSYCHIATRIC CLINICS
OF NORTH AMERICA

Index

Note: Page numbers of article titles are in **boldface** type.

1056-4993/08/$ - see front matter © 2008 Elsevier Inc. All rights reserved.
doi:10.1016/S1056-4993(08)00010-2